ELEMENTS OF
Anatomy and Physiology

SECOND EDITION

Stanley W. Jacob, MD, F.A.C.S.

Gerlinger Associate Professor of Surgery, School of Medicine,
Oregon Health Sciences University, Portland, Oregon
First Kemper Foundation Research Scholar,
American College of Surgeons
Markle Scholar in Medical Sciences

Clarice Ashworth Francone

Medical Illustrator,
Formerly Head of the Department of Medical Illustrations,
Oregon Health Sciences University, Portland, Oregon

1989
W.B. SAUNDERS COMPANY
Harcourt Brace Jovanovich, Inc.

Philadelphia   London   Toronto
Montreal   Sydney   Tokyo

W. B. SAUNDERS COMPANY
Harcourt Brace Jovanovich, Inc.

The Curtis Center
Independence Square West
Philadelphia, PA 19106

Library of Congress Cataloging-in-Publication Data

Jacob, Stanley W. (Stanley Wallace), 1924 –
  Elements of anatomy and physiology / Stanley W. Jacob, Clarice
Ashworth Francone. — 2nd ed.
    p. cm.
  Includes index.
  1. Human physiology. 2. Anatomy, Human. I. Francone, Clarice
Ashworth. II. Title.
  [DNLM: 1. Anatomy. 2. Physiology. QS 4 J16e]
QP34.5.J28 1989
612 — dc19
DNLM/DLC
ISBN 0-7216-5089-9   89-4203

Editor: Michael Brown
Developmental Editor: Lisa Konoplisky
Designer: Lawrence DiDona
Production Manager: Peter Faber
Manuscript Editor: Roger Wall
Illustration Coordinator: Peg Shaw
Indexer: Julie Palmeter
Cover Photo: CompStock Inc./Tom Grill

Elements of Anatomy and Physiology   ISBN 0-7216-5089-9

Last digit is the print number: 9   8   7   6   5   4   3   2   1

To my children,
Stephen, Jeff, Darren, Rob, and Elyse,
with love
STANLEY W. JACOB

To my grandchildren
CLARICE ASHWORTH FRANCONE

Preface

The human body is still much more complex than the most involved computer mechanism ever produced. Moreover, scientists from all parts of the world are constantly adding to our knowledge of physiology and anatomy. It is not possible for any one person to absorb all of these facts or even to understand the immense ramifications of this explosion in knowledge. It is, however, possible for even a beginning student to master enough information so as to appreciate the major components and activities of the body. In this text we have tried to describe the structure and function of the human body in a manner that the student with no prior preparation in the sciences will find interesting and comprehensible.

To help the student understand and retain new terms and ideas, we have incorporated a number of special features. For example, because most students using this text will be participating in some way in the care of patients, we have taken pains to mention the clinical implications of disordered physiology. Pronunciations are provided for unfamiliar terms, and Latin and Greek roots are included as memory cues. Major headings in the text are presented as questions —What Does a Neuron Look Like? How Does It Work?—that focus attention on what is to be learned.

New in this second edition is the Glossary, enabling the student to review terminology at any time without having to relocate the subject in the primary text.

There has been a continuing increase in basic knowledge of the cell and of the role of DNA and RNA in heredity and control of cellular life functions. Because these functions are so intimately involved in the workings of the body in both health and illness, all persons who contribute to patient care need to know about them. We have therefore dealt with cellular physiology more extensively than is common in a beginning textbook but have presented the information as simply as possible.

Within the last few years we have experienced dramatic advances in the understanding of the immune system. Furthermore, because of advances in transplantation techniques and the spread of the AIDS virus, the importance of understanding the immune system has increased enormously for all health care professionals. The new Chapter 10, The Immune System, offers a clear and simple introduction, appropriate for the broad range of students who use this text.

v

Special appreciation is due Terry Bristol, adjunct professor at the Linfield College School of Nursing, who has now moved on to become Director of the Institute for Science, Engineering and Public Policy, for his extraordinary and untiring efforts in overseeing the critical review, scholarly research, and appropriate revisions for this second edition. We wish also to express our indebtedness to our many colleagues as well as teachers and students who have read the manuscript for this text and have contributed valuable and constructive criticisms.

The authors wish to acknowledge the editorial assistance of the W.B. Saunders Company. A particular note of gratitude goes to Michael Brown, whose advice and encouragement contributed significantly to the completion of this work.

Contents

O N E

The Body As A Whole

O B J E C T I V E S

The aim of this chapter is to enable the student to do the following:

- Define anatomy and physiology.

- Explain the relation between structure and function in the body.

- Construct a diagram of the body and label it with respect to anatomic directions, planes, and cavities.

- Use the systems of anatomic reference to locate and to identify accurately areas and structures of the body.

- Define and relate the cell, tissue, organ, and system as structural units.

- Identify the two major types of communication mechanisms (and systems) involved in the coordination of the body.

- Define health and contrast it with disease and injury.

- Distinguish between acute and chronic as well as hereditary and infectious disease.

STUDYING THE HUMAN BODY

The human body may be viewed as a collection of thousands of billions of minute living units called *cells*. These cells are marvelously combined and organized to operate as a harmonious whole—the living body. The simplest structures formed by the cells are known as *tissues*, and these tissues combine to form larger more sophisticated structures known as *organs*. The organs work together as *systems*, such as the respiratory system, the digestive system, and the circulatory system.

When looked at in this way, the human body is an awe-inspiring phenomenon. Its highly organized design and the fine balance and interdependence of the various parts are the underlying bases

of the tremendous adaptability and diverse capabilities of human beings. An understanding of the structures and functions of the human body will greatly expand the student's appreciation of the magnificence of life.

What Is Human Anatomy

Anatomy is the science that studies the shape and structure of living organisms and their parts. *Human anatomy* is the study of the shape and structure of the human body and its parts.

Gross anatomy, or gross human anatomy, deals with the large, macroscopic structures that can be observed by normal dissection and with normal, unaided vision.

1

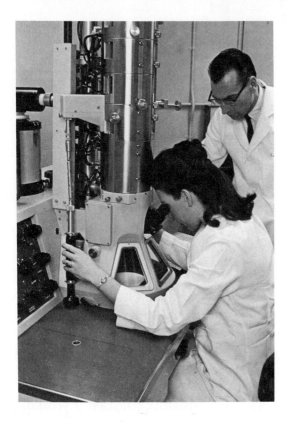

Figure 1–1 The electron microscope is now being employed to study structures at a magnification of 200,000×.

Microscopic anatomy deals with structures that can be seen only with the use of the light microscope. The modern electron microscope, which was developed during the 1940s, is 400 times more powerful than the light microscope (Figs. 1–1 and 1–3) and has become an important instrument of research in current anatomic investigation.

What Is Human Physiology?

Physiology (from the Greek, *physis*, meaning natural science, and *-logy*, meaning study of) is the science that deals with the functions of living organisms and their parts. It is the study of what the parts do and why. *Human physiology* is the study of the functions of the human body and its parts. Some physiologists specialize in the study of the functions of systems, such as the circulatory system, whereas others may center their attention on a particular organ, such as the heart or kidneys.

Cellular physiology, the most prominent branch of modern physiology, is the study of the *how* and *why* of the activities of individual cells and their internal parts.

How Are Anatomy and Physiology Related?

The structure and the function of any part of a living organism are always related. For instance, the heart is a specially designed muscular pump whose main function is to keep the blood moving continuously throughout the body. The design of the heart is very much different from the design of a lung, whose function is the exchange of carbon dioxide for oxygen between the outside environment and the blood.

The structure of a part can provide a clue to its function. Likewise, knowing the function of a part helps us properly to understand its size, shape, and structural organization. Just as structure and function are related in the practical study of the body and its parts, so are anatomy and physiology always closely related. Consequently, the use of the terms "anatomy" and "physiology" is best thought of as indicating an emphasis rather than a sharp division in what is being studied.

SYSTEMS OF REFERENCE

How Are the Structures of the Body Accurately Identified?

Because of the great complexity of the human body, anatomists have developed several *systems of reference* over the years to aid in the rapid and accurate identification of the part or area of the body to be described or discussed.

Directions in the Body Perhaps the most common approach involves the use of the general terms of anatomic direction (Fig. 1–2). The 10 main terms of direction are as follows:

Superior—means above or upper portion. For example, the head is superior to the neck.

Inferior—means lowermost or below; the foot is inferior to the ankle; the neck is inferior to the head.

Anterior (or Ventral)—means toward the front; the breasts are on the anterior chest wall.

Posterior (or Dorsal)—means toward the back; the spinal cord is posterior to the internal organs (heart, lungs, intestines, and so on).

Medial—means nearest the midline of the body; the ulna is on the medial side of the forearm.

Lateral—means toward the side, away from the midline; the radius is lateral to the ulna.

Proximal—means nearest the point of attachment or origin; the elbow is proximal to the wrist.

Distal—means away from the point of attachment or origin; the wrist is distal to the elbow.

Superficial—means on or near the surface of the body; an injury involving only the skin is superficial.

Deep—means inward away from the body surface; a lacerated liver is a deep injury.

What Are the Reference Planes of the Body?

The body is also discussed with respect to planes passing through it.

Midsagittal—refers to the plane that vertically divides the body through the midline into right and left halves.

Sagittal—refers to any plane parallel to the midsagittal plane.

Transverse—refers to any plane dividing the body into superior and inferior portions; sometimes called a horizontal plane.

Coronal—refers to any plane dividing the body into anterior (or ventral) and posterior (or dorsal) portions at right angles to the sagittal plane.

What Are the Main Reference Cavities of the Body?

A second common anatomic reference system involves viewing the body as being made up of several "rooms" or *cavities* (Fig. 1–4). The body has two major cavities, each of which is made up of smaller cavities. The larger of the two major cavities is usually referred to as the *ventral cavity*, and the

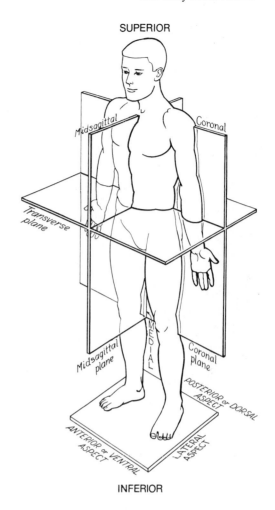

Figure 1–2 Anatomic position of body (anterior view, palms forward) with reference systems.

smaller is called the *dorsal cavity*. How might these be identified by alternative terms?

Ventral Cavity   The ventral cavity contains the internal organs, which maintain the basic life processes. These include the heart, lungs, kidneys, stomach, and intestines as well as several other organs. The ventral cavity is frequently distinguished into three smaller cavities.

The uppermost (superior) of the smaller cavities contains the heart and lungs and is referred to as the *thoracic* (tho-ras'-ik) *cavity* or, more commonly, as the chest. The thoracic cavity also contains the *pleural cavity*, which contains the lungs, and the *pericardial cavity*, which contains the structures of the heart. The middle cavity is the *abdominal cavity*,

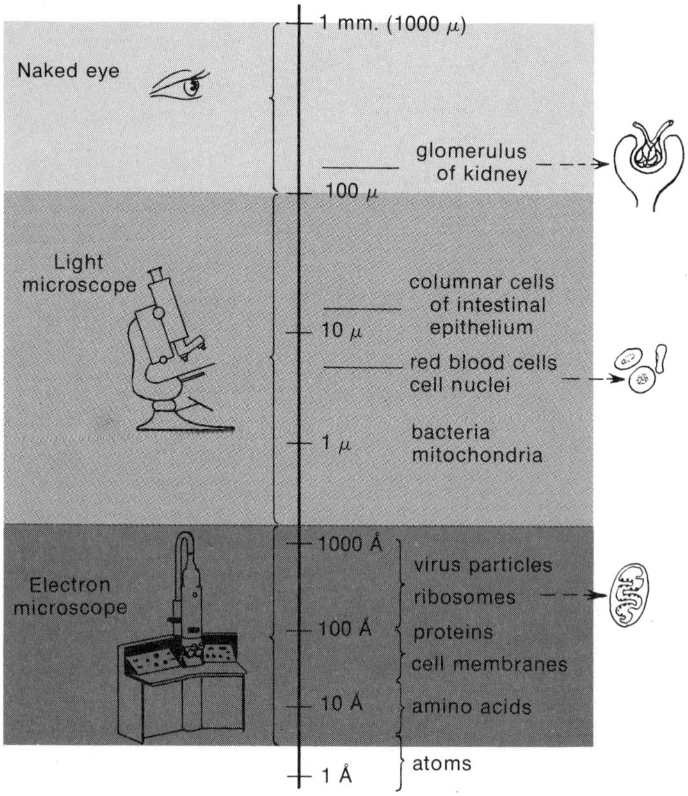

Figure 1-3 The limits of resolution of the electron microscope as contrasted to those of the eye and the light microscope. A millimeter, mm, is equal to 1/1000 meter, or 0.03937 inch; a micrometer, μm, 1/1000 millimeter; an angstrom, Å, 1/10,000 micrometer.

which contains the liver, kidneys, and most of the digestive tract, including the stomach. The lowermost (inferior) cavity is referred to as the *pelvic cavity*, since it is bounded on the outside by the pelvic bones; it contains the lower digestive tract and the bladder.

Dorsal Cavity   The dorsal cavity contains the brain and spinal cord. It is commonly distinguished into the *cranial cavity*, containing the brain, and the *spinal cavity*, containing the spinal cord.

What Is the "Structural Unit" Reference System?

In studying the physiology of an organism, the most useful system of anatomic reference is that based on the *structural units* approach. In this approach, the body is described in four levels of detail —the cellular level, the tissue level, the organ level, and the systems level. As previously mentioned,

these four levels are related in an organized fashion as follows: The cells combine to form tissues; the tissues combine to form organs; and the organs work together to form systems.

The Cellular Level   All living matter is composed of cells; tiny microscopic units that are the smallest living parts of all organisms. All cells are made up of three basic parts—the *cell membrane*, which envelops the other parts; the *cytoplasm* (si'to-plazm"), which is the body substance of the internal portion; and the *nucleus* (nu'kle-us), which is the control center, located near the center of the cell. However, beyond this basic common structure, different cells vary in size, shape, and composition according to what they do. For instance, muscle cells differ from nerve cells, and both of these differ from bone cells, although all (muscle, nerve, and bone cells) have a cell membrane, cytoplasm, and nucleus. Cytoplasm is derived from the Greek, *cyto-*, meaning cell, and *-plasm*, meaning formed material. The word nucleus is derived from the Latin word *nucis*, meaning kernel.

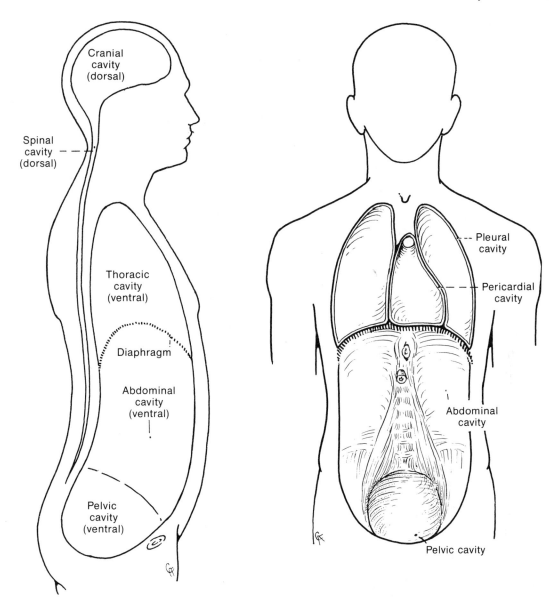

Figure 1–4 *Left*, The body has two major cavities, dorsal and ventral, each subdivided into lesser cavities. *Right*, Frontal view of body cavities.

The Tissue Level Collections of similar cells combine to form particular types of tissues. The term "tissue" is derived from the Latin word *textura*, meaning texture, or something woven together. Cells hold themselves together in tissues by weaving a network or matrix of soft glue-like substance, known as the intercellular matrix. The prefix "inter-" means between. Anatomists usually refer to four main categories of tissues that make up most of the organ structures of the body. These are epithelial (ep"i-the'le-al) tissues, connective tissues, muscular tissues, and nervous tissues. These four types also correspond to the four main types of cells— epithelial, connective, muscle, and nerve. *Epithelial tissues* are found covering all surfaces of the body, both internally and externally; for instance, the cov-

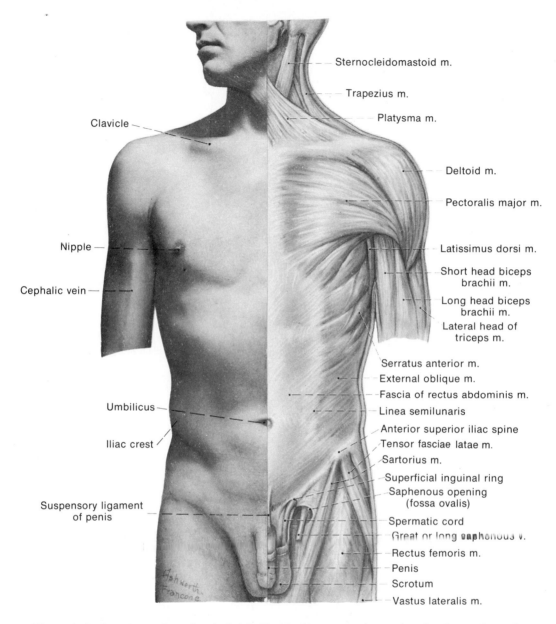

Sternocleidomastoid m.

Trapezius m.

Platysma m.

Clavicle

Deltoid m.

Pectoralis major m.

Nipple

Latissimus dorsi m.

Short head biceps
brachii m.

Long head biceps
brachii m.

Lateral head of
triceps m.

Cephalic vein

Serratus anterior m.

External oblique m.

Fascia of rectus abdominis m.

Linea semilunaris

Umbilicus

Anterior superior iliac spine

Tensor fasciae latae m.

Iliac crest

Sartorius m.

Superficial inguinal ring

Saphenous opening
(fossa ovalis)

Suspensory ligament
of penis

Spermatic cord

Great or long saphenous v.

Rectus femoris m.

Penis

Scrotum

Vastus lateralis m.

Figure 1–5   Anterior surface of male, left half with skin removed to expose first layer of muscles.

erings on the organs and digestive tract and the skin covering the whole body. *Connective tissues* are harder—containing much more intercellular matrix substance—and function in holding things together; for example, bones, tendons, and cartilage.

Muscular tissues make up muscles but are also found wherever movement occurs; for instance, besides arm and leg muscles, muscular tissue is found in the stomach and digestive tract as well as in association with the skin. *Nervous tissues* make up the

brain and spinal cord and all the millions of nerves that carry signals throughout the body.

The Organ Level   An organ is a somewhat independent structure within the body made up of several types of tissues, *all serving a common function*. For instance, the stomach is an organ made up of layers of epithelial, connective, and muscular tissues, all working together as a whole to break up food into tiny particles for digestion. The stomach is

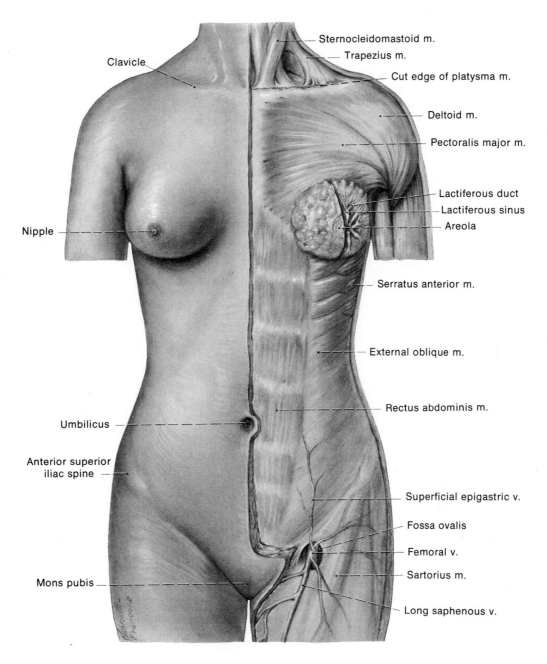

Clavicle

Sternocleidomastoid m.

Trapezius m.

Cut edge of platysma m.

Deltoid m.

Pectoralis major m.

Lactiferous duct

Lactiferous sinus

Areola

Nipple

Serratus anterior m.

External oblique m.

Rectus abdominis m.

Umbilicus

Anterior superior
iliac spine

Superficial epigastric v.

Fossa ovalis

Femoral v.

Sartorius m.

Mons pubis

Long saphenous v.

Figure 1–6 Anterior surface of female, left half with skin removed to expose first layer of muscles.

connected to the brain centers by nerves (nervous tissue). Other organs are the liver, heart, lungs, and skin.

The Systems Level The highest level of structural unit used for purposes of reference is the system. A system is a group of organs acting together to accomplish some overall bodily function. For in-

stance, the circulatory system is made up of the heart, arteries, veins, and capillaries, all serving to circulate the blood throughout the body. The skeletal system is made up of bones, tendons, and cartilage, all serving the functions of support and movement. Figures 1–5 through 1–14 are representative anatomic diagrams showing a variety of bodily structures with their identifying names.

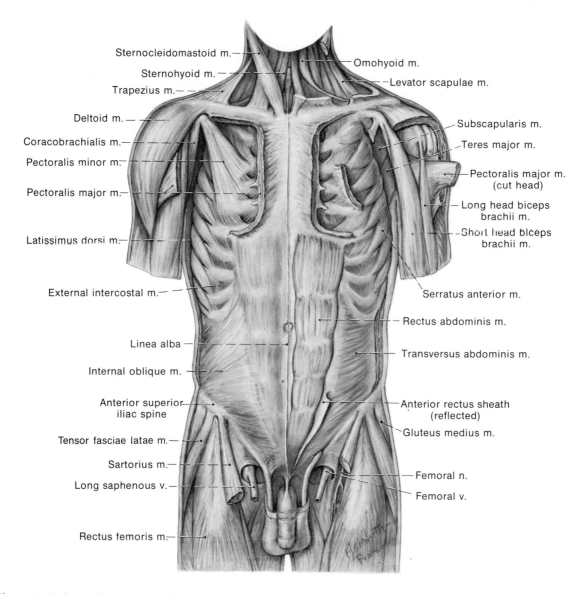

Figure 1–7   Pectoralis major muscle removed on right side, pectoralis minor on left side; second and third layers of abdominal muscles exposed.

THE COORDINATED WHOLE

How Are the Parts of the Body Functionally Related?

The human body is not simply a collection of substances or parts; it is a highly organized and precisely coordinated whole that functions as a harmonious unit. Each cell (or tissue, or organ, or system) benefits from its own activity as well as helping and benefiting from the activity of the cells of the other organs and systems. They all work to *help* themselves and one another as well as to *control* themselves and each other.

The overall coordination of the body and its parts is so important that two special organ systems

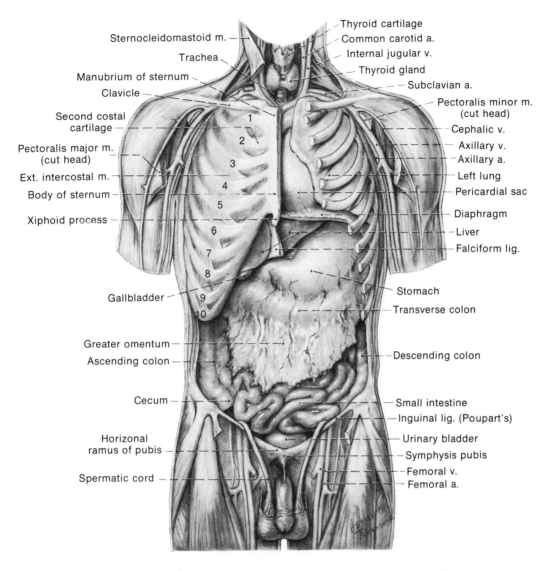

Figure 1-8 Anterior muscles of chest and abdomen removed, showing underlying viscera.

have evolved to handle this special function. These are the nervous system, which operates by sending and receiving electrical signals throughout the body, and the endocrine system, a system of eight glands, each of which keeps track of chemical substances in the body and sends out, when needed, stimulating chemical messengers known as *hormones* (from the Greek, *hormaein*, meaning to set in motion). These two systems are responsible for maintaining the symphony of activities of the individual cells, tissues, organs, and systems.

CLINICAL CONSIDERATIONS

What Is Health?

Health is a state of soundness of the organism when all systems of the body are functioning in harmony with vitality. Health is also characterized by the lack of any evidence of disease or abnormality.

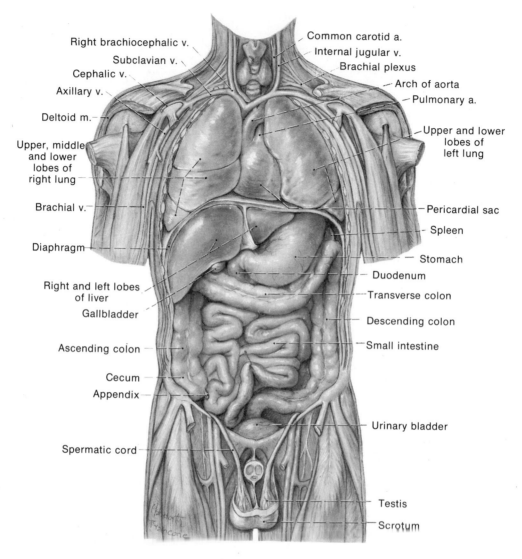

Figure 1-9 Rib cage and omentum removed, showing visceral relations.

What Is a Disease? An Injury?

The most general definition of a disease is any impairment (hindrance) of normal bodily activity, which affects the performance of the vital functions. In diagnosing a disease, it is most important to gain an understanding of the origin or cause of the abnormal conditions or symptoms of the body. An *acute disease or illness* is one with a sharp onset and having a short and relatively severe course. A *chronic disease or illness* is one that persists over a long period of time.

Hereditary diseases are abnormalities that are usually handed down from generation to generation. It is generally agreed today that these problems can be traced, in the final analysis, to some abnormality of the chromosomes or the DNA that composes them.

Infectious diseases are those that can be transmitted from one individual to another. These diseases are due to the invasion and growth in the body

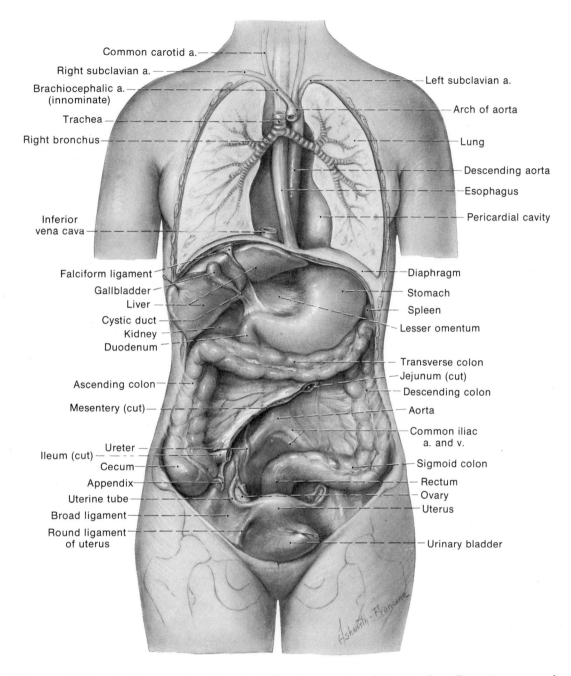

Figure 1–10 Female, demonstrating visceral relations; lungs sectioned, heart and small intestine removed.

of either viruses or bacteria. The invasion of larger parasitic organisms can also disrupt normal functioning.

Injuries can be classified into two general types. Immediate traumatic injuries, or *traumas*, result from some physical or chemical interference. This includes physical forces that result in broken bones and bruises as well as contact with or ingestion of poisons. *Long-term injuries* can occur from many different aspects of our relation to our environment.

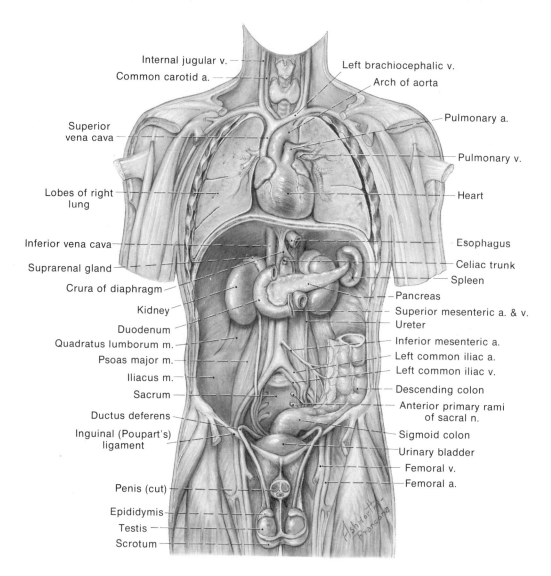

Figure 1–11   Male, with stomach, small intestine, most of colon, and anterior parts of lungs removed.

Included in this category are injuries or abnormalities resulting from long-term use of cigarettes and alcohol and a variety of dietary excesses or deficiencies.

SUMMARY

A. Anatomy is the study of the shapes and structures of the parts of living organisms.

1. Gross anatomy deals with large, macroscopic structures.
2. Microscopic anatomy deals with structures only visible through a microscope.

B. Physiology is the study of the functions of the parts of living organisms.

C. Anatomy and physiology are always related.
1. Structures provide clues to functions.
2. Knowing the function helps to understand the importance of specific structures.

D. Systems of reference allow us to identify accurately the areas and structures of the living organism.

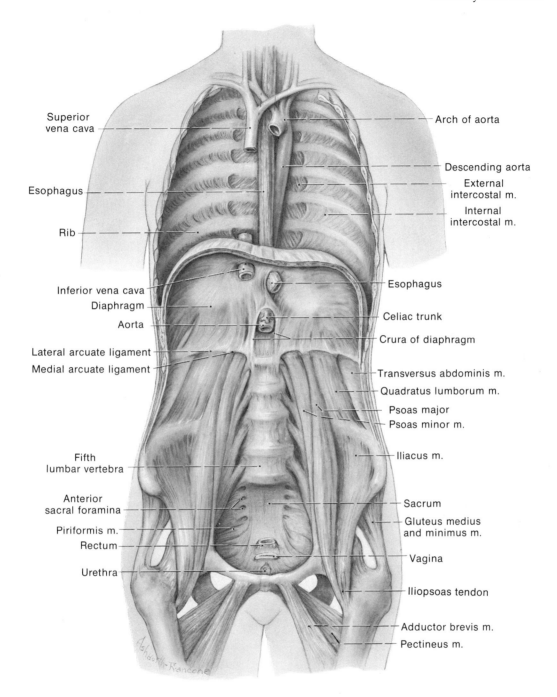

Superior vena cava

Esophagus

Rib

Inferior vena cava

Diaphragm

Aorta

Lateral arcuate ligament

Medial arcuate ligament

Fifth lumbar vertebra

Anterior sacral foramina

Piriformis m.

Rectum

Urethra

Arch of aorta

Descending aorta

External intercostal m.

Internal intercostal m.

Esophagus

Celiac trunk

Crura of diaphragm

Transversus abdominis m.

Quadratus lumborum m.

Psoas major

Psoas minor m.

Iliacus m.

Sacrum

Gluteus medius and minimus m.

Vagina

Iliopsoas tendon

Adductor brevis m.

Pectineus m.

Figure 1–12 Female, with all the viscera removed, exposing the internal posterior walls of chest and abdominal and pelvic cavities.

1. Directions are specified by several pairs of terms.
   a. Superior/inferior means up and down.
   b. Anterior (ventral)/posterior (dorsal) means front and back.
   c. Medial/lateral means toward and away from the midline.
   d. Proximal/distal means near and away from the point of attachment.
   e. Superficial/deep means near and in-

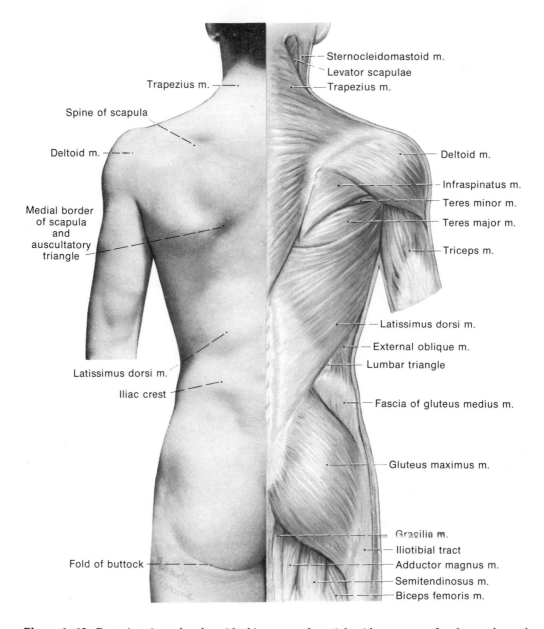

Figure 1-13 Posterior view of male, with skin removed on right side to expose first layer of muscles.

wardly away from the surface of the body.

2. There are three distinct orientations of reference planes.

   a. Sagittal planes divide the body into left and right portions.

   b. Transverse (horizontal) planes divide the body into superior and inferior portions.

   c. Coronal (vertical) planes divide the body into anterior and posterior portions.

3. There are two main cavities: the ventral and the dorsal.

   a. The ventral cavity is made up of the thoracic, abdominal, and pelvic cavities.

   b. The dorsal cavity is made up of the cranial and spinal cavities.

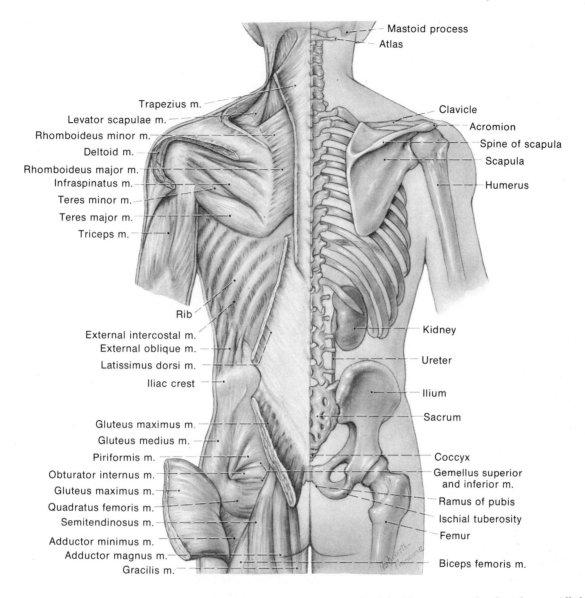

Figure 1-14 Most of the superficial muscles have been removed on the left side to expose the deep layers. All the muscles have been removed on the right side, exposing the skeletal framework.

4. The structural units reference system is based on cells, tissues, organs, and systems.
5. All living matter is composed of cells—the smallest living unit. Cells are woven together to form tissues: epithelial, connective, muscular, and nervous.
   a. Epithelial cells cover surfaces; for instance, the skin.
   b. Connective tissues function to support shape and structure; for instance, bones and cartilage.
   c. Muscular tissues are found where there is movement; for instance, biceps.
   d. Nervous tissues respond to stimuli and transmit impulses. They make up the brain, spinal cord, and millions of nerves reaching out to all areas of the body.
6. An organ is a structure made up of several

types of tissues, all serving a common function; for instance, the stomach.

    7. A system is a group of organs acting together to accomplish some overall body function; for instance, the respiratory system.

E. The human body is a highly organized and precisely coordinated whole that functions as a harmonious unit.

    1. Each cell, tissue, and organ makes at least some contribution to the harmonious coordination.

    2. Two special systems have evolved to orchestrate coordination.

      a. The nervous system sends, receives, and processes signals traveling through nerves.

      b. The endocrine system, an assortment of integrated glands, coordinates and communicates using stimulating chemical messengers called hormones.

F. Health is a state of soundness of the organism and exists when all systems are functioning with vitality without evidence of disease or abnormality.

G. A disease is any impairment of normal body activity affecting the performance of the vital functions.

    1. An acute disease (or illness) has a sharp onset and a short and relatively severe course.

    2. A chronic disease (or illness) persists over a long period of time.

    3. Hereditary diseases are traceable to the genetic code and can be handed down from generation to generation.

    4. Infectious diseases can be transmitted from one person to another and are due to bacteria or viruses.

    5. Injuries are of two types.

      a. Traumas are immediate traumatic injuries.

      b. Long-term injuries are due to repeated insults to the body.

REVIEW QUESTIONS

1. Define cells, tissues, organs, and systems and explain the relation among them.

2. What is anatomy? Characterize and distinguish gross anatomy and microscopic anatomy.

3. What is physiology? Characterize cellular physiology.

4. How are the two distinct types of study, anatomy and physiology, related? How can advances in one field help the other?

5. Define the main terms of direction used in anatomy: superior, inferior, anterior (ventral), posterior (dorsal), medial, lateral, proximal, distal, superficial, and deep.

6. Construct and label a diagram of the human body in anatomic position.

7. Name each of the main reference cavities of the body.

8. Construct and label a diagram showing the major cavities of the body.

9. What are the subcavities of the ventral cavity? What are the subcavities of the dorsal cavity?

10. Explain the "structural unit" approach to reference, giving examples of the structures at each level.

11. What are the two special systems that have evolved to handle overall coordination of the body and its parts?

12. Define health.

13. Define and distinguish an injury and a disease.

14. When is a disease chronic and when is it acute?

15. Distinguish between a hereditary disease and an infectious disease.

T W O

The Cell and Its Environment

O B J E C T I V E S

The aim of this chapter is to enable the student to do the following:

- Identify the main structures and primary activities of all living cells.

- Describe the characteristics and functions of the cell membrane.

- List the organelles found in the cytoplasm and explain the activities of each in the life of the cell.

- Describe, with illustrations, the structure and function of DNA and three types of RNA molecules.

- Outline the process of protein synthesis.

- Describe, with illustrations, the four phases of mitosis.

- Describe the cellular environment.

- Describe the distribution of body fluids.

- Define and distinguish between osmosis and diffusion.

- Define homeostasis.

- Define and distinguish between positive and negative feedback.

WHAT IS A CELL?

Cells are the tiny building blocks of the body. Unlike simple substances or collections of substances, cells are *living units*. This is shown by their ability to *grow* and *reproduce*, their need for *nourishment* and disposal of *waste products*, and their ability to *respond* and *adapt* to changes in the environment.

Human cells are so small that 2000 of them would have to be lined up to measure one inch, with each cell being about 1/2000th of an inch across. They are so small that individual human cells cannot even be seen without the aid of a microscope.

The microscope was developed only about 135 years ago, and only since then have we known that large living organisms are made up of cells.

Cells come in many different shapes. Some are shaped like long hot dogs, some are like square bricks, some are like flat tiles, and many are of various, irregular shapes.

What Are the Three Main Divisions of the Cell?

For study purposes, the three main divisions of each cell are the cell membrane, the cytoplasm, and the nucleus (Figs. 2–1 and 2–2).

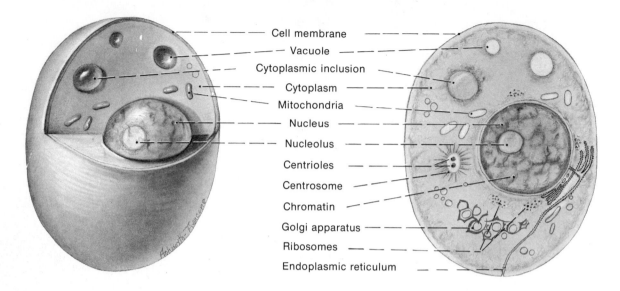

Figure 2-1 Two views of a cell based on what can be seen through the electron microscope.

The cell membrane is the extremely thin covering of the outer surface of each cell. It operates in both cellular ingestion (eating) and cellular excretion (of waste products) and generally serves to control the exchanges of air, water, and chemical substances between the cell and its environment.

The cytoplasm is the main body substance of the cell. It is made up of water and contains many microminiature "factory" units, discussed below.

The nucleus is contained in its own separate membrane, which floats in the cytoplasm, usually toward the center of the cell. The nucleus is the control center of the cell, directing and coordinating the activities of all parts of the cell.

How Does the Cell Membrane Function?

The cell membrane controls what substances pass into or out of the cell. This control is selective and is very important for maintaining the proper makeup of the cellular material. Tiny holes in the cell membrane allow some substances, such as oxygen and carbon dioxide and water, to pass in either direction fairly freely. But larger substances are restricted from moving into or out of the cell. When the cell wants to ingest some larger nutrient (food) substances, such as proteins or sugars, it forms little incuppings and "swallows" these substances into

the cell. *Pinocytosis* (pi"no-si-to'sis) (pino- from the Greek, *pinein*, meaning to drink, + *kytos*, cell, + *osis*, process) is the process in which the cell membrane forms a channel and "swallows" nutrient molecules (into little packets, which are called vacuoles) in its environment (Fig. 2-3). *Phagocytosis* (fag"o-si-to'sis) is the process of ingesting large particles, in which the cell surrounds and engulfs the particles. Figure 2-4 shows a white blood cell (neutrophil) engulfing some bacteria. (Phago- is derived from the Greek, *phagein*, to eat).

What Are the Cytoplasmic Organelles? What Do They Do?

The cytoplasm of all cells has been found to be highly organized, containing several types of functioning "factory" units, which are like miniature cellular organs. These are referred to as *organelles* (or"gan-els'); this term means, literally, "little organs." These include the mitochondria, lysosomes, ribosomes, and the endoplasmic reticulum.

Mitochondria (mit"o-kon'dre-ah) These are commonly referred to as the "powerhouses" of the cell. Their main function is to change small food molecules into other forms of energy that can be used by the cell for a variety of activities. Mitochon-

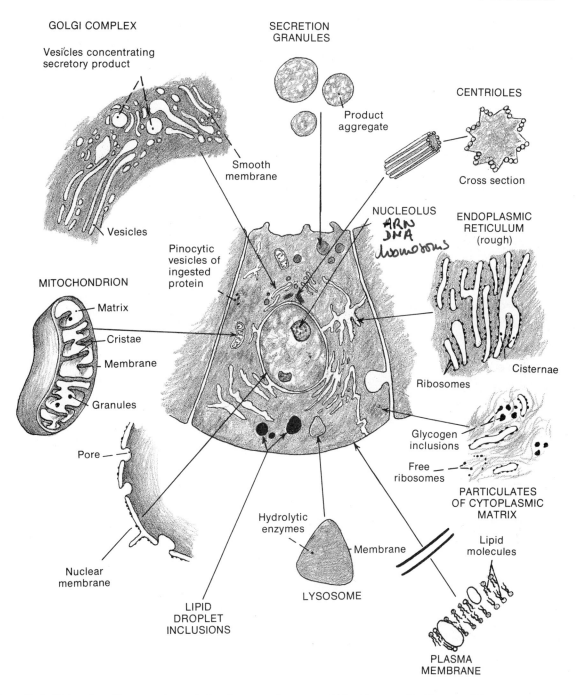

Figure 2–2 Parts of a cell as seen through the electron microscope. (After Fawcett, D.: *Bloom and Fawcett: A Textbook of Histology,* 8th ed. Philadelphia, W. B. Saunders Co., 1962.)

dria look like tiny, sausage-shaped bodies and are made up of a double membrane that is formed into several "inner folds."

When simple food molecules, such as the sugar glucose, enter the mitochondria, they are broken into small pieces. This process releases energy. The energy is then stored in a very important, special molecule called *ATP*. The abbreviation ATP stands for *adenosine* (ah-den'o-sen) *triphosphate*. The ATP molecules, with their stored energy (They can be

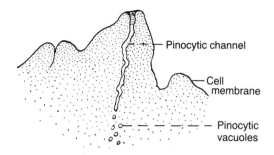

Figure 2–3 Pinocytosis.

thought of as storage batteries or universal energy transporters.) move out of the mitochondria and supply energy wherever it is needed in the cell (Fig. 2–5).

The number of mitochondria in a cell depends on its energy need. Muscle cells use a great deal of energy in their daily activity, and each cell contains several thousand mitochondria. Skin cells often have less than a hundred.

Lysosomes (li′so-soms) Sometimes referred to as the digestive organs (or organelles) of the cell (probably because of their Greek origin; *lyso-*, meaning to dissolve, and *-some*, meaning body), lysosomes are tiny units, even smaller than mitochondria, containing several powerful enzymes. (An *enzyme* is a chemical substance that causes a chemical reaction to take place.) When large, complex food molecules are taken into the cell, the lysosomes act to break down the particles into simple substances. These simple food molecules can then enter the mitochondria for energy processing.

Ribosomes (ri′bo-soms) These are still smaller granules of ribonucleic acid, or RNA, and protein and are usually attached to the endoplasmic reticulum. The ribosomes are the specific sites at which cells construct new protein molecules. These new molecules are used for many purposes within the cell, and some are passed out of the cell to act in other parts of the body.

Endoplasmic Reticulum (re-tik′u-lum) This is one organelle that is spread through the cytoplasm. It is a cellular membrane arranged to form complex networks of channels and surfaces throughout the cytoplasm. In some parts of the endoplasmic reticulum one finds thousands of ribosomes; here is

where new proteins are made. The channels of the endoplasmic reticulum serve also to carry substances to different parts of the cell and sometimes function in storage.

How Does the Nucleus Function?

The nucleus of the cell controls and coordinates cellular activity by controlling the chemical makeup of the cytoplasm.

How Does the Nucleus Control and Coordinate Cellular Activities?

When some process or activity of the cell needs to be increased, the nucleus (or, more specifically, the DNA molecules in the nucleus) sends out directions by messenger (messenger RNA molecules) to produce specific *proteins* that will then act to speed up the process or activity. In order to slow down some cellular activity, the DNA can either stop sending out directions for production of the key substances or else send out new directions for construction of a protein-blocking substance, or inhibitor, which rapidly slows down the activity.

How Does the Nucleus Direct Protein Manufacture?

The easiest way to understand the function of the nucleus is by using an analogy. Imagine the cell to be a large carpentry workshop. The director of the workshop sits in a separate office—this office would be the nucleus. The director himself has all the plans and designs needed to construct objects in the workshop; the director, with all the different

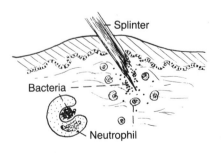

Figure 2–4 Phagocytosis.

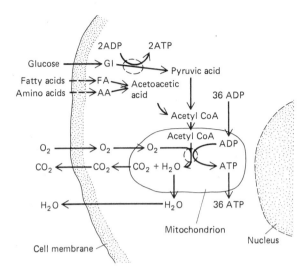

Figure 2–5 Formation of ATP in the cell. (From Guyton, A. C.: *Basic Human Physiology*. Philadelphia, W. B. Saunders Co., 1971.)

plans and designs, corresponds to the special *DNA molecules* in the nucleus. Since the director is always very busy deciding which products should be made in the work area, he never leaves his office. So, in order to get the plans and designs from his office (the nucleus) to the working area (cytoplasm), a messenger is needed. The messengers in the cell are special *RNA molecules*, known appropriately as *messenger RNA*. These messenger RNA molecules take the plans or designs for the specific products the director wants manufactured and carry them from the director's office (nucleus) to the workbenches. The workbenches, where the products are to be assembled, correspond to the *ribosomes*. The ribosomes are composed of another very large type of RNA known simply as *ribosomal RNA*. So far, we have the plans and designs (brought by or contained in the messenger RNA) at the workbenches (ribosomes), but we lack the materials needed to construct the product specified in the plans.

The materials needed to manufacture the specified product must be gathered and brought to the workbenches. This job requires another worker. In the cell, this worker is another type of RNA, known as *transfer RNA*, since it functions to transfer the basic building materials from around the working area (cytoplasm) to the ribosomes (workbenches). All the objects produced in the cell's workshop, at

the direction of the director (DNA) are *proteins*; proteins are made up of *amino acids*. The amino acids, then, are the basic building materials that need to be gathered by the transfer RNAs and brought to ribosomes. At the ribosomes, the amino acids are assembled into proteins, according to the plans brought by the messenger RNA.

Just how the materials (amino acids) are assembled to form the products (proteins) is still somewhat of a mystery. Some scientists think the ribosomes do it and, therefore, according to our analogy, should be thought of as automatic workbenches, which receive design plans and materials and then automatically construct the right objects. Others feel that the messenger RNA and transfer RNA participate in the construction process. In any case, we can generalize and say that the DNA, which always remains in the nucleus, is the ultimate director—it selects the plans to be sent and the number of products of that type to be manufactured. The various types of RNA (messenger, transfer, and ribosomal) are the workers; they operate to carry the plans, gather the materials (amino acids), and construct the products (proteins).

What Is DNA?

DNA is the main substance found in the nucleus of every cell; it is rarely if ever found outside the nucleus. It is a very large molecule whose full name is *deoxyribonucleic* (de-ok″se-ri″bo-nu′kle′ik) *acid*, or deoxyribonuclease, and is abbreviated as DNA. There are thousands of these large DNA molecules in the nucleus of every cell. Some of the DNA in the nucleus simply holds information or directions for production (referred to as *synthesis*) of protein molecules, whereas other DNA operates in coordinating and selecting which directions should be sent out (by messenger) and when. The protein molecules are made in the cytoplasm (at the ribosomes), but the directions on how to synthesize them are kept stored in the nucleus, in the DNA molecules.

The DNA molecules are extremely long and thin, and are composed of surprisingly few basic chemical compounds (Fig. 2–6). These include *phosphoric acid*, a sugar called *deoxyribose*, and four nitrogenous bases: *adenine, guanine, thymine,* and *cytosine.* The structure of the molecule is easily de-

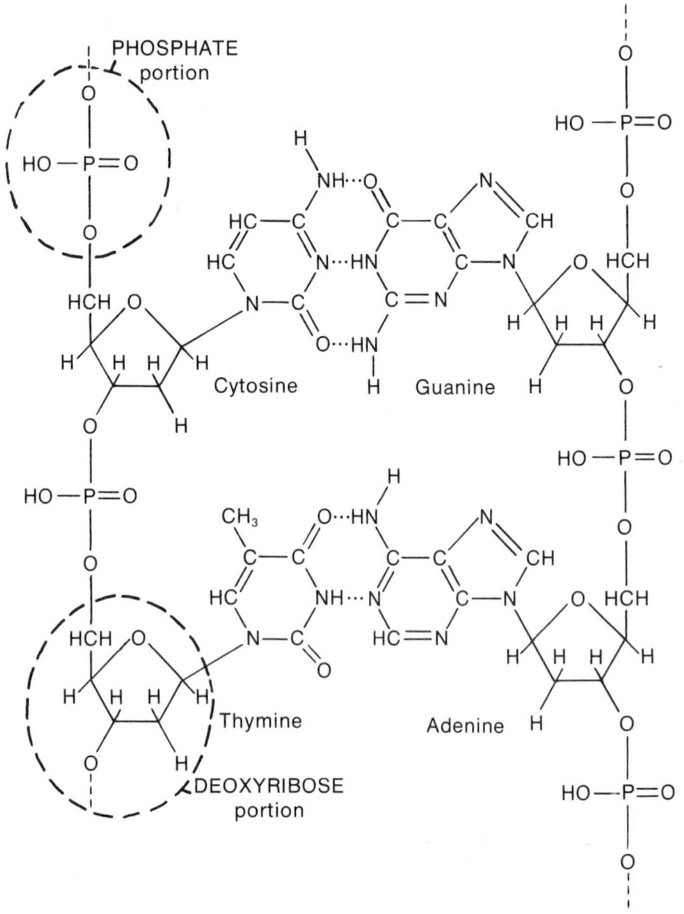

Figure 2-6 Chemical structure and diagrammatic representation of a segment of a DNA molecule and its components. (Courtesy of Richard Lyons, M.D.)

scribed by first noting that it has two very long strands of alternating deoxyribose and phosphoric acid (d-p-d-p-d). The number of each of these molecules in each strand is well into the thousands. Attached to each deoxyribose molecule is one of the four nitrogenous bases. The specific sequence of bases along the strands makes up a code—the genetic code.

The nitrogenous bases of each strand face each other and are loosely bonded in opposite matching pairs. The deoxyribose and phosphoric acid sequences serve as the sides of a ladderlike structure. The two strands (on the ladder) are twisted to form the double spiral, or helix (Fig. 2–7). The opposite pairing of the bases is quite specific; guanine (gwan'in) and cytosine bond only with each other; likewise, adenine and thymine are exclusive complements. Therefore, if there is a sequence of bases on one strand (G-A-A-C-T-G), then matching it re-

spectively on the opposite strand is the complementary sequence (C-T-T-G-A-C).

What Is the Language of DNA?

Within the last decade, biochemists have managed to decipher the coding system of the DNA molecule—the code by which DNA molecules store the information on how to make all the various proteins produced by cells. This code, most interestingly, is the same for all living organisms. The code itself turns out to be extremely simple and straightforward. The letters of the code are represented by the nitrogenous bases, which we can abbreviate as above: C, for cytosine; G, for guanine; T, for thymine; and A, for adenine.

These letters go to make up words or to code words. The key to understanding the language of DNA turns out to be the fact that each code word

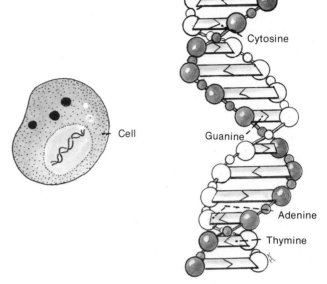

Figure 2-7 Diagrammatic representation of DNA helix.

contains only three letters. For instance, CAT, TAC, or GAA. Each of these words names, in the language of DNA, one of the amino acids. The amino acids are the building blocks of the proteins. So, if the DNA wants to give the code or information for making some protein, it simply sends out protein; that is, it sends out the messenger (RNA) with the words or sentence that specifies that particular protein. For instance, CAT-CAT-TAC-GAA-CAT would specify one very small protein made up of five amino acid units (only three different kinds of amino acids, however). Most proteins are larger than this, ranging from 25 or more amino acid units up to several thousand for complex proteins. The protein hemoglobin, which operates in red blood cells to carry oxygen, is known to be made up of about 575 amino acid units. Insulin, the protein involved in the maintenance of the blood sugar level (and given artificially to diabetics), contains about 51 amino acid units.

What Is RNA?

The RNA molecules, or ribonucleic acids, are a group of molecules found mostly in the cytoplasm; however, their functions are to be understood in relation to the organization and coordination activities of DNA.

The basic building blocks of RNA molecules are quite similar to those of DNA; however, RNA contains the sugar *ribose*, instead of deoxyribose, and the base *uracil* (u'rah-sil), in place of thymine. RNA is usually *single stranded*; in all other ways it resembles DNA in molecular structure.

There are three different types of RNA found in the cell, each with a specific function related to protein synthesis. These are *messenger RNA* (abbreviated mRNA), *transfer RNA* (tRNA), and *ribosomal RNA* (rRNA).

Messenger RNA   The name is quite appropriate, since this molecule carries the information from the DNA molecule in the nucleus out into the cytoplasm, where the actual protein synthesis takes place. mRNA is formed when the two strands of the DNA molecule separate and the paired building blocks for RNA match up against the code of the exposed DNA. Then an enzyme stimulates the building blocks to combine into one RNA molecule. The mRNA that has been formed then contains the information in the gene (genetic sentence) of the DNA (Table 2-1). The messenger RNA then moves to the cytoplasm.

Transfer RNA   This is the smallest RNA molecule. It circulates around the cytoplasm, where it captures stray amino acids and brings them to a specific site in the cytoplasm, to be combined into

Table 2–1 SOME BIOLOGICALLY IMPORTANT AMINO ACIDS AND THEIR RNA CODE WORDS

AMINO ACIDS	RNA CODE WORDS			
Alanine	CCG	UCG		
Arginine	CGC	AGA	UCG	
Asparagine	ACA	AUA		
Aspartic acid	GUA			
Cysteine	UUG			
Glutamic acid	GAA	ACU		
Glutamine	ACA	AGA	AGU	
Glycine	UGG	AGG		
Histidine	ACC			
Isoleucine	UAU	UAA		
Leucine	UUG	UUC	UUA	UUU
Lysine	AAA	AAG	AAU	
Methionine	UGA			
Phenylalanine	UUU			
Proline	CCC	CCU	CCA	CCG
Serine	UCU	ICC	UCG	
Threonine	CAC	CAA		
Tryptophan	CGU			
Tyrosine	AUU			
Valine	UGU			

protein molecules. There is one type of transfer RNA for each type of amino acid.

Ribosomal RNA The site of the actual protein synthesis is at the ribosomes, which are made up of ribosomal RNA and special ribosomal proteins. *Ribosomal RNA* is a very stable molecule of high molecular weight, which probably determines the alignment of the messenger RNA when it reaches the ribosome from the nucleus.

How Is the Protein Synthesized?

The process by which a particular protein comes to be synthesized within the cell is most easily viewed as beginning with the uncoiling of a specific DNA molecule in the nucleus. RNA parts then move to line up along the code strand of the uncoiled DNA molecule, according to the base-pair rule. By action of an enzyme, the messenger RNA molecule is formed. The mRNA then migrates out of the nucleus to the ribosomes in the cytoplasm (Fig. 2–8).

In the meantime, transfer RNAs have collected the amino acids and carried them to the ribosomes for synthesizing the protein molecule.

As the messenger RNA arrives at the ribosome, it is sequentially "read," or "translated," and the amino acids are properly lined up, ready for formation of the protein.

In some unknown manner, the ribosome then stimulates the now properly ordered amino acids to form the indicated protein—the protein whose code was contained in the DNA and mRNA.

THE CELL

What Are Relative Sizes in the Cell?

In order to help visualize the relative sizes of the parts of a cell, we can imagine a cell enlarged to a point at which its diameter is 100 yards—the length of a football field.

Each of the *mitochondria*, or energy factories of the cell, would be about the size of an automobile. You could fit 30 of these, end-to-end, across the length of the football field—100 yards. Glucose molecules, which in our enlarged cell would be about 1/8 inch in diameter, enter the mitochondria and are processed. ATP molecules (1/2 inch) carrying the stored energy migrate out of the mitochondria to various parts of the cell, where they release the energy as needed for cellular activities.

The *lysosomes*, which are the cell's digestive organs, would be about the size of small sports cars.

The *ribosomes* would be about the size of baseballs (3.6 inches in diameter), and they would be scattered throughout the cytoplasm.

The *cell membrane* would be only 1 1/2 inches thick. Similarly, the endoplasmic reticulum would be constructed of a membrane about 1 1/2 inches thick.

An average *bacterium* that might invade the cell would be about the size of a mitochondrion (the size of an automobile).

On the *molecular level*, the water molecules would be only 1/18 inch in diameter, or smaller than the ball in a ballpoint pen. You could fit 780,000 of these balls into a teacup. The large protein molecules, those that make up many of the

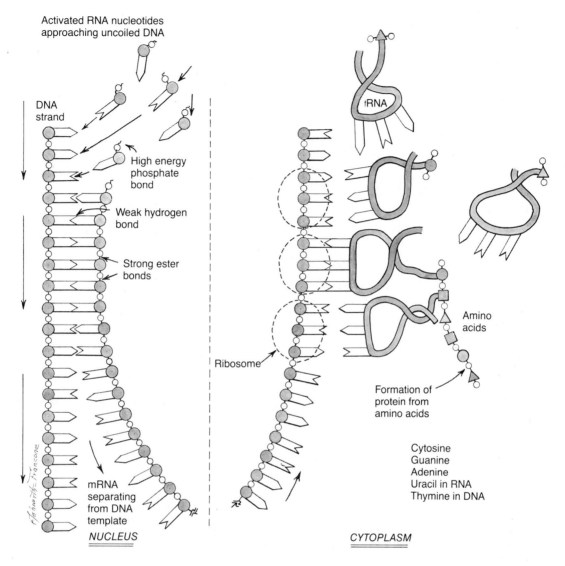

Figure 2–8 Messenger RNA duplicates the information encoded in the DNA molecule and attaches itself to the ribosomes. Amino acids, carried by loops of transfer RNA, are bonded together, move away, and become a three-dimensional protein.

structures of the cell and take part in most cellular chemical processes, would be 1 to 2 inches in diameter.

Perhaps the most interesting features of our enlarged cell are the long DNA molecules. They would appear as lengths of relatively thin rope (1/3 inch in diameter). There is so much DNA in the nucleus that if we put all the DNA end-to-end it would make a thin rope 5500 *miles* long. When this is wound-up, as it is in the nucleus, it would make a tight ball about 10 yards in diameter.

The whole *nucleus*, which contains some special nuclear proteins as well as the DNA, would be about 17 yards in diameter.

How Do Cells Reproduce?

All body cells reproduce by a process of division called *mitosis* (mi-to'sis). In the process of mitosis the original cell self-duplicates its internal constituents and then divides, producing two *daughter* cells, which are identical to the parent type.

It is through the self-duplication of the material in the nucleus—the DNA molecules—that it is possible for the parent cell to divide into two identical daughter cells. The DNA is the crucial hereditary (or genetic) material.

DNA self-duplication begins when the DNA molecules split apart lengthwise into two long strands (just as in mRNA formation). Next, DNA building blocks line up along the two strands to form, in each case, the complementary strand. The result is the production of the two new, identical DNA molecules. When the cell divides, one goes to one daughter cell and the other to a second daughter cell. Each new DNA (and each new daughter cell) contains one strand from the original DNA of the mother cell.

What Are the Four Main Stages of Mitosis?

Normal mitosis is usually described in four stages (Fig. 2–9). The normal functioning state of the cell is the *interphase*, or "resting" state. During this phase, the DNA molecules are somehow stimulated to self-duplicate. Also, during this phase, the cell stores up many cytoplasmic constituents that will later be divided between the two daughter cells. (The factors that stimulate a cell to divide in an adult are not well understood. However, this is the subject of intensive research, since it is believed to involve the key to understanding the uncontrolled growth found in cancerous tumors.)

In the *prophase*, the DNA complex becomes tightly coiled, forming the rodlike *chromosomes* (kro'mo-soms). *Microtubules* (mi"kro-tu'buls) begin to develop around each of the *centrioles* (sen'tri-ols) like the spokes of a wheel. Some of these microtubules penetrate the nucleus and apparently attach to the individual, coiled chromosomes at their midpoint, or *centronucleus*. During this process, the nuclear membrane disintegrates, and the nucleoli disappear.

Next, in *metaphase* the chromosomes move toward the center of the cell and arrange themselves in a plane perpendicular to the line connecting the

centrioles. The structure formed is usually referred to as the *equatorial plate*.

Then, in *anaphase* the duplicated chromosomes begin to separate; one set moves to one pole, and the duplicate set moves to the opposite pole. One chromosome from each of the 46 chromosomes found in human cells finds its way into each daughter cell, giving each cell an identical set of chromosomes.

Finally, in *telophase* the chromosomes reach the general location of the centrioles. Then the chromosomes uncoil, the nuclear membrane reappears, and an equatorial membrane appears at the former site of the metaphase plate, dividing the cytoplasm into two parts.

By this process, one cell with 23 pairs of chromosomes (or 46 individual chromosomes) becomes two cells, each of which has 23 pairs, or 46 individual chromosomes

THE CELLULAR ENVIRONMENT

What Is the Internal Environment?

A cell can live within a certain range of conditions or environments. There must be a certain amount of food, water, and oxygen present, and waste products must be taken away regularly. This situation is quite similar to that for each human being. However, the individual can move around and seek environments in which survival is possible, unlike the cell, which is limited in its movement.

To understand the problem of cellular environment, you might ask yourself what you would need to survive if you were sealed in a large jar. How would you obtain fresh air? Where would you obtain your food? How would you get rid of your waste products? How would you protect yourself from heat and cold?

Living organisms solve these problems partly by their movement within the external environment and partly by maintaining a fairly constant *internal environment* for each cell. If this internal environment changes too much, either over the whole body or in particular areas, then the cells in that area are going to begin to act abnormally and, eventually, die.

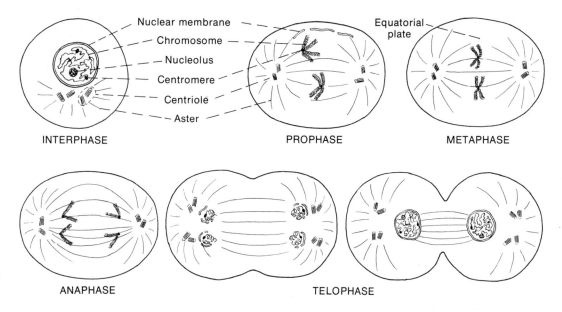

Figure 2-9 Mitosis, showing details of division. Shown are a pair of identical (homologous) chromosomes. Prior to the onset of mitosis, DNA replicates, giving rise to the double-stranded chromosomes that become apparent during mitosis. In prophase the two strands of each chromosome, attached to a common centromere, can be clearly seen. In metaphase the centromeres of the double-stranded chromosomes are lined up along the equatorial plate. The centromeres divide, and during anaphase the single strands move toward the centrioles at opposite poles of the cell. The end results of mitosis are two daughter cells with the same genetic composition as the original parent cell.

What Is the Distribution of Water in the Body?

In the human body, about 60 to 70 per cent of the lean body weight is water (Table 2-2). About two thirds of this is contained inside the individual cells as part of the cytoplasm. This is called the *intracellular* (inside the cell) water. The remaining one third is called the *extracellular* (outside of the cell) water (Table 2-3).

This extracellular water is very important. A large part of it is a major component of the blood. What is not contained in the blood is found slowly circulating between the cells as part of their environment.

What Is the Extracellular Fluid?

The extracellular water, both in the blood stream and between the cells, contains many dissolved substances. This water, together with its dissolved substances, is called the *extracellular fluid*.

The extracellular fluid is made up of water, salts, dissolved sugars (such as glucose), proteins, and a variety of substances in smaller amounts. It is very important that the concentrations of substances in this extracellular fluid remain fairly constant. This is a part of the homeostatic environment of the cells. If the concentration changes, so as to contain too much or too little of these substances, the cells will become sick and act abnormally and eventually begin to die.

What Are Osmosis and Diffusion?

The transportation of water and dissolved substances at the cellular level occurs in large part through two passive processes: osmosis and diffusion. Osmosis is the natural movement of water through a semipermeable membrane from a dilute

Table 2-2   PERCENTAGE COMPOSITION OF REPRESENTATIVE MAMMALIAN TISSUES*

TISSUE	WATER	SOLIDS	PROTEINS	LIPIDS	CARBOHYDRATES
Striated muscle	72–78	22–28	18–20	3.0	0.6
Whole blood	79	21	19	1	0.1
Liver	60–80	20–40	15	3–20	1–15
Brain	78	22	8	12–15	0.1
Skin	66	34	25	7	present
Bone (marrow-free)	20–25	75–80	30	low	present

* Source: White, A., Handler, P., Smith, E., and Stetten, D.: *Principles of Biochemistry.* New York, McGraw-Hill, 1954.

to a concentrated solution. A semipermeable membrane, like the cell membrane, allows only certain substances to pass through (i.e., permeate), and some do this much more easily than others. The direction of flow across the membrane is always two way, but the net flow is such that water moves from a dilute to a more concentrated solution.

If the concentration of dissolved substances is the same both inside and outside the cell, then there is not net movement of water between the intracellular and extracellular compartments. However, if the intracellular environment becomes more concentrated (as after the cell has ingested something) there will be a net flow of water into the cell until the intracellular and extracellular concentrations are the same. Similarly, if the extracellular compartment becomes overly concentrated perhaps due to perspiration on a hot day, then there will be a net flow from the intracellular compartment until the concentrations are even.

Diffusion is the natural microscopic mixing of all substances. Diffusion always results in dissolved substances moving from areas of higher concentration toward areas of lower concentration until all concentrations are the same, at which time mixing is completed. Diffusion is a natural process that promotes homeostasis. It is also important in bringing nutrients to all parts of the body and in removing waste products from all parts of the body. Diffusion is important in the exchange of gases in the lungs:

Table 2-3   CHEMICAL COMPOSITION OF BODY FLUIDS

	EXTRACELLULAR FLUID	INTRACELLULAR FLUID
Na^+	137 mEq/liter	10 mEq/liter
K^+	5 mEq/liter	141 mEq/liter
Ca^{++}	5 mEq/liter	0 mEq/liter
Mg^{++}	3 mEq/liter	62 mEq/liter
Cl^-	103 mEq/liter	4 mEq/liter
HCO_3	28 mEq/liter	10 mEq/liter
Phosphates	4 mEq/liter	75 mEq/liter
SO_4	1 mEq/liter	2 mEq./liter
Glucose	90 mg%	0 to 20 mg%
Amino acids	30 mg%	200 mg%
Cholesterol Phospholipids Neutral fat }	0.5 g%	2 to 95 g%
P_{O_2}	35 mm Hg	20 mm Hg ?
P_{CO_2}	46 mm Hg	50 mm Hg ?
pH	7.4 mm Hg	7.1 ?

Positive and Negative Feedback

Rather than thinking of the body exclusively as a clockwork mechanism of causes and effects—although this is clearly part of the true picture of how the body works—scientists have found it helpful in understanding biologic systems to think of the body also in terms of purposes and "intelligent" communication among the parts carrying out those purposes. One very important concept in understanding how the body works is feedback.

The coordination of activities and the maintenance of homeostasis in the body depend on the communication among the various systems, organs, tissues, and cells. This communication, or feedback, although often causal, directs the purposes.

The simplest example of a nonbiologic feedback system can be seen in the regulation of room temperature (purpose) by a thermostat. As long as the room is too cold, the thermostat tells the furnace to produce more heat. If the room becomes too warm the thermostat tells the furnace to slow down or perhaps even to shut off. The thermostat measures the temperature, the information, and then transmits the signal to the furnace.

Positive feedback occurs when the signal tells the furnace to produce more heat.

Negative feedback takes place when the signal tells the furnace to produce less heat. The balanced regulation of these two options can keep the room more or less at the same temperature.

The intelligent regulation, or balancing, of positive and negative feedback in biologic systems is what produces life-sustaining coordination and homeostasis. Throughout the body one finds physiologic processes (and corresponding anatomic structures) organized, at least in part, to regulate and to be regulated by positive and negative feedback. For instance, the brain senses the temperature of the body and sends out signals to the cells to produce more or less heat as needed.

Short-lived chemical messengers are sent out from a wide range of organs and tissues to other parts of the body, asking for some sort of assistance. These messengers increase in number as the need increases. As the need is met, the number of messengers decreases.

As you learn about the anatomy and physiology of the human body, always ask yourself how the process is turned on and how it is turned off. This applies equally to understanding fully the activity of the individual cell as well as that of each organ and at the system level.

The high concentration of carbon dioxide in the blood—building up as a waste product from cells—diffuses to the lower concentration in the lungs and outside environment. Likewise, the higher concentration of oxygen in the lungs and in the outside environment diffuses into the blood and oxygenates it.

What Is Homeostasis?

The process of keeping the cellular internal environment fairly constant, or within a "normal" range, is known as *homeostasis* (ho"me-o-sta'sis). The term homeostasis was derived from the Greek words, *homoios*, meaning to keep the same or to maintain, and *stasis*, a standing still.

In order to accomplish homeostasis, the various systems of the body must be able to respond to the important changes in the environment, before these changes begin to harm the cells. Four major organ systems are responsible for maintaining a homeostasis of the primary factors in the internal environment of each cell. These are the *respiratory system*, which operates to maintain an oxygen supply and to remove carbon dioxide; the *digestive system*, which supplies all solid nutrients and salts; the *urinary system*, which regulates the water content and the concentration of many substances in the fluid surrounding each cell; and the *circulatory system*, which connects each individual cell with the other organ systems. In this way, the circulatory system holds a central place of importance in maintaining the internal environment of each cell.

SUMMARY

A. Cells are the microscopic living units that make up large organisms.
1. Each individual cell is alive as demonstrated by their activities.
   a. Cells grow, reproduce, and die.
   b. They need nourishment and require disposal of waste products.
   c. They are able to respond and adapt to changes in the environment.
2. Cells come in different shapes and sizes.
B. The three main divisions of the cell are the cell membrane, the cytoplasm, and the nucleus.
1. The cell membrane is the extremely thin outer covering of the cell.
   a. It functions in both ingestion and excretion.
   b. It controls exchanges of air, water, and chemical substances.
2. The cytoplasm is the main body contents of the cell.
   a. Cytoplasm is composed primarily of water.
   b. It contains "factory" units called organelles.
3. The nucleus is contained in its own thin membrane.
   a. The nucleus floats in the cytoplasm.
   b. It is the control center, directing and coordinating the activities of cell parts.
C. The cell membrane controls which substances pass into and out of the cell.
1. Tiny holes allow water, oxygen, and carbon dioxide to pass freely back and forth.
2. Active ingestion of small proteins and sugars is called pinocytosis.
3. Ingesting larger particles is accomplished by a process called phagocytosis.

D. The cytoplasm is highly organized with miniature cellular "factories," which are called organelles.
1. Mitochondria, the "powerhouses," transfer the energy from food molecules to special ATP molecules.
   a. ATP is the abbreviation for adenosine triphosphate.
   b. The cells use ATP molecules to store and transport energy.
   c. Mitochondria are most abundant in muscle cells, which use a great deal of energy.
2. Lysosomes break down, or digest, large food molecules.
   a. The digestive process uses enzymes to break down food particles chemically into simple substances.
   b. The simpler food molecules are then able to enter the mitochondria.
3. Ribosomes, usually attached to the endoplasmic reticulum, are the specific sites at which cells construct new types of molecules.
4. The endoplasmic reticulum is an internal network of channels.
   a. Its surfaces are formed out of a thin cellular membrane, spread throughout the cytoplasm.
   b. The channels serve to transport and store substances.
E. The nucleus controls and coordinates cellular activities.
1. DNA molecules in the nucleus send out messenger RNA molecules with directions ("blueprints") for producing specific proteins.
2. The proteins are assembled from amino acid building blocks at the ribosomes.
3. Ribosomes are composed of ribosomal RNA.
4. The amino acid building blocks are brought to the ribosomal assembly sites by transfer RNA molecules.
F. DNA molecules (or deoxyribonucleic acid), the main substance of every cell nucleus, are very large double-stranded molecules made up of only a few basic chemical compounds.
1. The double backbone of the molecule is thousands of alternating molecules of phosphoric acid and deoxyribose: d-p-d-p-d-p-d-p-d.
2. Attached to each deoxyribose is one of

the four nitrogenous bases: adenine, guanine, thymine, and cytosine. The opposite strand has the exact opposite sequence of bases.

3. The specific sequence of these bases reads like a code and is called the genetic code, which specifies the structure of all the proteins of a particular living organism.

4. The two strands fit together to form a ladderlike structure that is twisted to form a double spiral, or helix.

5. The genetic code is written in sets of three bases.

   a. Each set specifies one of the amino acids.

   b. Larger groupings of these sets specify particular proteins.

   c. The coding system is the same for all living organisms.

G. RNA molecules (or ribonucleic acid), located primarily in the cytoplasm, are single-stranded molecules (similar to DNA) made up of only a few basic chemical compounds. There are three different types.

1. Messenger RNA (mRNA) carries information from the DNA molecules in the nucleus out into the cytoplasm where protein synthesis takes place.

2. Transfer RNA (tRNA) gathers amino acids in the cytoplasm and brings them to the ribosomes to be assembled into proteins.

3. Ribosomal RNA (rRNA) is the main constituent of the ribosomes and operates in protein synthesis.

H. Protein synthesis begins with the uncoiling of a specific DNA molecule.

1. A mRNA forms to encode the DNA sequence.

2. The mRNA migrates to the ribosome, while the tRNAs are collecting the amino acids.

3. The mRNA is sequentially "read," and the protein, specified by the original DNA coding, is formed.

I. Cells reproduce by a process of division called mitosis. Through self-duplication, the original parent cell divides to produce two daughter cells, each identical to the original parent. There are four main stages.

1. Interphase is the normal, "resting" state.

2. Prophase is marked by the DNA becoming tightly coiled, forming the rodlike chromosomes.

3. In metaphase the chromosomes move toward the center.

4. In anaphase the duplicated chromosomes begin to separate, giving each new cell an identical set of chromosomes.

5. In telophase the chromosomes uncoil, the nuclear membrane reappears, and the cytoplasm divides into two parts.

J. The internal environment of each cell (primarily food, water, oxygen, and waste removal) must be maintained within certain limits to sustain life and health.

K. Of the lean body weight, 60 to 70 per cent is water.

1. Two thirds of this water is contained inside cells as part of the cytoplasm and is called intracellular water.

2. The remaining one third is extracellular water, a large portion of which makes up the blood.

3. The extracellular fluid contains many dissolved substances.

   a. These substances include salts, sugars, proteins, and a variety of trace chemicals.

   b. The concentration of these dissolved substances must remain fairly constant through homeostasis.

L. The transportation of water and other substances at the cellular level occurs primarily through two passive physical processes.

1. Osmosis is the natural movement of water through a semipermeable membrane from a dilute to a concentrated solution.

   a. A semipermeable membrane, like the cell membrane, allows only certain substances to pass through (i.e., permeate), with some substances permeating much more easily than others.

   b. Water is the most active osmotic substance transported between the cellular and extracellular compartments, always from a dilute toward a more concentrated solution.

2. Diffusion is the natural mixing of substances.

   a. The result is that substances move from areas of higher concentration toward areas of lower concentration.

   b. For instance, the exchange of gases in the lungs occurs in part through diffusion.

      i. The high concentration of carbon

dioxide in the blood diffuses to the lower concentration in the lungs and outside environment.
    ii. The higher concentration of oxygen in the lungs and the outside environment diffuses into and oxygenates the blood.
M. Homeostasis is the process of keeping the internal environment within a fairly constant "normal" range.
    1. The body must be able to respond to changes in the environment.
    2. The four main systems dedicated to homeostasis are the respiratory, digestive, urinary, and circulatory systems.

REVIEW QUESTIONS

  1. What are the common functional abilities of all living cells?

  2. What are the three main divisions of the cell?

  3. Describe the general functions of the cell membrane.

  4. Describe the makeup of the cytoplasm.

  5. Describe the general location and function of the cell nucleus.

  6. Explain how small molecules enter and leave the cell.

  7. Characterize and distinguish both pinocytosis and phagocytosis.

  8. How does the increased production of specific proteins serve to direct the activities of the cell?

  9. How does the nucleus slow down some cellular activity?

10. Explain the process by which the nucleus directs the manufacture of proteins from their amino acid building blocks.

11. Identify the elementary constituent molecules that make up the DNA molecule. Name the four nitrogenous bases associated with DNA.

12. Construct and label a diagram of a portion of a DNA molecule showing the constituents and their structural relationships.

13. What is the complementary sequence to T-T-T-C-G-A?

14. What is the relation between the base sequence of the DNA molecule and the amino acids that reveal the genetic code?

15. Identify the elementary constituent molecules that make up all RNA molecules. Name the four nitrogenous bases associated with RNA.

16. Construct and label a diagram of a portion of an RNA molecule showing the constituents and their structural relationships.

17. What are the three types of RNA found in each cell?

18. Explain how the formation of messenger RNA reads the exposed code sequence on the DNA.

19. What is the function of transfer RNA? What is the function of ribosomal RNA?

20. Summarize the process of protein synthesis.

21. Construct and label a diagram of the cell that shows the relative sizes of the cell and its parts.

22. Outline the process of cellular reproduction by cell division. Briefly describe each of the four main stages of mitosis.

23. What is meant by the internal environment?

24. What portion of the lean body weight is water? How much of this is intracellular and how much is extracellular?

25. Describe the osmotic movement of water between intracellular and extracellular compartments when a cell is placed in a surrounding environment of higher salt concentration? What occurs when a cell is placed in an environment of lower salt concentration?

26. Characterize diffusion and give an example in the biologic setting.

27. Define homeostasis.

28. Name the four major organ systems responsible for maintaining homeostasis of the internal environment of each cell. Explain how each of these systems serves that purpose.

29. Define feedback and distinguish between positive and negative feedback.

T H R E E

Tissues and the Skin

O B J E C T I V E S

The aim of this chapter is to enable the student to do the following:

- Identify the four basic types of tissues and describe their functions.
- List the types of specialized epithelial, connective, muscular, and nervous tissues and identify their functions.
- Describe, with illustrations, the layers of the skin and its appendages.

- Classify the four main functions of the skin.
- List six common skin problems seen clinically.
- Distinguish among first, second, and third degree burns.

TISSUES

What Is a Tissue?

A tissue is a network of similar cells woven together. The cells hold themselves together by producing an intercellular (between the cells) substance, to which they all attach themselves. The precise amount and composition of these intercellular "cementing" substances vary, depending on the type of tissues, as will be seen.

There are four main types of tissues in the body: *epithelial, connective, muscular,* and *nervous.*

Epithelial Tissues These tissues function in protection, absorption, and secretion. When serving a *protective* function, epithelial tissue is found in sheets, covering a surface such as the skin (Fig. 3–1). In the absorptive function, the epithelial tis-

sues form specialized surfaces, as in the tiny air sacs of the lung tissue, where oxygen is absorbed into the blood. In the functions of secretion there are two specialized epithelial tissues—mucous membrane and glandular epithelium. *Mucous membrane* lines the digestive, respiratory, urinary, and reproductive tracts, secreting mucus as well as other special substances. Glands are incuppings of special epithelial tissue; they function to produce and secrete a wide variety of important substances. The glands include simple sweat glands, mammary glands, and large salivary glands (Fig. 3–2) as well as the endocrine gland group, which includes the thyroid, pituitary, ovaries, and testes. (The endocrine glands are discussed in Chapter 7.)

Connective Tissues These tissues allow movement and provide support. In this type of tissue there is an abundance of fiberlike intercellular material, which the cells produce and deposit in order to give great strength to the connective tissues (Fig.

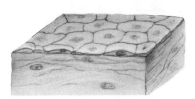

Simple squamous

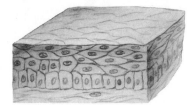

Stratified squamous

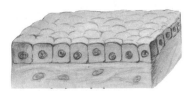

Cuboidal

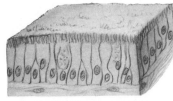

Pseudostratified ciliated columnar

Figure 3–1 Types of epithelial tissue, classified according to shape and arrangement of cell layers.

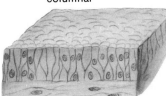

Simple columnar

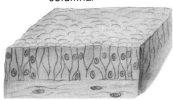

Pseudostratified columnar

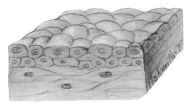

Transitional

3–3). The two main types of *loose connective tissue* are known as areolar (ah-re′o-lar) tissue and adipose tissue. *Areolar tissue* is the most widely distributed connective tissue; it resists tearing and is somewhat elastic. Its main function is to connect other tissues and to provide support when needed. *Adipose tissue* is specialized areolar tissue, with many fat-containing cells. Its functions are in fat storage and as a cushion between organs and other structures in the body.

Dense connective tissue makes up the main parts of tendons, ligaments, and various tough tissue sheaths, which hold various parts of the body in position. For instance, dense connective tissue holds joints together and holds muscles and organs in position.

There are a number of specialized connective tissues. *Cartilage,* which is a special connective tissue, is the flexible material found on the outer ear and nose; it is also found between bones at the joints, where it serves to cushion shocks to the body. *Bone,* which is also a special connective tissue, has the important property of rigid strength. This property arises from the fact that bone cells surround themselves with large stores of inorganic salts—primarily *calcium phosphate. Blood* and blood-forming tissue are also considered to be special connective tissues. This is because blood cells are born and

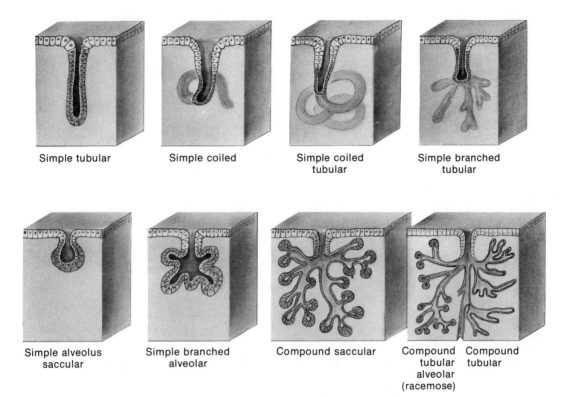

Simple tubular   Simple coiled   Simple coiled tubular   Simple branched tubular

Simple alveolus saccular   Simple branched alveolar   Compound saccular   Compound tubular alveolar (racemose)   Compound tubular

Figure 3–2 Exocrine glands. These glands may be tubular, coiled, saccular, or racemose (resembling a bunch of grapes on a stalk).

grow to maturity in the bone marrow, which is the tissue in the center of most bones (Fig. 3–4). Blood is a fluid tissue that circulates through the body, carrying nutrients to cells and removing waste products.

Muscular Tissue   The main function of muscle tissue is to produce movement through contraction and relaxation. The voluntary muscles are made up of a particular type of muscle tissue. The internal, involuntary muscles are made up of another specialized type of muscle tissue. Finally, the heart, which is the most important muscular organ of the body, contains its own special type of muscle tissue (Fig. 3–4).

Nervous Tissue   This is the most highly organized tissue in the body. It functions to control and coordinate all the many complicated activities of the body. In nervous tissue, the specialized conducting cells are called *neurons*. Neurons are linked together to form nerve pathways (Fig. 3–4).

THE SKIN

What Is the Skin?

The skin is an organ (or group of organs) that covers the external surface of the body. It functions as a protective surface, keeping out bacteria and harmful substances. It also operates in the regulation of body temperature and in the disposal of water (through sweat). Figure 3–5 shows a three-dimensional view of the skin.

What Are the Epidermis and the Dermis?

The skin is composed of two distinct kinds of tissue. The outer surface, known as the *epidermis*

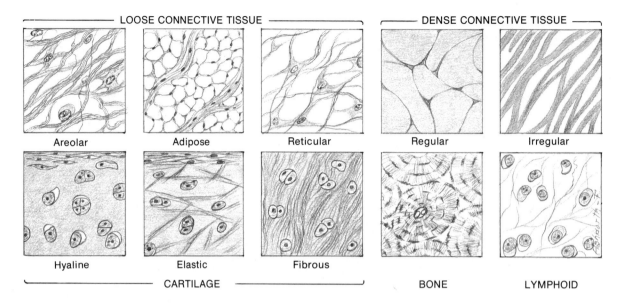

Figure 3-3 *Loose connective tissue:*
Areolar: loosely arranged fibroelastic connective tissue.
Adipose: regions of connective tissue dominated by aggregations of fat cells.
Reticular: makes delicate connecting and supporting frameworks, enters into the composition of basement membranes, produces macrophages, and plays important roles as scavenger and agent of defense against bacteria.
Dense connective tissue:
Regular: fibers that are oriented so as to withstand tension exerted in one direction.
Irregular: fibers that are arranged so as to withstand tensions exerted from different directions.
Cartilage:
Hyaline: the most fundamental kind of cartilage, consisting of a seemingly homogeneous matrix permeated with fine white fibers.
Elastic: specialized cartilage with elastic fibers in the matrix.
Fibrous: specialized cartilage emphasizing collagenous fibers in its matrix.
Bone: a tissue consisting of cells, fibers, and a ground substance, the distinguishing feature of which is the presence of a ground substance of inorganic salts.
Lymphoid tissue: a tissue consisting of two primary tissue elements—reticular tissue and cells, chiefly lymphocytes—intermingling in intimate association in the reticular interstices

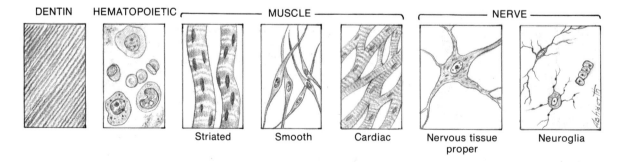

Figure 3-4 *Dentin,* like bone, consists of a collagenous mesh and calcified ground substance; unlike bone, it contains neither vessels nor total cells. *Hematopoietic tissue:* blood-forming tissues, i.e., red bone marrow. *Muscle tissue* has the properties of contractility and excitability (see Chapter 5). *Nervous tissue* has the properties of excitability and conductivity (see Chapter 6).

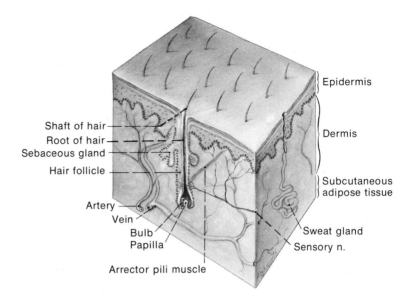

Figure 3-5 Three-dimensional view of the skin.

Shaft of hair
Root of hair
Sebaceous gland
Hair follicle
Artery
Vein
Bulb
Papilla
Arrector pili muscle

Epidermis
Dermis
Subcutaneous adipose tissue
Sweat gland
Sensory n.

(*epi*, meaning upon), is made up of several layers of a special epithelial tissue. The deeper layer of tissue is known as the *dermis* (Greek for skin) and consists of a tough connective tissue (Figs. 3–6 and 3–7).

The innermost cells of the epidermis are continually reproducing and replacing the cells of the outer surface, which flake off by the millions each day. One of the factors that determine the skin color is the amount of a dark pigment substance called *melanin* (mel'ah-nin), which is produced by the epidermal cells. Melanin production increases with exposure to strong ultraviolet light (creating a suntan).

The dermis (or corium) lies directly beneath the epidermis and is composed of strong fibrous connective tissues. Within the dermis are hundreds of nerve endings, sweat glands, and hair roots. About one third of the body's blood normally flows

through the dermis. Heat or motion can increase this flow and give the skin a reddened appearance.

What Are the Appendages of the Skin?

The main appendages of the skin are hair, nails, sebaceous glands, and sweat glands (Fig. 3–8).

Hair covers the entire body, except the palms, soles, and portions of the genitalia. The visible portion of the hair is the *shaft*. The *root* is situated in an epidermal tube known as the hair *follicle*, which consists of an outer connective tissue sheath and an inner epithelial membrane. When the *arrector pili* (Latin, "raiser of the hair") muscles contract, the skin assumes a so-called "goose flesh" appearance,

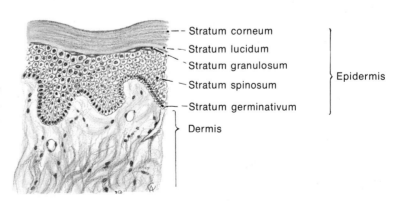

Figure 3-6 The epidermis (consisting of five distinct layers) and the dermis compose the protective covering of the body.

Stratum corneum
Stratum lucidum
Stratum granulosum
Stratum spinosum
Stratum germinativum
Epidermis
Dermis

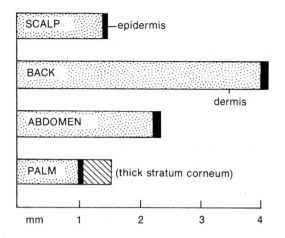

Figure 3-7 Graphic representation of skin thicknesses from various body sites.

and the hairs tend to "stand on their ends," to a certain degree (see Figs. 3-5 and 3-8).

Around each hair follicle is a *sebaceous* (se-ba'shus) *gland,* which produces *sebum* (se'bum), the oily substance primarily responsible for lubrication of the surface of the skin.

Sweat glands are simple, tubular glands that are found in most parts of the skin; they are most prominent in the palms and soles. It has been estimated that there are 3000 sweat glands per square inch on the palm of the hand. Sweating leads to loss of heat in the body.

The *nails* are composed of hard *keratin* (ker'ah-tin), the same protein substance that makes up a major part of the hair shaft. Air mixed with keratin forms the white crescent, or *lunula* (lu'nu-lah), of each nail. Each nail grows about 1 mm per week. Regeneration of a lost nail occurs in 4 to 8 months.

What Are the Four Main Functions of the Skin?

The skin functions are *sensation, protection, thermoregulation,* and *secretion.*

Sensation   Located in the skin are specific receptors, which are sensitive to the four basic sensations of pain, touch, temperature, and pressure. Upon stimulation of a receptor, a nerve signal is sent to the brain, where it is interpreted.

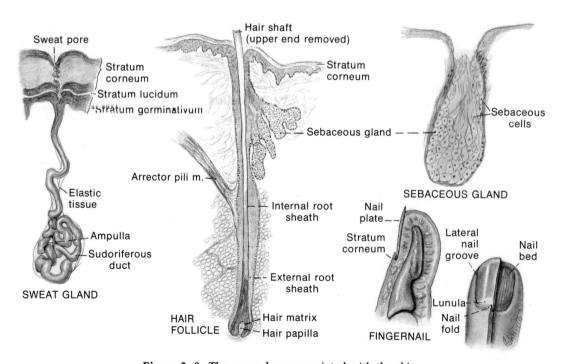

Figure 3-8 The appendages associated with the skin.

Protection   The skin forms an elastic, resistant covering that protects the person from a complex environment. This covering prevents the passage of harmful physical and chemical agents and prevents excess loss of water and salts.

Temperature Regulation   As the body needs to dissipate heat, blood vessels of the skin dilate (expand), allowing more blood to come to the surface, with a resulting loss of heat; also, the evaporation of sweat from the skin surface leads to a loss of body heat.

Secretion   The skin plays a part in the secretory functions of the body. Sebum, secreted by sebaceous glands, fights fungus and bacterial growth on the skin surface and also helps maintain the texture of the skin. Sweat is a secretion.

Clinical Aspects of the Skin

What Does Skin Appearance Tell Us?

The appearance of the skin can be an important sign in the diagnosis of various disorders. For instance, the skin may be red in hypertension (high blood pressure) and in other conditions in which the blood vessels of the skin are dilated. A pale skin suggests anemia (too few red blood cells or too little hemoglobin). The color of the skin may be blue or purple (a condition known as cyanosis) in severe heart disease and in lung-related diseases such as pneumonia (in which the blood is not being adequately supplied with oxygen). A yellow skin (jaundice) indicates the presence of larger than normal amounts of bile pigments in the blood.

What Are Some Common Skin Problems?

Acne (pimples) is an inflammatory disease of the sebaceous glands that occurs mainly over the face, neck, upper chest, back, and shoulders. It may occur at any time from puberty through the period of sexual development and remain for years.

Hives is a skin condition characterized by the sudden appearance of raised patches that are white in the center and itch severely. Hives often occur after ingestion of certain foods, such as strawberries or seafood, to which the individual is sensitive.

Psoriasis (so-ri'ah-sis) is a chronic inflammatory disease that is neither infectious nor contagious; its cause is unknown. Psoriasis is characterized by patches of dry, whitish scales.

Bed sores are caused by areas of pressure on the body of a bedridden person. Frequent turning and

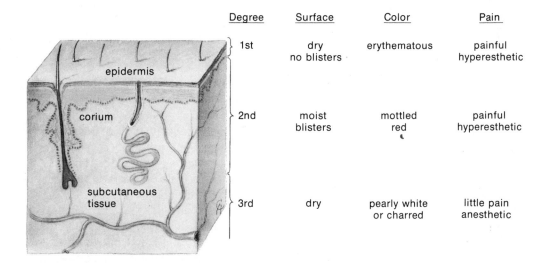

Degree	Surface	Color	Pain
1st	dry no blisters	erythematous	painful hyperesthetic
2nd	moist blisters	mottled red	painful hyperesthetic
3rd	dry	pearly white or charred	little pain anesthetic

Figure 3-9 Extent of burn injury — first, second, and third degrees. In a first degree burn only the epidermis is injured (as in sunburn); a second degree burn extends into the dermis; and a third degree burn involves the full thickness of skin, epidermis and dermis, extending into subcutaneous tissue. (Courtesy of Parke-Davis.)

alcohol rubs help to prevent this distressing condition.

Sunburn is a condition in which the skin is swollen and red after excessive exposure to the sun, especially its ultraviolet rays, and can happen even on a cloudy day.

Boils are localized inflammations of the dermis and underlying tissue; they are caused by bacteria that enter through the hair follicles.

How Are Burns Rated?

It is important to be able to determine the extent of a burn injury before any therapy is undertaken.

In a *first degree* burn, only the epidermis is injured (as in sunburn). A red coloration appears on the surface. A *second degree* burn extends into the dermis and forms blisters on the surface. A *third degree* burn involves both the epidermis and dermis as well as the underlying tissues; complete destruction of all layers of the skin results (Fig. 3–9).

SUMMARY

A. Tissues are networks of similar cells bound together by an intercellular "cementing" substance.
B. Epithelial tissues function in protection, absorption, and secretion.
   1. In the protective function they are found in sheets covering a surface, for instance, the skin.
   2. In the absorptive function they form special surfaces, as in the tiny air sacs that absorb oxygen in the lungs.
   3. In the functions of secretion there are two types of specialized epithelial tissue.
      a. Mucous membrane lines the digestive, respiratory, urinary, and reproductive tracts.
      b. Glands are incuppings of special epithelial tissue. These glands range from simple sweat glands to sophisticated endocrine glands like the thyroid and pituitary.
C. Connective tissues function to provide support and to make movement possible. This type of

tissue contains an abundance of fiberlike intercellular material.
   1. There are two main types of loose connective tissue.
      a. Areolar tissue functions to connect other tissues, provides general structural support, is somewhat elastic, resists tearing, and is widely distributed.
      b. Adipose tissue functions to store fat and to provide cushioning.
   2. Dense connective tissue makes up the main parts of tendons, ligaments, and tough tissue sheaths. It holds together joints and maintains muscles and organs in position.
   3. Cartilage, a specialized connective tissue, is the flexible material found on the outer ear and nose.
      a. It serves as a shock absorber between bones in the joints.
      b. It also helps to give shape to various parts of the body.
   4. Bone, another specialized connective tissue, provides rigid strength by means of large deposits of calcium phosphate.
   5. Blood and blood-forming tissues found in the bone marrow are also considered to be special connective tissues.
      a. Blood cells are born and mature in the marrow.
      b. Blood is a fluid tissue that circulates through the body, carrying nutrients to cells and removing waste products.
D. Muscular tissues function to provide movement through contraction and relaxation.
   1. There are two main types of muscular tissue: the voluntary and the involuntary.
   2. The heart contains its own type of muscular tissue.
E. Nervous tissues, through their highly organized system of neurons, function to control and coordinate all the complicated activities of the body.
F. The skin functions as an organ or system that covers the external surface of the body.
   1. The skin serves as a protective shield.
   2. The skin helps regulate body temperature and, through sweat, disposes of water.
G. The skin has two main layers.
   1. The epidermis, made up of several thicknesses of epithelial tissue, is the outermost layer.

2. The dermis (or corium), made up of strong fibrous connective tissue, is the deeper layer.

H. There are several main appendages of the skin.

1. Hair, found over most of the body, is composed of the visible shaft, with a root situated in the follicle.

2. The arrector pili muscle makes hair stand on end.

3. A sebaceous gland surrounds each hair follicle, producing the oily substance that lubricates the surface of the skin.

4. Sweat glands are simple tubular glands most prominent on the palms of the hands and the soles of the feet.

5. The nails are composed of keratin, a protein substance.

I. The skin has four main functions.

1. Sensation: The four types of special sensors in the skin are sensitive to pain, touch, temperature, and pressure.

2. Protection: The skin forms an elastic resistant covering for the body.

3. Temperature Regulation: By increasing blood flow to the surface, the skin produces a loss of heat. Evaporation of sweat (a secretion) also produces loss of body heat.

4. Secretion: Sebum, secreted by the sebaceous glands, fights fungus and bacterial growth and maintains skin texture.

J. Important signs of various disorders can be seen in the appearance of the skin.

K. Six common problems of the skin:

1. Acne is an inflammation of the sebaceous glands.

2. Hives, which are raised, itchy patches, most often occur as a reaction to certain foods.

3. Psoriasis is a chronic inflammatory disease characterized by patches of dry, whitish scales.

4. Bed sores (decubiti) are caused by areas of pressure on the body of a bedridden person.

5. Sunburned skin is red and swollen because of excessive exposure to the sun.

6. Boils are caused by bacteria and result in a localized inflammation of the dermis around a hair follicle.

L. The extent of a burn injury is rated as follows:

1. First degree burns involve the epidermis only.

2. Second degree burns involve the dermis and result in blisters in the epidermis.

3. Third degree burns result in damage that destroys the skin and involves underlying tissues.

REVIEW QUESTIONS

1. What holds cells together to form tissues?

2. Name the four main types of tissues.

3. What are the three functions of epithelial tissue? Give one or more example of each.

4. What sort of tissue are glands made of?

5. What are the main functions of connective tissue?

6. Characterize and distinguish the two main types of loose connective tissue.

7. Identify the body parts composed primarily of dense connective tissue.

8. What is the specialized connective tissue that makes up the firm, flexible material of the nose and outer ear?

9. What substance gives bone its rigidity?

10. Is blood a tissue? What is its function?

11. Where are blood cells born and where do they mature?

12. Describe the function of muscular tissue and the two mechanical operations to accomplish that function.

13. Distinguish three types of muscular tissue.

14. Characterize nervous tissue and describe its function.

15. Name the two layers of the skin and outline their relation.

16. What are the appendages of the skin?

17. List and explain the four main functions of the skin.

18. What diseases might be indicated by exceptionally red, blue or yellow skin?

19. List and characterize six clinically common skin problems.

20. How is the degree of a burn rated in terms of skin damage?

F O U R

The Skeletal System

The aim of this chapter is to enable the student to do the following:

- Describe the functions of bone.

- Describe the formation and growth of the skeleton.

- Distinguish the two types of bone tissue.

- Identify the major anatomic areas of the long bone.

- Explain the function of the bone marrow.

- Explain the role and regulation of calcium salts.

- Identify the bones of the axial and appendicular skeletons.

- Name the three types of joints and compare the amount of movement allowed by each.

- Construct and label diagrams showing the gross anatomy of the knee joint.

- Distinguish and explain the types of fractures.

- Identify two separate causes of bone and joint disorders.

- Define osteoporosis.

WHAT DOES THE SKELETAL SYSTEM DO?

The skeletal system provides the rigid framework that supports and gives shape to the body. It also serves to protect delicate internal organs such as the brain, heart, and lungs. Together with the muscular system, the skeletal system enables the body to accomplish a wide range of movements.

Two lesser known functions of the skeletal system are the manufacture of blood cells and the storage of mineral salts, especially calcium.

HOW DOES THE SKELETON DEVELOP?

The complete skeleton is first formed in the fetus at the end of the third month of pregnancy. At that time it is composed entirely of cartilage tissue —like the flexible material of your outer ear and nose. The cartilage is gradually replaced by bone tissue. This process, known as *ossification* (os"i-fi-ka'shun), occurs when dormant bone cells are stimulated to mature. During the initial phase, the bone cells produce a matrix or membrane system. Later the bone cells and the matrix absorb calcium phosphate crystals in a regular pattern to form the typical hardened network of bone tissue. The early patterns of the solid network are not final but rather are being constantly remade and modified as the bone cells multiply and adapt.

Longitudinal (lengthwise) growth of bones continues in a definite sequence until approximately 15 years of age in the female and 16 years in the male. Longitudinal growth should not be confused with bone maturation (the process of maturing) and remodeling, which are processes that continue until the age of 21 in both the male and female. This pattern of maturation is so regular that an individual's age can be determined with amazing accuracy from radiologic (using x-ray pictures) examination of his or her bones (Fig. 4–1).

THE NATURE OF BONE

What Does a Typical Bone Look Like?

The parts and structure of bones in general can be seen by examining a typical long bone, such as the humerus of the upper arm. There are two distinct types of bone tissue: one is referred to as *compact* and is dense and strong; the other is referred to as *cancellous* (kan'se-lus) and is more spongy and porous (Figs. 4–2 and 4–3). A long bone consists of a central shaft referred to as the *diaphysis* (di-af'i-sis), which is composed primarily of compact bone. Careful examination by x-rays (radiology) shows that the central shaft has more compact bone in the middle. This is appropriate, since mechanical strain is greatest in the middle. The overall strength of the long bone is further ensured by a slight curvature of the shaft. The interior of the central shaft is called the *medullary* (med'u-lar"e) *canal* and is filled, for the most part, with yellow marrow (see below).

The two ends, or extremities, of the long bone, each called an *epiphysis* (e-pif'i-sis), have a thin covering of compact tissue overlying cancellous tissue. The cancellous tissue normally contains *red marrow,* which manufactures blood cells. The extremities of the long bone are generally broad and expanded when compared with the shaft. This allows for easy jointing (articulation) with other bones and provides a larger surface for muscle attachment.

What Is the Function of Bone Marrow?

In the normal adult, the ribs, vertebrae, sternum, and bones of the pelvis contain red marrow in cancellous tissue. Red marrow within the ends of the humerus and femur is plentiful at birth but decreases in amount throughout the years. The primary function of red marrow is to form red and white blood cells and platelets. The technical name for this process is called *hematopoiesis* (hem"ah-to-poi-e'sis). The red blood cells, white blood cells, and platelets all originate from the same type of bone marrow cell, the *hemocytoblast* (he"-mo-si'to-blast), or stem cell. Red blood cells (erythrocytes) and white blood cells (leukocytes) in various stages of maturation are the main constituents of red bone marrow.

Yellow bone marrow is not very active in blood cell production. It consists chiefly of fat cells and is found primarily in the central shafts of long bones. As a person ages, red marrow is slowly replaced by the less active yellow marrow. Only a small fraction of the original red marrow remains in the bones of elderly persons. This helps to explain the difficulty they often have in replacing lost blood.

CALCIUM

What Is the Function of Calcium in the Body?

Ninety-nine per cent of the total calcium of the body exists in solid deposits of calcium phosphate (a salt crystal) in the bone tissue. The small but important remainder is dissolved (in ionized form) in the blood plasma and other body fluids, where it actively participates in vital chemical reactions (Fig. 4–4).

The solid deposits of calcium salts in the bone tissue serve to give the bones strength and stability of shape. In addition, these solid deposits help to supply body needs during periods such as preg-

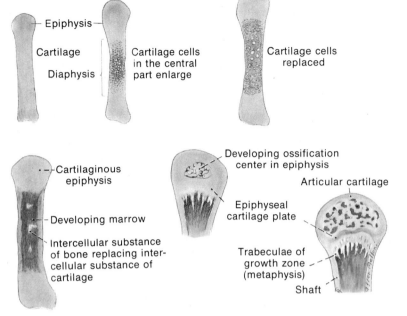

Epiphysis

Cartilage

Diaphysis

Cartilage cells in the central part enlarge

Cartilage cells replaced

Cartilaginous epiphysis

Developing marrow

Intercellular substance of bone replacing intercellular substance of cartilage

Developing ossification center in epiphysis

Articular cartilage

Epiphyseal cartilage plate

Trabeculae of growth zone (metaphysis)

Shaft

Figure 4-1 The bony deposit laid down around the diaphysis spreads toward the epiphysis, where ossification is also occurring. Gradual replacement of cartilage by bone occurs, and an increase in lengthwise direction of the bone accompanies this process. Growth in diameter of the bone occurs primarily with the deposit of bony tissue beneath the periosteum.

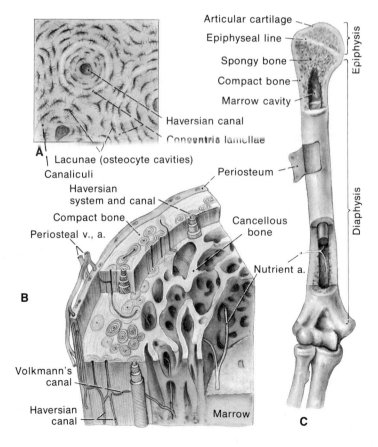

Articular cartilage

Epiphyseal line

Spongy bone

Compact bone

Marrow cavity

Epiphysis

Haversian canal

Concentric lamellae

Lacunae (osteocyte cavities)

Canaliculi

Haversian system and canal

Compact bone

Periosteal v., a.

Periosteum

Cancellous bone

Nutrient a.

Diaphysis

Volkmann's canal

Haversian canal

Marrow

A

B

C

Figure 4-2 *A,* Cross section of bone, showing relation of osteocytes to haversian system. *B,* This section has been magnified out of proportion to show haversian system and lamellae. (Note communication between periosteal vessels and haversian canal vessels by way of Volkmann's canals.) *C,* Diagram of the structure of a long bone. (After Lockhart.)

nancy when normal mineral intake is deficient or body demand is great.

The small amount of dissolved calcium is necessary for the proper operation of both nerve and muscle cells. Because too much or too little dissolved calcium in the body fluids causes serious abnormalities in the operation of both nerve and muscle cells, it is crucial that the concentration be carefully regulated.

How Is Calcium Concentration in the Body Fluids Regulated?

The movement of small amounts of calcium between the bone deposits and the body fluids occurs through two opposite processes controlled by the bone cells. They are appropriately referred to as *deposition,* in which calcium from the body fluids is added to bone, and *reabsorption,* in which solid calcium in the bone dissolves back into the fluids.

The total amount of calcium in the body can change a great deal, depending on intake and loss, with no serious health problems developing. During pregnancy, for instance, the total body calcium of the mother can change considerably, but this only leads to problems when her calcium intake is grossly deficient.

Even though such changes may occur in the total amount, the small amount dissolved in the body fluids must remain very nearly constant. This concentration of calcium in the body fluids is kept at a constant (homeostatic) level primarily through the alternating actions of deposition and reabsorption, controlled by the bone cells.

The parathyroid gland, which will be discussed more fully in Chapter 7, The Endocrine System, is known to be important in stimulating the deposition and reabsorption activities of the bone cells. Generally speaking, the parathyroid gland monitors (keeps track of) the concentration of calcium in the fluids, and when the concentration begins to decrease, the parathyroid releases a *hormone* (chemical stimulant or messenger) that stimulates the bone cells to release more calcium into solution. Less hormone is secreted when reabsorption is called for.

Vitamin D has been shown to be necessary in the process by which ingested calcium is absorbed from the intestines. Parathyroid hormone seems also to regulate the rate of intestinal absorption but cannot operate if vitamin D is not present.

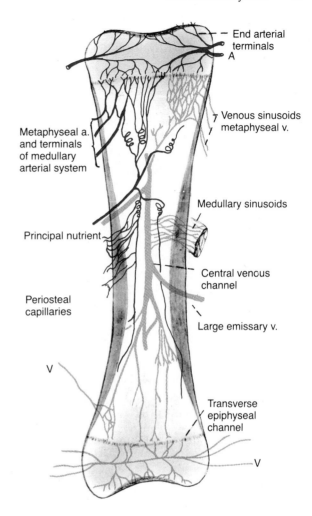

Figure 4–3 Blood supply to long bone.

WHAT ARE THE TWO MAIN SUBDIVISIONS OF THE SKELETON?

The human skeleton has two main subdivisions, known as the axial (ak'-se-al) skeleton and the appendicular (ap"en-dik'u-lar) skeleton. The axial skeleton makes up the central axis, or axle, to which the parts of the appendicular (from appendage, addition to the main body) skeleton are attached. Together they contain a total of 206 bones (Figs. 4–5 and 4–6, and Table 4–1).

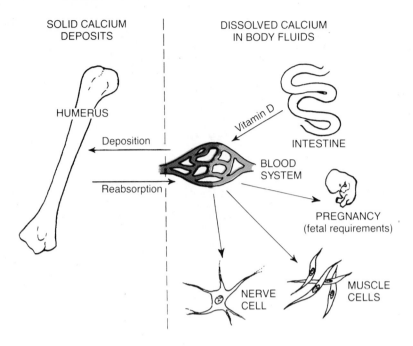

SOLID CALCIUM DEPOSITS

DISSOLVED CALCIUM IN BODY FLUIDS

HUMERUS

Deposition

Vitamin D

INTESTINE

Reabsorption

BLOOD SYSTEM

PREGNANCY (fetal requirements)

NERVE CELL

MUSCLE CELLS

Figure 4–4 Most of the calcium in the body is in solid bone deposits. The dissolved calcium in the body is regulated by the balancing of deposition and reabsorption. All calcium enters the body through the intestine; vitamin D is essential for uptake into the blood. Calcium is needed in large amounts during pregnancy for the formation of the fetal skeletal framework; if insufficient calcium is ingested by the mother, calcium is removed from the mother's bones to supply the fetus. Nerve cells and muscle cells are extremely sensitive to the calcium concentration in the body fluids, necessitating very sensitive homeostasis of dissolved calcium concentration.

The *axial skeleton* includes the bones of the cranium and face, the spinal column, and the chest (ribs and sternum).

The *appendicular skeleton* includes the shoulder girdle and the upper extremities (arms and hands) as well as the hip (pelvic) girdle and the lower extremities (legs and feet).

The Axial Skeleton

What Is the Skull?

The skull is made up of both the facial and cranial bones. Among the bones of the face are the maxilla and mandible. The bones of the cranium are those that enclose and protect the brain and its associated structures, including the eyes and ears. The muscles of mastication (chewing), as well as the muscles for head movement, are attached to the cranial bones. At certain locations within the cranial structure are spaces or cavities (cavelike) usually referred to as air sinuses. These are connected to the nasal (nose) cavity (Figs. 4–7 to 4–19).

Although the cranium looks as if it might be just one large bone enclosing the brain, it is actually several bones that have grown together. During infancy and early childhood, the articulations (joints) between these bones are composed of cartilage, which gradually disappears as the bones grow together, or ossify. The bones actually seem to grow toward each other and eventually meet at what are called juncture (from junction) or suture (from sewn, because of appearance) lines.

These joints between the cranial bones do not allow for any movement

What Are the Bones of the Torso?

The torso, or trunk portion of the axial skeleton, is made up of the *thorax* (tho'raks), or rib cage, and the vertebral, or spinal, column.

What Is the Thorax?

That portion of the torso consisting of the sternum, the costal cartilages, the ribs, and the bodies of the thoracic (from thorax) vertebrae is properly called the thorax. This bony cage encloses and protects the lungs and other structures of the chest cavity. The thorax also provides support for the bones of the shoulder girdle and upper extremities. At

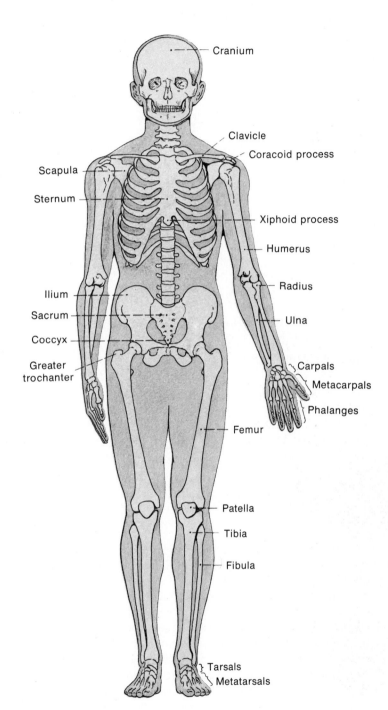

Cranium

Clavicle

Coracoid process

Scapula

Sternum

Xiphoid process

Humerus

Radius

Ilium

Sacrum

Ulna

Coccyx

Greater trochanter

Carpals

Metacarpals

Phalanges

Femur

Patella

Tibia

Fibula

Tarsals

Metatarsals

Figure 4–5 Anterior view of the skeleton.

Table 4–1 BONES

BONE	NUMBER	LOCATION
1. Skull	28 bones	
Cranium	8 bones	
Occipital	1	Posterior cranial floor and walls
Parietal	2	Forms the greater part of the superior lateral aspect and roof of the skull between frontal and occipital bones
Frontal	1	Forms forehead, most of orbital roof, and anterior cranial floor
Temporal	2	Inferior lateral aspect and base of the skull, housing middle and inner ear structures
Sphenoid	1	Midanterior base of the skull; forms part of floor and sides of orbit
Ethmoid	1	Between nasal bones and sphenoid, forming part of anterior cranial floor, medial wall of orbits, part of nasal septum, and roof
Face	14 bones	
Nasal	2	Upper bridge of nose
Maxillary	2	Upper jaw
Zygomatic (malar)	2	Prominence of cheeks and part of the lateral wall and floor of the orbits
Mandible	1	Lower jaw
Lacrimal	2	Anterior medial wall of the orbit
Palatine	2	Posterior nasal cavity between maxillae and the pterygoid processes of sphenoid
Vomer	1	Posterior nasal cavity, forming a portion of the nasal septum
Inferior nasal conchae (inferior turbinates)	2	Lateral wall of nasal cavity
Auditory Ossicles	6 bones	
Malleus (hammer)	2	Small bones in inner ear in temporal bone, connecting the
Incus (anvil)	2	tympanic membrane to the inner ear and functioning in
Stapes (stirrup)	2	sound transmission
Hyoid	1 bone	Horseshoe shaped, suspended from styloid process of temporal bone
2. Trunk	51 bones	
Vertebrae	26 bones	
Cervical	7	Neck
Thoracic	12	Thorax
Lumbar	5	Between thorax and pelvis
Sacrum	1 (5 fused)	Pelvis—fixed or false vertebrae
Coccyx	1 (4 fused)	Terminal vertebrae in pelvis—fixed or false vertebrae

birth the thorax is spherical, while in adult life it is more cone shaped, with a broad base.

The 12 pairs of ribs (costae) are named according to how they are attached in front to the sternum. The upper seven pairs articulate (or connect) directly with the sternum and are called *true ribs.*

The lower five pairs (8, 9, 10, 11, 12), which join with the sternum either indirectly or not all, are called *false ribs.* The eighth, ninth, and tenth pairs are attached to the sternum indirectly through the costal cartilages of the above ribs (Figs. 4–20 and 4–21). The eleventh and twelfth "false" ribs are also called *floating ribs,* since their anterior ends are completely unattached.

What Is the Vertebral Column?

The vertebral column provides protection for the delicate and vital spinal cord contained within

Table 4-1   BONES *Continued*

BONE	NUMBER	LOCATION
Ribs	24	True ribs—upper seven pairs fastened to sternum by costal cartilages; false ribs—lower five pairs; eighth, ninth, and tenth pairs attached to the seventh rib by costal cartilages; last two pairs do not attach and are called floating ribs
Sternum	1	Flat, narrow bone situated in median line anteriorly in chest
3. Upper Extremity	64 bones	
Clavicle	2	Together, clavicles and scapulae form the shoulder girdle; the clavicle articulates with the sternum
Scapula	2	
Humerus	2	Long bone of upper arm
Ulna	2	The ulna is the longest bone of forearm, on medial side of radius
Radius	2	Lateral to ulna, shorter than ulna, but styloid process is larger
Carpals	16	Two rows of bones comprising the wrist
Scaphoid		
Lunate		
Triangular		
Pisiform		
Capitate		
Hamate		
Trapezium		
Trapezoid		
Metacarpals	10	Long bones of the palm of the hand
Phalanges	28	Three in each finger and two in each thumb
4. Lower Extremity	62 bones	
Pelvic	2	Fusion of ilium, ischium, and pubis
Femur (thigh bone)	2	Longest bone in body
Patella	2	Kneecap; located in quadriceps femoris tendon; a sesamoid bone
Tibia	2	Shin bone; anteromedial side of the leg
Fibula	2	Lateral to tibia
Tarsals	14	Form heel, ankle (with distal tibia and fibula), and proximal part of the foot
Calcaneum		
Talus		
Navicular		
Cuboid		
First cuneiform (medial)		
Second cuneiform (intermediate)		
Third cuneiform (lateral)		
Metatarsals	10	Long bones of the foot
Phalanges	28	Three in each lesser toe and two in each great toe

its jointed channel. It has a remarkable combination of properties, being rigid enough to provide adequate support for the body, yet being highly flexible in many directions, allowing for considerable upper body movement.

The vertebrae are numbered by regions from the top down. There are 7 *cervical,* 12 *thoracic,* and 5 *lumbar* vertebrae. These remain separate through-out life and are called moveable vertebrae. In addition, there are five *sacral* vertebrae, which by adulthood have become fused to form a single *sacrum,* and four *coccygeal* (kok-sij'e-al) vertebrae, which unite firmly into a single *coccyx* (kok'siks). The vertebrae of these last two regions are called fixed, and, consequently, the complete vertebrae are referred to as being 26 in number rather than 33 (Fig. 4-22).

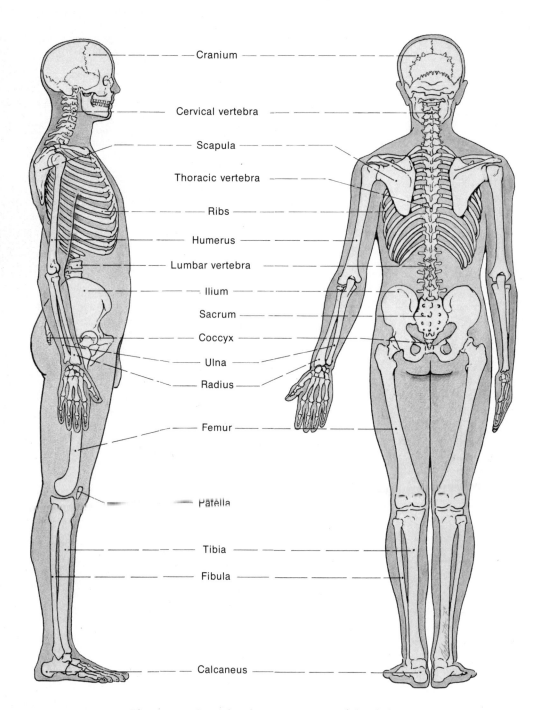

Cranium

Cervical vertebra

Scapula

Thoracic vertebra

Ribs

Humerus

Lumbar vertebra

Ilium

Sacrum

Coccyx

Ulna

Radius

Femur

Patella

Tibia

Fibula

Calcaneus

Figure 4-6 Lateral and posterior views of the skeleton.

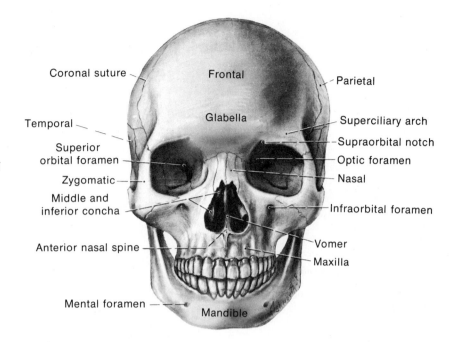

Figure 4-7 Frontal aspect of the skull.

Labels: Coronal suture, Frontal, Parietal, Temporal, Glabella, Superciliary arch, Superior orbital foramen, Supraorbital notch, Optic foramen, Zygomatic, Nasal, Middle and inferior concha, Infraorbital foramen, Anterior nasal spine, Vomer, Maxilla, Mental foramen, Mandible

Why Is the Vertebral Column Curved?

In the fetus, the vertebral column shows a single, C-shaped curve. After birth, raising of the head creates the beginning of an S-curve in the neck. Later, the erect posture involved in standing and walking creates the beginning of a similar inward curve in the lumbar region.

The normal curves of the spine can become exaggerated as a result of injury, poor body posture, or disease. When the posterior curvature is exaggerated in the thoracic area, the condition is called *ky-*

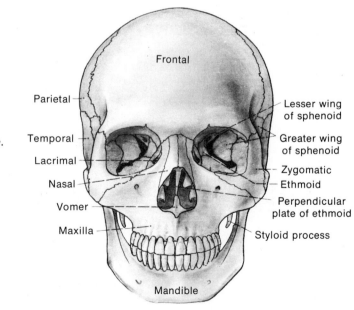

Figure 4-8 Bones of the face.

Labels: Frontal, Parietal, Lesser wing of sphenoid, Temporal, Greater wing of sphenoid, Lacrimal, Nasal, Zygomatic, Ethmoid, Vomer, Perpendicular plate of ethmoid, Maxilla, Styloid process, Mandible

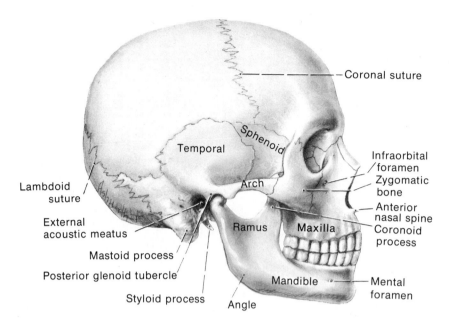

Figure 4-9 Right side of the skull.

phosis (ki-fo′sis) or, more commonly, *hunchback.* The word *kyphos* is Greek and means hump. When the lower anterior curvature in the lumbar region is exaggerated it is known as *lordosis* (from the Greek, meaning bending backward) or, commonly, as swayback. A sideways curve, which involves rotation of some of the vertebrae, is termed *scoliosis* (sko″le-o′sis) (from the Greek word *skolios,* meaning crooked).

Appendicular Skeleton

What Are the Bones of the Upper Extremities?

The bones of the upper extremities can be separated into three groupings.

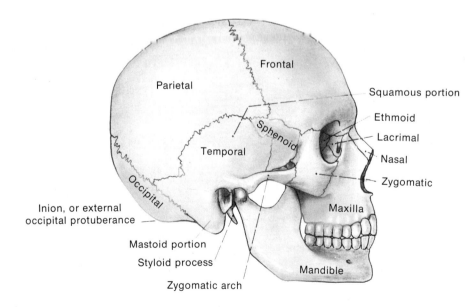

Figure 4-10 Bones of the right side of the skull.

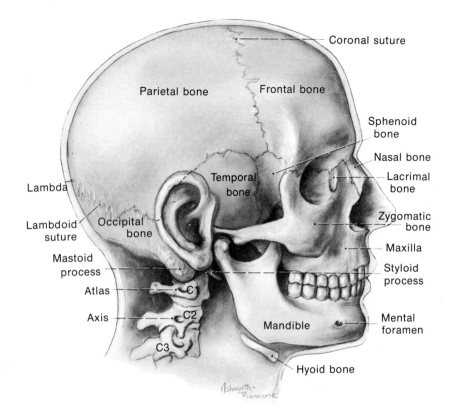

Figure 4-11 Relationship of skull and cervical vertebrae to face.

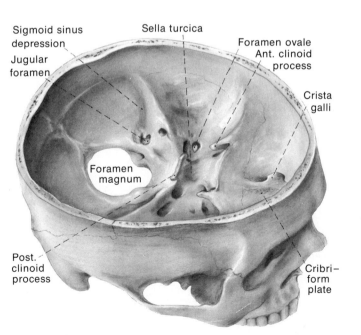

Figure 4-12 Interior of the brain case.

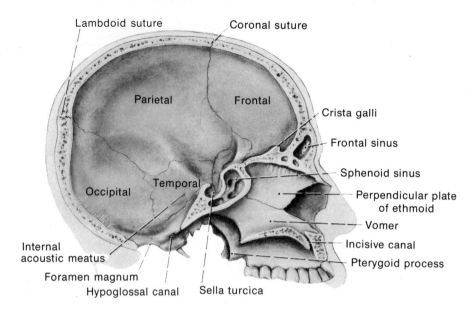

Figure 4–13 Sagittal section of skull.

1. The *shoulder girdle,* or pectoral girdle, is made up of two major bones, the *collar bone,* also called the clavicle, and the *shoulder blade,* or scapula (skap'u-lah) (Fig. 4–23).
2. The bones of the *arm* proper are the humerus, ulna, and radius. The *humerus* connects at the top with the scapula and at the elbow with the two forearm bones. The forearm bones are the *ulna,* on the little finger side, and the *radius,* on the thumb side (Figs. 4–23 and 4–24).
3. The bones of the wrist are called *carpals* (kar-pals) and are situated in two rows of four each. The palm of the hand consists of five metacarpal bones, each with a base, shaft, and head. The metacarpals radiate from the wrist line like spokes from a wheel, rather than being parallel, and join with the proxi-

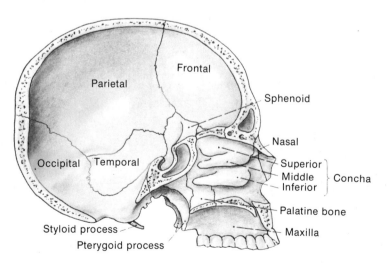

Figure 4–14 Sagittal view showing bones of skull.

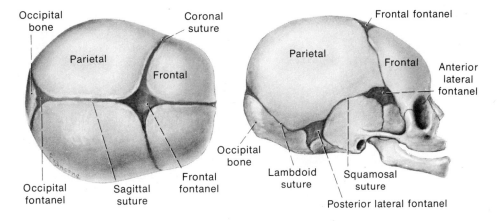

Figure 4-15 Fetal skull, demonstrating that ossification is not complete at birth. The occipital, or posterior, fontanel closes at about 6 to 8 weeks after birth; the anterior lateral, or sphenoid, fontanel closes at about 3 months after birth; the frontal, or anterior, fontanel closes at about 18 months of age; and the posterior lateral, or mastoid, fontanel closes at about 2 years of age.

mal phalanges (fa-len'jez) of the fingers. Each finger (excluding the thumb) has three phalanges —a proximal, a middle, and a terminal (or distal) phalanx. The thumb has only two phalanges (see Fig. 4–24).

What Are the Bones of the Lower Extremities?

The bones of the lower extremities can also be separated into three groupings.

Figure 4-16 Sinuses of the skull.

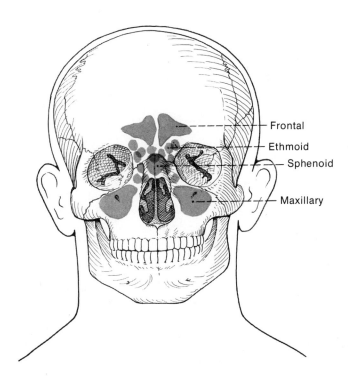

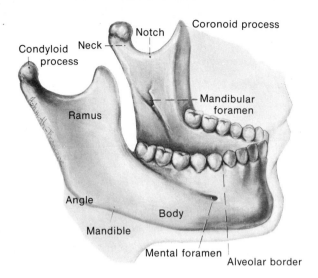

Figure 4–17 Mandible.

has bigger bones but forms a narrower structure overall. The female pelvis is shaped like a basin (the word pelvis is from the Greek word *pyelos*, meaning basin) (Fig. 4–25).

2.   The *femur* is the bone of the thigh. It is the largest and heaviest bone in the body. Notice that the femur is *not* in a vertical line with the axis of the erect body. Rather, it is positioned at an angle, slanting downward and inward. From the point of view of the skeleton, the two femurs appear as a ''V.'' Because of the female's greater pelvic breadth, the angle of inclination of the femurs is greater than in the male (Fig. 4–26). The *patella* (pah-tel'lah), or kneecap, is a small, flat, and somewhat triangular bone lying in front of the knee joint and enveloped within the tendon that attaches to the large, rectus femoris muscle of the anterior upper leg. The patella is moveable and serves to increase the leverage of the muscles that straighten the knee.

The *tibia* (shin bone) is the larger of the two bones forming the lower leg. The *fibula* (calf bone) is the smaller of the bones in the lower leg and in proportion to its length is the most slender bone in the body, lying parallel with and on the lateral (toward the outside) side of the tibia (Fig. 4–26).

3.   The ankle and foot are composed of the tarsal

1.   The *pelvic girdle* supports the trunk and provides attachment for the legs. The paired *os coxae* (pelvic bone or ''hipbone'') originally consist of three separate bones, the ilium, ischium, and pubis. These names are retained as descriptive regions for areas of the fused adult pelvic bone. The male pelvis

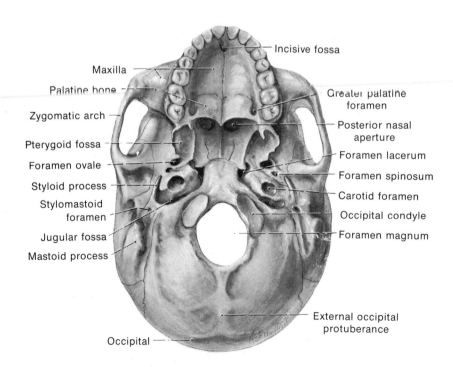

Figure 4–18 Inferior surface of the skull.

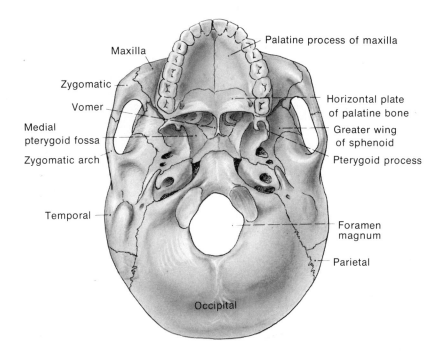

Figure 4-19 Inferior surface of skull, showing the various bones composing it.

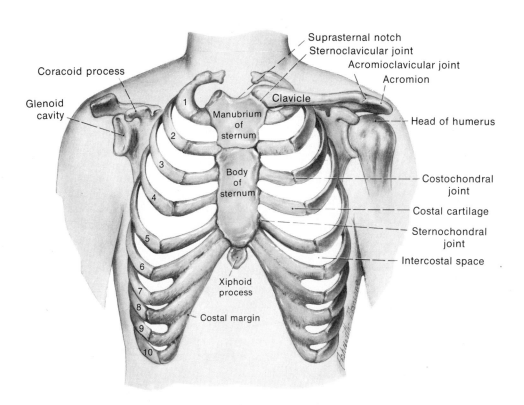

Figure 4-20 Anterior view of the rib cage.

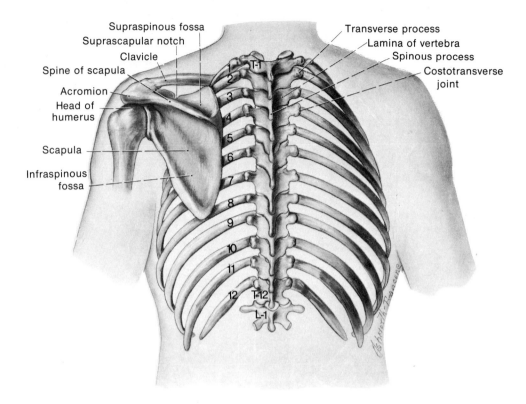

Figure 4-21   Posterior view of the rib cage and scapula.

(tahr'sal) and metatarsal bones as well as the phalanges. The general design is very similar to that of the wrist and hand. Can you find any differences? You can remember that the tarsals are in the foot and the carpals are in the hand by associating the "t" of tarsal with the "t" of toes (Fig. 4-27).

ARTICULATIONS

What Are the Three Types of Joints?

The joints, or articulations (ar-tik"u-la'shuns), of the skeletal system may be defined as the region of union of two or more bones. Every bone of the human body, with one exception, articulates with at least one other bone; the exception is the hyoid in the neck, to which the tongue is attached. Joints may be distinguished into three classes on the basis of the amount of movement possible at the point of connection (Fig. 4-28). The *fixed* joints, such as those found between the bones of the cranium, allow no movement. There are a few *slightly moveable* joints, such as the one between the radius and the ulna in the forearm. The vast majority of joints in the body allow considerable movement— sometimes in many directions and sometimes in only one or two directions; these are the *freely moveable* joints. Figure 4-29 shows the types of movements permitted by some freely moveable joints.

What Is the Structure of a Typical Joint?

All freely moveable joints are bound together by a *capsule*, which fits like a tight sleeve. This capsule is made from strong, fibrous cartilage and is

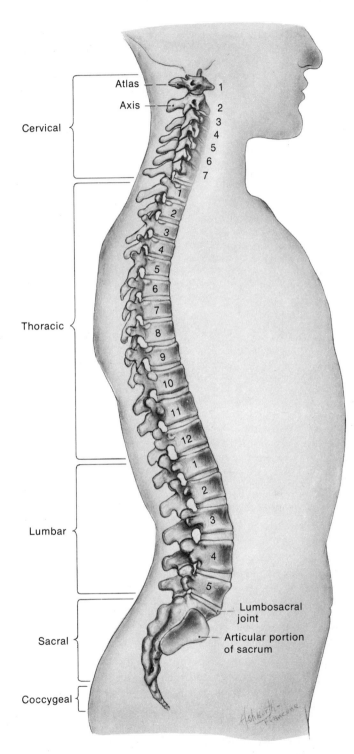

Atlas

Axis

Cervical

1
2
3
4
5
6
7

Thoracic

1
2
3
4
5
6
7
8
9
10
11
12

Lumbar

1
2
3
4
5

Lumbosacral joint

Articular portion of sacrum

Sacral

Coccygeal

Figure 4-22 Vertebral column in relation to body outline.

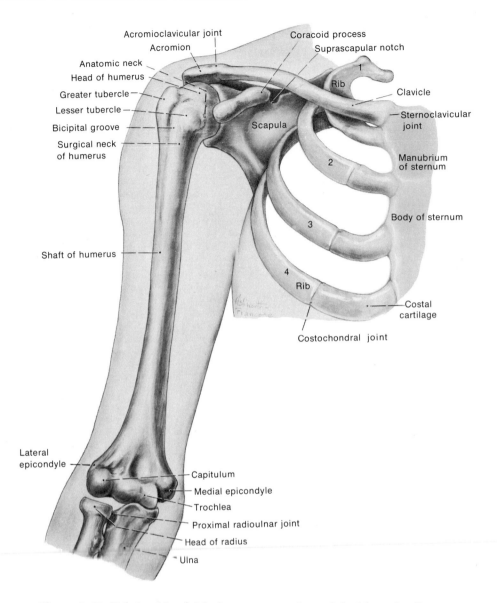

Figure 4-23 Relationship of right humerus, scapula, and clavicle to the rib cage.

lined with smooth, slippery synovial (si-no've-al) membrane. The capsule sleeve holds the bones securely together and yet permits free movement of the joint. Closely associated with the capsule are the *ligaments*, which are tough fibrous cords or bands that bind and reinforce the capsule (Figs. 4–30 and 4–31).

The ends of the bones in all joints are covered by a smooth layer of cartilage. This layer of articular cartilage acts like the rubber heel of a shoe, softening the impact of jolts. The joint space or cavity is filled with synovial fluid, which lubricates the joint.

What Is a Bursa?

A bursa (ber'sah) is a closed sac containing a small amount of synovial fluid and having a synovial membrane lining similar to that of a joint. A bursa can be found between tendons, ligaments, and bones or generally where friction would otherwise develop. Bursae facilitate the gliding of muscles or tendons over bony or ligamentous surfaces (Figs. 4–32 and 4–33).

CLINICAL CONSIDERATIONS

What Is Rickets?

Rickets is a disorder that occurs when there is too little vitamin D in a child's system. Without adequate vitamin D both absorption of calcium from the small intestine and deposition of calcium in the child's bones are inhibited. As a result, the bones fail to harden and the child may develop curved legs and spine. When a baby with this condition begins to walk, the bones bend in response to the mechanical stresses; various deformities, such as bowed legs, result.

Rickets was first described in England about 1650, when the use of soft coal had become prevalent. It was caused, it is now known, by a deficiency in the ultraviolet radiation of sunlight in factory towns, where the coal smoke and dark alleys created a sunless environment. Ultraviolet radiation activates the conversion of a natural substance in the skin to vitamin D.

What Are Two Types of Fractures?

The breaking of a bone or cartilage is known as a *fracture*. A fracture is usually accompanied by an injury to the surrounding soft tissue. A fracture is called *compound* if the broken bone protrudes through the skin or *simple* if it does not. Because of the greater possibility of infection, a compound fracture is the more dangerous of the two. Bone healing occurs best when the fracture ends are repositioned accurately and tightly.

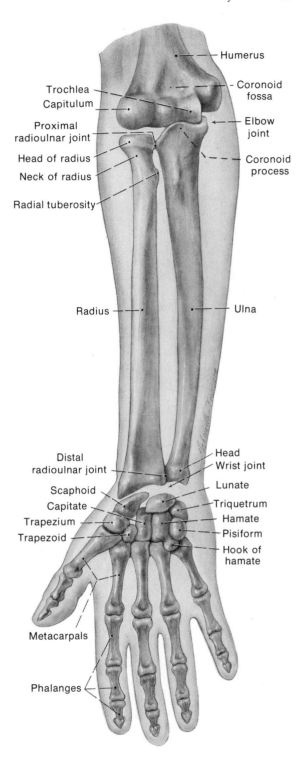

Figure 4–24 Anterior view of bones of the right forearm and hand.

Osteoporosis

Osteoporosis (osteo, meaning bone, and porosis, meaning porous) is a disorder characterized by loss of calcium from the bones. This reduction in the quantity of bone occurs primarily in postmenopausal women and elderly men. As a result, the bones become very porous. This loss of bony substances makes the bones brittle (easily broken) as well as soft (less strong), often leading to a decline in posture. The two most important contributing factors to osteoporosis are believed to be a progressive loss of sex hormone output and lack of exercise.

The female sex hormone estrogen facilitates calcium absorption from the digestive tract. Women past childbearing age no longer produce the estrogen they did when they were younger. Consequently, their ability to absorb calcium decreases. When the intestine absorbs insufficient calcium from the diet, the blood robs bones of calcium the body needs for other vital functions.

According to current estimates by the National Institutes of Health (NIH), approximately 25 per cent of women over 65 years of age develop osteoporosis. It affects 15 to 20 million people in the United States, and approximately 40,000 older women die every year from complications arising from hip fractures due to osteoporosis.

Currently, scientists believe that maintaining adequate calcium levels throughout a lifetime may be the key to preventing osteoporosis. NIH recommends 1500 mg per day for postmenopausal women; some recent research suggests that up to 2500 mg per day may be appropriate.

The best dietary source of calcium is dairy products, followed by leafy green vegetables such as turnip greens, broccoli, and kale. Canned salmon and sardines containing bones are also excellent calcium sources.

In addition to adding calcium to the diet, NIH strongly recommends weight-bearing exercises such as walking, jogging, and aerobic dance, which will strengthen bones by increasing their density and serve directly to prevent bone degeneration.

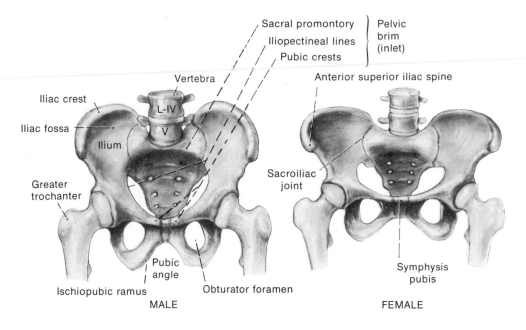

Figure 4–25 Comparison in proportions of the male and female pelves.

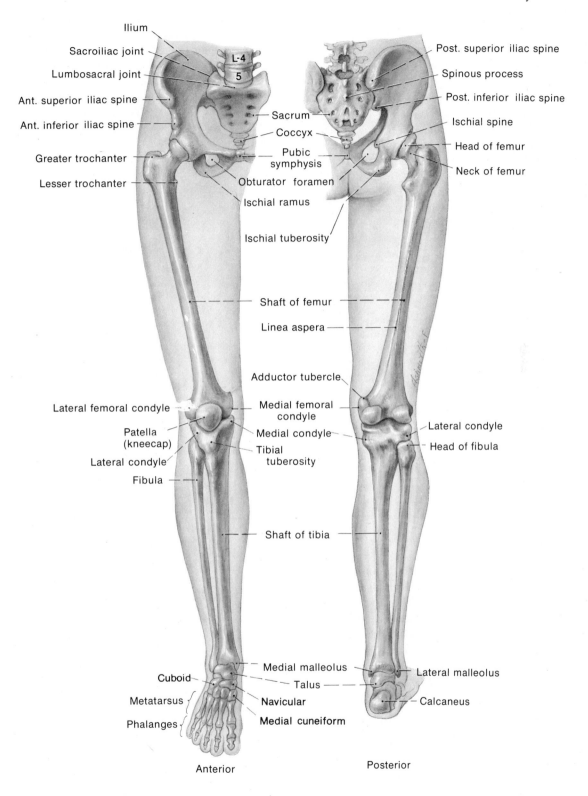

Ilium

Sacroiliac joint

Lumbosacral joint

Ant. superior iliac spine

Ant. inferior iliac spine

Greater trochanter

Lesser trochanter

L-4

5

Sacrum

Coccyx

Pubic symphysis

Obturator foramen

Ischial ramus

Ischial tuberosity

Post. superior iliac spine

Spinous process

Post. inferior iliac spine

Ischial spine

Head of femur

Neck of femur

Shaft of femur

Linea aspera

Adductor tubercle

Lateral femoral condyle

Patella (kneecap)

Lateral condyle

Fibula

Medial femoral condyle

Medial condyle

Tibial tuberosity

Lateral condyle

Head of fibula

Shaft of tibia

Cuboid

Metatarsus

Phalanges

Medial malleolus

Talus

Navicular

Medial cuneiform

Lateral malleolus

Calcaneus

Anterior

Posterior

Figure 4–26 Anterior and posterior views of bones of the right leg and foot.

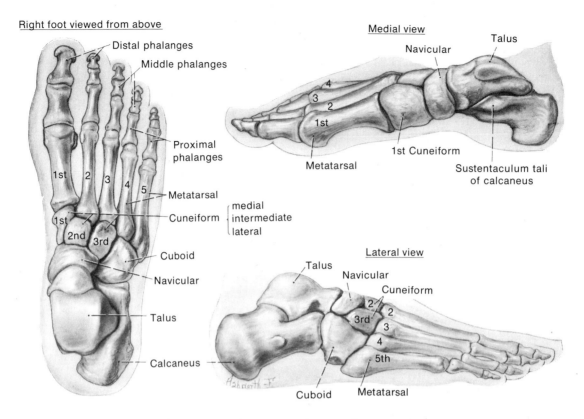

Figure 4–27 Three views of bones of the right foot.

What Are Three Common Disorders of the Joints?

Arthritis (ar-thri'tis), or joint inflammation, significantly immobilizes thousands of people every year. Nearly everyone suffers from some kind of arthritis in some part of the body sooner or later. *Rheumatoid* (roo'mah-toid) *arthritis* is a systemic disease with widespread involvement of connective tissue. Inflammation of the synovial membrane leads to damage and degeneration of cartilage; finally calcification of the damaged cartilage results in joint immobility. *Osteoarthritis* involves a slow wearing away of weakened cartilage, with the underlying bone around the joints developing ivory-like calcium growths called "spurs" or "marginal lippings." These result in a joint stiffness and eventual immobility.

Gout is a metabolic disorder that leads to the deposition of uric acid crystals in and about the joint tissues and, together with inflammation of the synovium, results in damage to the articular cartilage and eventual gouty arthritis.

Bursitis (ber-si'tis) is an inflammation of the bursa that may result from excess stress or tension having been placed on the bursa or from some local or systemic inflammatory process. The most frequent location is in the shoulder, where movement of the joint becomes limited and painful. Eventually, with the inflammation, abnormal deposits of calcium occur and further interfere with joint movement.

SUMMARY

A. The skeletal system has five important functions.

NONSYNOVIAL

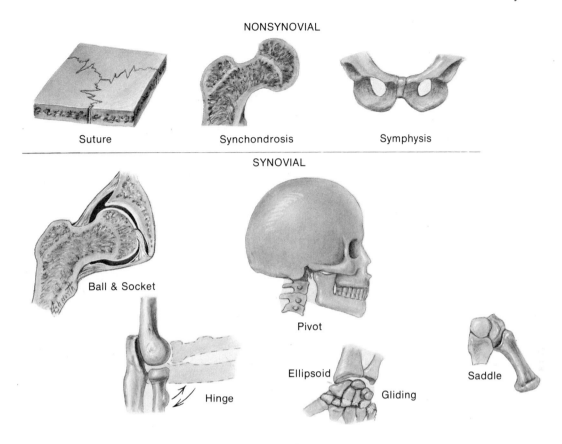

SYNOVIAL

Figure 4–28 Joints are placed in two general groups on the basis of their mechanical properties—nonsynovial and synovial. Nonsynovial joints are subdivided primarily on the basis of the type of connective tissue that joins the articulating surfaces. Synovial joints are classified on the basis of the shapes of the articulating surfaces and the kinds of movements that occur.

1. The skeleton provides the support framework for the body.
2. It protects organs, like the brain, heart, and lungs.
3. It allows a wide range of movements.
4. In the bone marrow, blood cells are manufactured.
5. Calcium salts are stored in the bone matrix.
B. The cartilage skeleton forms in the third month of life.
  1. Hardening or ossification occurs as bone cells develop a matrix system and absorb calcium phosphate crystals.
  2. Longitudinal growth continues to age 15 to 16.
  3. The early patterns are constantly remade until age 21.

C. There are two distinct types of bone tissue.
  1. Compact bone is dense and strong.
  2. Cancellous bone is more spongy and porous.
D. A long bone has several important features.
  1. The strong central shaft is called the diaphysis.
  2. The interior of the twisted central shaft, which is called the medullary canal, is filled with yellow marrow.
  3. Each of the two broad ends is called an epiphysis.
    a. Each epiphysis is composed of cancellous tissue.
    b. These ends are filled with red marrow.
    c. Each epiphysis is covered by hard compact tissue.
E. The primary function of red marrow is hemato-

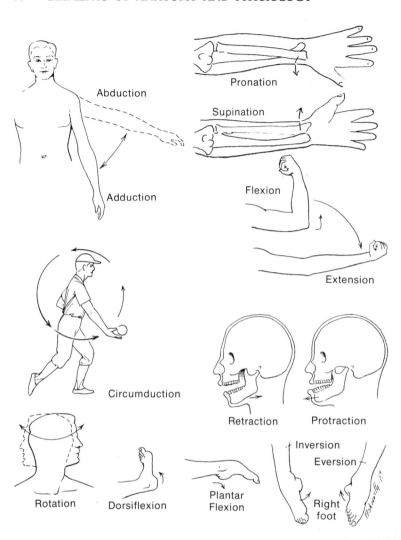

Figure 4-29 Types of movement permitted by synovial joints.

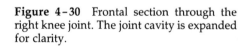

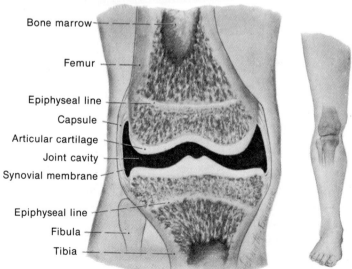

Figure 4-30 Frontal section through the right knee joint. The joint cavity is expanded for clarity.

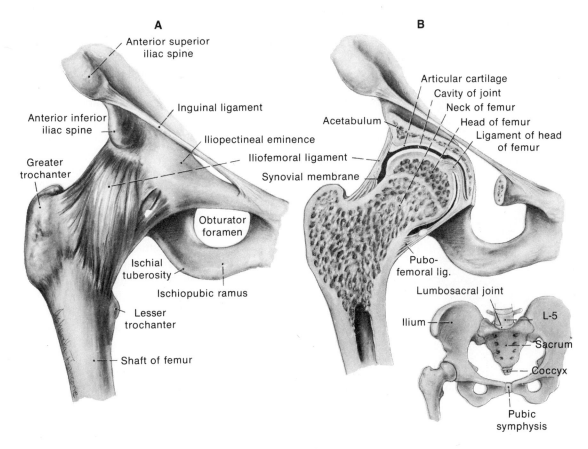

Figure 4–31 Hip joint, showing ligaments between femur and pelvic bone; intact *(A)* and sectioned *(B)* to show attachments.

poiesis: the formation of red and white blood cells and platelets.

1. Red and white blood cells and platelets all originate and mature in their own direction from the same hemocytoblast, or stem cell.
2. Red marrow is made up primarily of red and white blood cells in various stages of maturing.
3. Yellow marrow is less active and more prevalent as a person ages.

F. The solid deposits of calcium phosphate (a salt crystal) serve to give bones strength and stability of shape.

1. These deposits supply body needs during pregnancy and when mineral intake is deficient.
2. The small amount of dissolved calcium (less

than 1 per cent) is necessary for nerve and muscle cell function.

G. The concentration of dissolved calcium must be carefully regulated.

1. The deposition of calcium from body fluids to bone is balanced by the reverse — reabsorption of solid calcium dissolving into the fluids.
2. The parathyroid gland is important in stimulating the deposition and reabsorption activities of the bone cells.
3. Parathyroid hormone, in the presence of adequate vitamin D, regulates intestinal absorption of calcium.

H. The human skeleton has two main subdivisions, the axial and the appendicular skeletons.

1. The axial skeleton makes up the body's central axis, or axle.

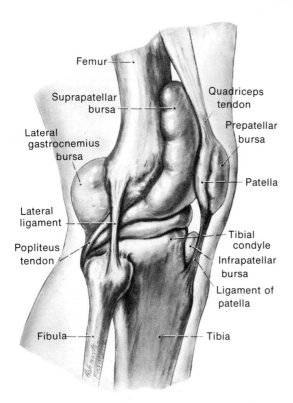

Figure 4–32 Lateral view of the right knee joint. The bursae have been expanded for clarity.

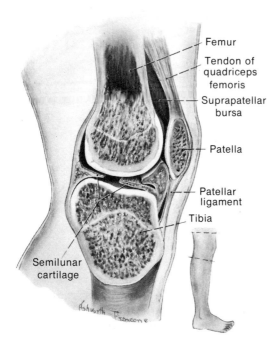

Figure 4–33 Lateral view of the right knee joint in sagittal section.

a. The upper portion includes the cranium and face.

b. The lower portion includes the spinal column and the chest (ribs and sternum).

2. The appendicular skeleton is made up of the attachments to the axial skeleton.

a. The upper portion includes the shoulder girdle and upper extremities (arms and hands).

b. The lower portion includes the hip (pelvic girdle) and the lower extremities (legs and feet).

I. The skull is made up of facial and cranial bones, including the maxilla and mandible.

1. The cranium is actually composed of several bones that have grown together. The joints do not allow for any movement.

2. The cranial bones enclose and protect the brain, eyes, and ears.

3. The air sinuses are localized spaces within the cranial bones connected to the nasal cavity.

J. The torso, or trunk, is made up of the thorax and vertebral column.

1. The thorax, or rib cage, includes the sternum, the costal cartilages, the ribs, and the bodies of the thoracic vertebrae.

a. The upper seven pairs of true ribs are attached directly to the sternum.

b. The lower five pairs of false ribs join the sternum indirectly or not at all.

2. The curved vertebral column consists of 26 vertebrae.

a. The moveable portion is made up of the 7 cervical, 12 thoracic, and 5 lumbar vertebrae.

b. There are five sacral vertebrae that by adulthood fuse to form the sacrum, which is counted as one.

c. Four coccygeal vertebrae unite firmly into the single coccyx, which is counted as one.

K. The bones of the upper extremities are made up of the shoulder girdle and the bones of the arm, wrist, and hand.

1. The shoulder girdle is made up of the clavicle (collar bone) and the scapula (shoulder blade).

2. The bones of the arm are the humerus, ulna, and radius.

3. The bones of the wrist are called the carpals,

the bones of the palm of the hand are called the metacarpals, and the bones of the hand are called the phalanges.

L. The bones of the lower extremities are made up of the pelvic girdle and the bones of the leg, ankle, and foot.
   1. The pelvic girdle consists of three fused bones, the ilium, ischium, and pubis.
   2. The bones of the leg are the femur (upper leg) and the tibia and fibula (lower leg).
   3. The ankle and foot are composed of the tarsal and metatarsal bones as well as the phalanges.

M. The three types of joints are the fixed, slightly moveable, and freely moveable.
   1. Freely moveable joints are bound together by a capsule, which is like a tight sleeve.
   2. The ligaments are tough fibrous cords that bind and reinforce the capsule, holding the bones of the joint together.
   3. The ends of the joints are covered by smooth cartilage, acting to soften impacts.
   4. The joint space is filled with a lubricating synovial fluid.

N. A bursa is a closed sac containing a small amount of synovial fluid with a synovial membrane lining.
   1. Bursae serve to lubricate between tendons, ligaments, and bones.
   2. Bursae facilitate the gliding of muscles or tendons over bony or ligamentous surfaces.

O. Rickets is disease resulting from a deficiency in vitamin D in the body.
   1. Without vitamin D absorption, deposition of calcium is inhibited.
   2. Rickets in England around 1650 was caused by a deficiency of ultraviolet light from the sun due to the smoky environment.

P. A fracture is called compound if the broken bone protrudes through the skin, or simple if it does not.

Q. Arthritis, or joint inflammation, significantly immobilizes thousands of people every year.

R. Bursitis is an inflammation of the bursa resulting from excess stress or is due to an inflammatory process.

S. Osteoporosis is a disorder characterized by a loss of calcium from the bones.
   1. Loss of calcium makes the bones soft and brittle.
   2. The two most important factors in loss of calcium are loss of sex hormone and lack of exercise.
   3. More calcium in the diet may help to counteract the problem.

REVIEW QUESTIONS

1. Identify three major and two minor functions of the skeletal system.

2. Describe the stages of skeletal formation from the third month of the fetus to age 21 years.

3. Differentiate the two types of bone tissue.

4. What is the strongest portion of the typical long bone? Identify two anatomic features of the bone that help provide this strength.

5. Construct and label a diagram of a typical long bone.

6. The ends of the long bones are larger around than the shaft. What function does this structure serve?

7. What are the main constituents of the red bone marrow? At what age is the amount of red marrow the greatest? Least?

8. What is yellow marrow? What are its main constituents?

9. What functions are served by the solid deposits of calcium phosphate?

10. What two processes maintain the proper homeostatic level of dissolved calcium? What gland and what hormones are most important in regulating these processes? How does vitamin D influence these processes?

11. Name the two main subdivisions of the skeleton.

12. Construct and label a diagram identifying the three major parts of the axial skeleton.

13. Name the eight bones of the cranium.

14. What are the bones of the upper and lower jaw?

15. What facial bones form the nose and cheeks?

16. Name the bones containing the paranasal sinuses.

17. Identify the bones of the cranium and face that form the orbital chambers for each eye.

18. Identify the bones of the cranium and face that form the middle and inner ear.

19. How does the skull of infancy and early childhood differ from the adult skull?

20. Name the two major portions of the trunk or torso.

21. Name the major components of the thorax.

22. What is a true rib? A false rib? Are floating ribs true or false?

23. What are the five major regions of the vertebral column?

24. Define kyphosis, lordosis, and scoliosis. Construct a diagram to show how each differs from normal spinal curvatures.

25. Name the three main groupings of the bones of the upper extremities.

26. Identify the bones of the shoulder girdle and explain how they are connected and anchored.

27. Name all the bones with which the radius articulates.

28. Name the three main groupings of the bones of the lower extremities.

29. What are the three descriptive regions of the fused adult pelvic bone?

30. Why is the angle of the femur, away from the axis of the erect body, greater in the female than in the male?

31. What is the heaviest bone in the body? What is the most slender bone in the body?

32. What one bone in the body does not articulate with any other bone?

33. Name the three classes of joints based on the amount of movement possible at the point of connection. Give an example of each class.

34. Describe the structures of the typical freely moveable joint. Construct and label a diagram of the knee joint.

35. Define and briefly characterize rickets.

36. What distinguishes a simple from a compound fracture?

37. Define and briefly characterize arthritis and bursitis. Distinguish rheumatoid arthritis from osteoarthritis.

38. What is osteoporosis? How might it be prevented?

F I V E

The Muscular System

O B J E C T I V E S

The aim of this chapter is to enable the student to do the following:

- Describe the similarities and differences in the three types of muscle tissue and note where the muscles are found in the body.
- Construct and label diagrams showing the microanatomy of muscle fiber and the mechanics of contraction.
- Distinguish the three types of muscle contraction.
- Explain the importance of exercise in keeping muscles healthy.
- Name and identify the major muscles

- of the human body on a diagram or chart and state the action of each.
- Distinguish the types of gross body movement and explain how the involved muscles are correspondingly named.
- Describe several of the major muscle disorders.
- Define aerobic exercise and explain its importance in maintenance of the muscular system.

THE MUSCLES: WHAT THEY DO, HOW THEY DIFFER

What Is the Function of the Muscular System?

The muscular system is responsible for producing all movements of the body. Every movement we make is the result of the contraction or relaxation of some muscle or group of muscles. For instance, all external or "action" movements, such as walking or turning one's head or swinging a golf club, are caused by coordinated contractions of our skeletal

muscles. Of equal importance are the internal or "life supportive" movements brought about by the activity of muscles, such as the circulation of the blood, the passage of food along the digestive tract, and the movement of the chest, diaphragm, and abdomen during respiration.

How Do the Three Types of Muscle Differ in Appearance, Location, and Function?

There are three main types of muscle cells: the *striated* (stri'at-ed), the *smooth*, and the *cardiac* (Fig.

5–1). They make up three corresponding types of muscle tissue—striated muscle tissue, smooth muscle tissue, and cardiac muscle tissue. These three types of muscle tissue, together with some special connective tissue known as fascia, make up the construction of the three basically different types of *muscle* (Fig. 5–2). This muscle may be formed into a single muscular organ, such as the biceps of the upper arm (striated muscle), or may compose only one of several layers of a more complex organ, such as the kidney or intestines (smooth muscle).

Striated Muscle   The cells of striated muscle are long and slender, their length being from 20 to 1000 times their width. Because of their exaggerated oblong shape, striated muscle cells are sometimes referred to as *muscle fibers.* Microscopic examination of these fibers reveals that they have many crosswise stripes or striations. The name *stri*-ated is derived from this striped appearance of the fibers. By using special staining techniques, it can also be shown that striated muscle cells (unlike the other two types) have several nuclei.

A *striated* muscle appears to be made up of bundles of fine threads (the fiberlike cells) held together with connective tissue. The striated muscles of the body are all attached to the skeleton and are sometimes called *skeletal muscles.* These muscles or muscular organs are all under conscious voluntary control and, with few exceptions, are the only muscles we can control consciously.

Smooth Muscle   The cells of smooth muscle are of various shapes but are usually several times longer than they are wide or thick and therefore are also often referred to as fibers. Unlike the striated muscle cells, the smooth muscle cells contain only one nucleus, and they are not striped or banded but appear smooth.

Smooth muscle tissue is found most typically in rolled layers, making up the muscular layers of the digestive tract and other internal (visceral) hollow structures such as the bladder and blood vessels. Smooth muscle is also a major component of the skin. These muscles normally cannot be influenced consciously. They are controlled by the unconscious or automatic parts of the nervous system.

Cardiac Muscle   Cardiac (heart) muscle is involuntary, like smooth muscle, but possesses the striated appearance of skeletal muscle. Interconnecting fibers of cardiac muscle are not single cells but are built up in a chainlike manner from cardiac muscle cells. These cardiac muscle cells are the most evenly proportioned of the three types of muscle cells.

The rapid rhythm of cardiac muscle is possible because this type of muscle tissue has a special ability to receive an impulse, contract, immediately relax, and receive another impulse. During normal daily activity all these events occur about 75 times each minute.

For simplicity, we will use the skeletal muscle as an example in explaining how muscles work. Other aspects of smooth and cardiac muscles will be discussed again in appropriate later chapters.

THE MUSCLES AT WORK

What Are the Three Types of Muscle Contraction?

There are three types of muscle contraction: two active, known as *isotonic* and *isometric contraction,* and one passive, called *tonic contraction.* The terms "isotonic" and "isometric" have been formed from Greek derivatives: *"iso-,"* meaning equal; *"tonz-,"* meaning put under tension; and *"metr-,"* meaning measure.

Isotonic (i"so-ton'ik) contraction occurs in *movements* of any part of the body and always involves a change in the length of the muscle; as for example, in lifting an object or doing exercises, such as jumping jacks. Figure 5–3 shows the latent period from stimulation to the beginning of contraction; the period it takes to contract and the period for relaxation total less than 1/10 second.

Isometric (i"so-met'rik) contraction does not produce any change in the overall length of the muscle and therefore does not lead to any movement; examples are holding an object in the air without moving it and pushing on an object that does not move.

The student may recognize the term "isometric" from exercise programs that recommended a group of exercises in relation to fixed objects; that is,

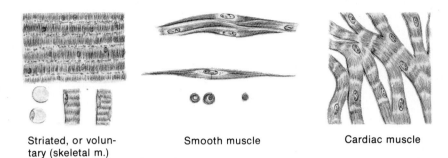

Figure 5-1 Types of muscle.

Striated, or volun-
tary (skeletal m.)

Smooth muscle

Cardiac muscle

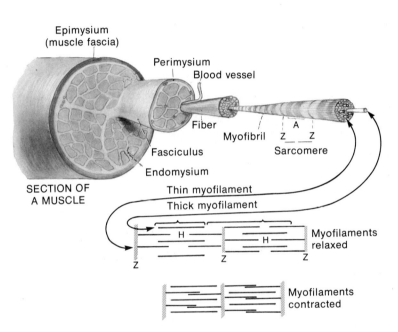

Figure 5-2 Detail of muscle showing structure and mechanics of muscular contraction.

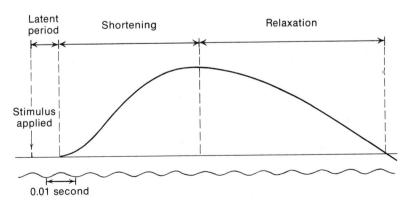

Figure 5-3 A single twitch recorded by attachment of a muscle to a moving lever. The rise in the lever records the shortening of the muscle. As the muscle relaxes, the fall in the lever records the return of the muscle to its original length. (After Carlson and Johnson.)

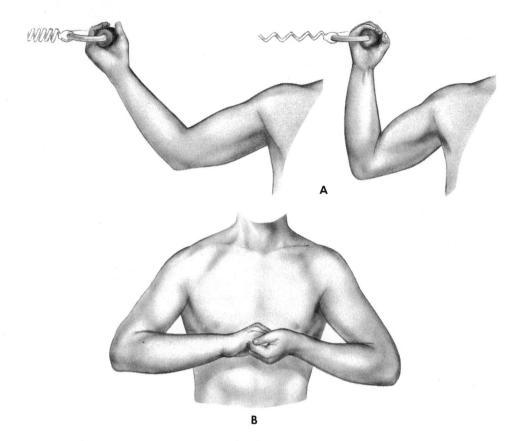

Figure 5–4 *A,* Isotonic contraction. Here there is movement, and the shape of the muscle alters to become shorter and wider or thicker. *B,* Isometric contraction. Here there is no movement of the skeletal framework, but there is exertion of the muscle. In isometric contraction the muscle will become slightly more compact as it is exerted and later may become slightly larger as it fills with blood.

one tightens or contracts one's muscles without producing any actual movement. Figure 5–4 illustrates isotonic and isometric contraction.

What Is Muscle Tone?

Muscle tone refers to the tone or tension of the muscular system. It is a measure of the degree of constant contraction of the muscles. We usually are not aware of this tonic contraction, since it does not require any conscious exertion; it is, in this sense, passive. The constant tonic contraction that maintains muscle tone is due to a continuous flow of nonconscious stimuli from the brain and spinal cord to each muscle. This constant stimulation increases

or decreases, depending on the level of activity of the nervous system. In times of excitement there is an increase in tone; during periods of restfulness, a decrease in tone occurs.

Besides serving to maintain a state of readiness of the muscular system, tonic contraction is the basis of good posture. As muscle tone decreases, posture deteriorates. This deterioration of posture causes abnormal pull on ligaments, joints, and bones, which in time may lead to permanent skeletal deformities. Persons with low muscle tone also tire much more easily.

Of primary clinical interest is the fact that individuals with good muscle tone will both look and feel better and almost invariably have an excellent response to disease or injury.

What Are the Benefits of Exercise?

The benefits of exercise have been well reported in both professional and popular literature. Properly planned and regularly practiced exercise greatly *increases muscle tone* and, as a consequence, improves health and the general ability of the individual to recover from disease or injury.

The general immobility of sick persons can often be as damaging as the primary illness or injury itself. The bedfast patient seems to recover more quickly when a program of regular exercise is maintained during convalescence. The nurse can help and encourage the bedridden to exercise regularly and by doing so have an enormously important effect on the recovery of the patient.

How Do Skeletal Muscles Produce Movements?

Most skeletal muscles are attached to two bones, with the muscle spanning the joint between the bones. One of the bones always moves more easily than the other in isotonic contraction (contractions producing movement) of any particular muscle. The muscle's attachment to the more stationary bone is called its *origin*. The attachment to the more easily moveable bone is called its *insertion*.

Most voluntary muscles are not inserted directly into bone but rather through the medium of a strong, tough, nonelastic cord called a *tendon*. Tendons vary in length from a fraction of an inch to more than a foot. In all cases, however, the arrangement is such as to allow the muscle the greatest leverage; that is, so that the muscle will get the most work or power from its activity. Skeletal muscles are sometimes categorized according to the type of action or work they perform. Muscles that bend a limb at a joint are called *flexors* (flek'sors); those that straighten a limb at a joint are called *extensors*. If the limb is moved away from the midline of the body, an *abductor* (ab-duk'tor) is at work; if the limb is brought toward the midline, *adductors* are responsible. There are also other muscles that rotate the involved limb.

LOCATION AND ACTION OF THE IMPORTANT SKELETAL MUSCLES

Figures 5–5 to 5–33 and Table 5–1 include most of the important muscles in the human body. Other organs that contain muscular tissue will be described in appropriate later chapters.

You will find it easier to remember the name, location, and action of each muscle if you keep in mind that muscles are named according to *action* (for example, adductor or extensor); according to *shape* (for example, quadrates); according to *origin* and *insertion* (for example, sternocleidomastoid); according to number of *divisions* (for example, quadriceps or triceps); according to *location* (for example, tibialis or radialis); and according to *direction of fibers* (for example, transversus).

In addition to listing the muscles, Table 5–1 describes the origin and insertion of each muscle and its principal action and nerve supply.

CLINICAL CONSIDERATIONS

What Are the Symptoms of Several Muscle Disorders?

The major symptoms of muscular disorders are paralysis, weakness, pain, atrophy (deterioration), and cramps.

The condition in which a muscle shortens its normal length in the resting state is known as *contracture* (kon-trak'tur). Contractures occur when an individual remains in bed for prolonged periods and the muscles are not properly exercised. Eventually, the muscles readjust to the resting length of a flexed arm or leg. Contractures are treated by the painful and slow procedure of exercising and relengthening the muscle. Contractures can be prevented by keeping the body in correct alignment when resting and by periodically exercising the muscles. Muscular exercise can be either active (by the patient himself) or passive (by someone else).

Text continues on page 81

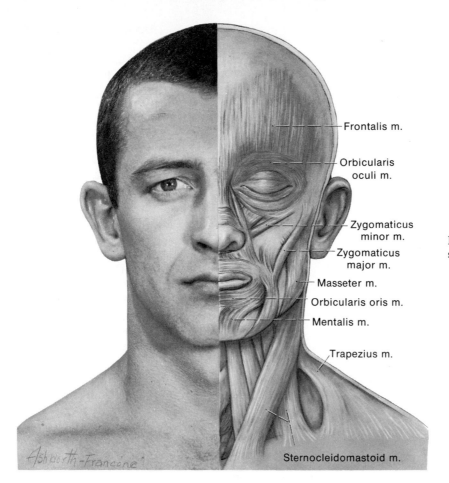

Frontalis m.

Orbicularis
oculi m.

Zygomaticus
minor m.

Zygomaticus
major m.

Masseter m.

Orbicularis oris m.

Mentalis m.

Trapezius m.

Sternocleidomastoid m.

Figure 5–5 Muscles of the face, superficial layer.

Figure 5–6 Muscles of the face, deep layer.

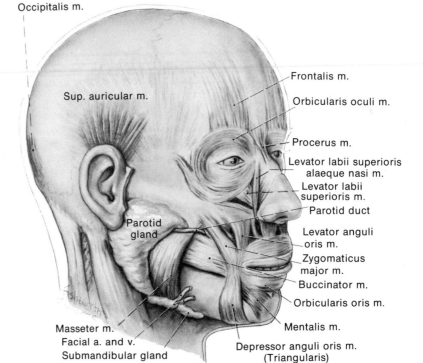

Occipitalis m.

Sup. auricular m.

Parotid gland

Masseter m.
Facial a. and v.
Submandibular gland

Frontalis m.

Orbicularis oculi m.

Procerus m.

Levator labii superioris alaeque nasi m.

Levator labii superioris m.

Parotid duct

Levator anguli oris m.

Zygomaticus major m.

Buccinator m.

Orbicularis oris m.

Mentalis m.

Depressor anguli oris m. (Triangularis)

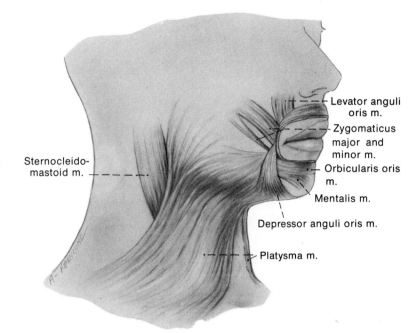

Figure 5–7 Superficial muscles of the neck and muscles around the mouth.

Levator anguli oris m.

Zygomaticus major and minor m.

Orbicularis oris m.

Mentalis m.

Depressor anguli oris m.

Sternocleido-mastoid m.

Platysma m.

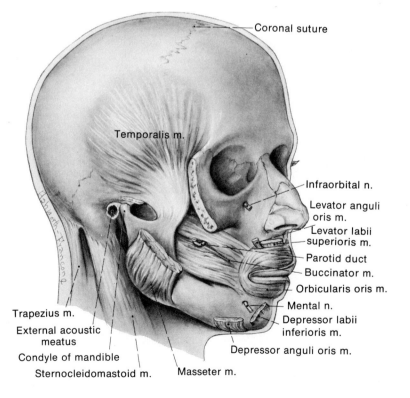

Coronal suture

Temporalis m.

Infraorbital n.

Levator anguli oris m.

Levator labii superioris m.

Parotid duct

Buccinator m.

Orbicularis oris m.

Mental n.

Depressor labii inferioris m.

Depressor anguli oris m.

Trapezius m.

External acoustic meatus

Condyle of mandible

Sternocleidomastoid m.

Masseter m.

Figure 5–8 Muscles of mastication.

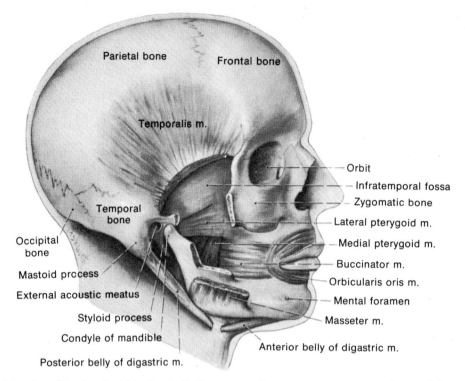

Figure 5–9 Muscles of the head within the skull. The temporalis, masseter, zygoma, and part of the mandible have been removed.

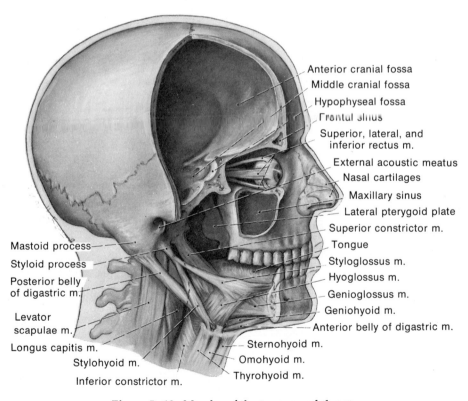

Figure 5–10 Muscles of the tongue and throat.

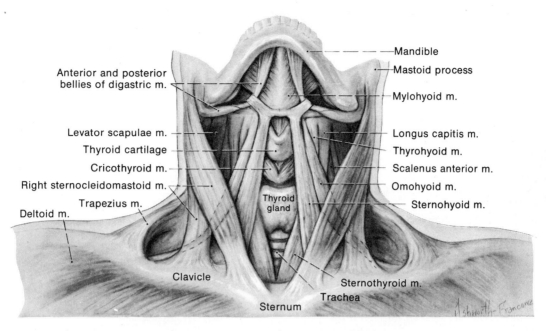

Figure 5-11 Muscles of the neck, superficial layer.

Mandible
Mastoid process
Anterior and posterior bellies of digastric m.
Mylohyoid m.
Levator scapulae m.
Longus capitis m.
Thyroid cartilage
Thyrohyoid m.
Cricothyroid m.
Scalenus anterior m.
Right sternocleidomastoid m.
Omohyoid m.
Trapezius m.
Sternohyoid m.
Deltoid m.
Thyroid gland
Clavicle
Sternothyroid m.
Trachea
Sternum

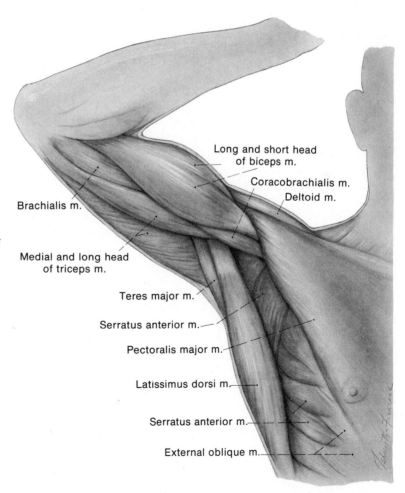

Figure 5-12 Muscles in the region of the axilla when the arm is raised.

Long and short head of biceps m.
Coracobrachialis m.
Deltoid m.
Brachialis m.
Medial and long head of triceps m.
Teres major m.
Serratus anterior m.
Pectoralis major m.
Latissimus dorsi m.
Serratus anterior m.
External oblique m.

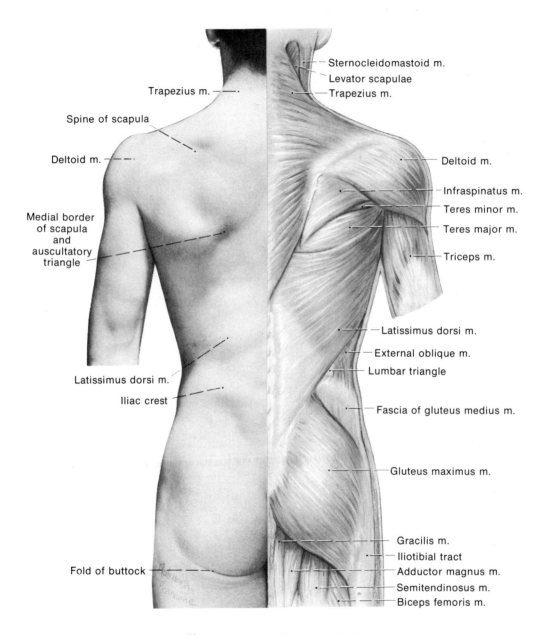

Figure 5–13 Muscles of the back.

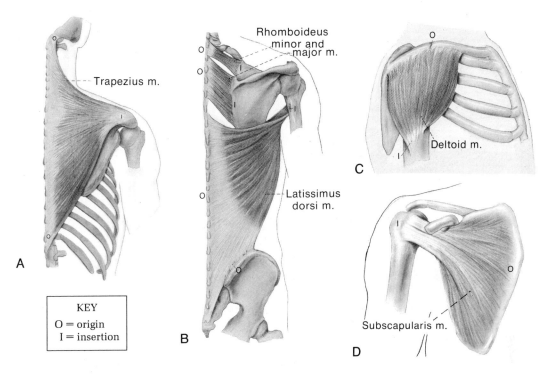

Figure 5-14 labels:

- Trapezius m. (A)
- Rhomboideus minor and major m. (B)
- Latissimus dorsi m. (B)
- Deltoid m. (C)
- Subscapularis m. (D)

KEY
O = origin
I = insertion

Figure 5-14 Deep muscles of the back.

Paralysis is a loss of responsiveness of muscles; this condition invariably results from disease or injury to the nervous system, usually damaging the brain or spinal cord. In cases of paralysis or lack of exercise, muscles tend to *atrophy* (at′ro-fe), meaning to deteriorate, shrink, and waste away. Muscle *hypertrophy* is the opposite of atrophy. Hypertrophy is an abnormal building up or increase in the size of the muscle; this may result from over-exercise.

Two other disorders of the muscular system are muscular dystrophy and myasthenia gravis. The exact cause and treatment of both are unknown. *Muscular dystrophy* (dys- means difficult, and trophy means to nourish) occurs most often in males and is a slowly progressive disorder that ends in complete helplessness. *Myasthenia gravis* (my- means muscle, *asthenia* means weakness, and *gravis* means heavy) is characterized by easy fatigability of muscles. It involves an impairment of conduction of

signals between the muscles and the nerves that normally serve them.

Where Should Intramuscular Injections Be Given? Why?

Figures 5–32 and 5–33 show the best locations for intramuscular injections. These areas are considered to be relatively safe because they are away from major blood vessels and nerves. When the needle has been inserted into the muscle, one should always *pull back* on the syringe plunger before injecting; this provides an immediate test of whether the needle is inside a vessel—if blood is drawn in, the needle is in a vessel and should be reinserted. If an injection goes directly into a major vessel or nerve, it can cause serious problems.

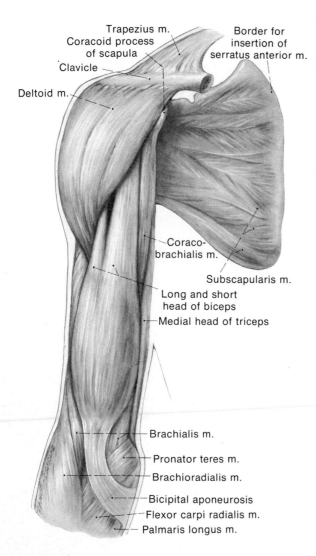

Trapezius m.
Coracoid process
of scapula
Clavicle
Deltoid m.
Border for
insertion of
serratus anterior m.
Coraco-
brachialis m.
Subscapularis m.
Long and short
head of biceps
Medial head of triceps
Brachialis m.
Pronator teres m.
Brachioradialis m.
Bicipital aponeurosis
Flexor carpi radialis m.
Palmaris longus m.

Figure 5-15 Muscles of the shoulder and the upper right arm, anterior view.

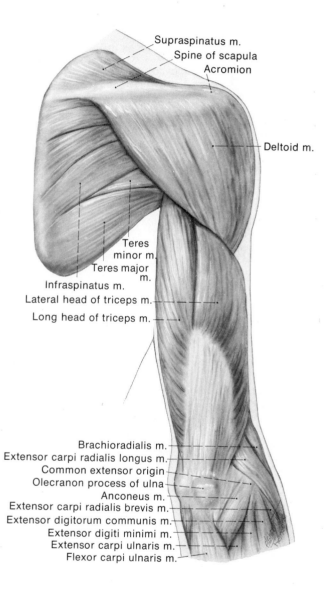

Supraspinatus m.
Spine of scapula
Acromion

Deltoid m.

Teres
minor m.
Teres major
m.
Infraspinatus m.
Lateral head of triceps m.
Long head of triceps m.

Brachioradialis m.
Extensor carpi radialis longus m.
Common extensor origin
Olecranon process of ulna
Anconeus m.
Extensor carpi radialis brevis m.
Extensor digitorum communis m.
Extensor digiti minimi m.
Extensor carpi ulnaris m.
Flexor carpi ulnaris m.

Figure 5-16 Muscles of the shoulder and upper arm, posterior view.

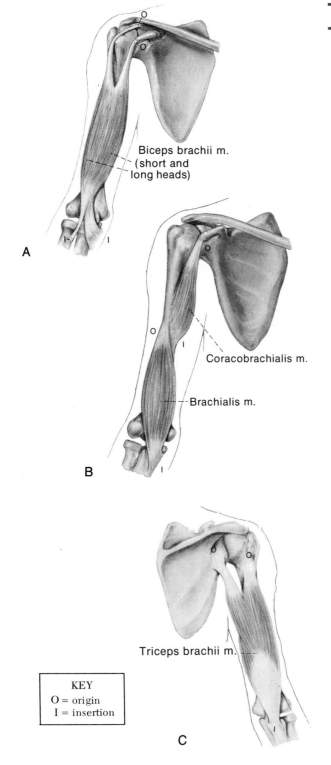

KEY
O = origin
I = insertion

Figure 5-17 Muscles that move the forearm.

SUMMARY

A. The muscular system produces all movement.
  1. External action movements are caused by co-ordinated contractions of the skeletal muscles.
  2. Internal life supportive movements, such as circulation, digestive passage, and respiration, are caused by cardiac and smooth muscles.
B. There are three main types of muscle cells: striated, smooth, and cardiac.
  1. They make up the corresponding three types of muscle tissue: striated, smooth, and cardiac.
  2. These three muscle tissues, together with special connective tissue known as fascia, make up the three types of muscle: striated, smooth, and cardiac.
C. The striated muscles are all attached to the skeleton. Also called skeletal muscles, they function to produce external movement.
  1. The cells of striated muscle are long and slender and are referred to as muscle fibers.
  2. The fiberlike cells are bound by connective tissue into bundles.
  3. Striated cells appear striped (thus the name) and unlike other types of muscle cells have many nuclei.
  4. These muscles are all under voluntary control.
D. Smooth muscles are found in rolled layers, making up the digestive tract and the bladder, the blood vessels, and the skin.
  1. The smooth cells are long and smooth (not striped).
  2. The muscles are controlled automatically by the unconscious parts of the nervous system.
E. Cardiac muscle is found only in the heart.
  1. Cardiac muscle is involuntary (like smooth) but striped (like skeletal).
  2. The interconnecting fibers are not single cells but are built up in a chainlike manner.
F. There are three types of muscle contraction: isotonic, isometric, and tonic.
  1. Isotonic contraction always involves movement and a change in the length of the muscles involved.

2. Isometric contraction does not involve movement or change of length—holding something up without moving it.
3. Tonic contraction produces muscle tone—the degree of constant contraction of the muscles.
   a. Muscle tone is the basis of good posture.
   b. People with good muscle tone look better, feel better, and have an excellent response to disease or injury.
G. Regular exercise greatly increases muscle tone and as a consequence improves health and the ability to recover from disease or injury.
   1. The immobility of sick persons can be as damaging as the primary illness or injury.
   2. Maintaining exercise during convalescence promotes recovery.
H. Skeletal muscles are attached to bones through the medium of a strong, tough, nonelastic cord called a tendon.
   1. The attachment of a skeletal muscle to the more stationary bone is called its origin.
   2. The attachment to the more easily moveable bone is called its insertion.
I. Skeletal muscles are often named by the type of action they perform, such as flexors, extensors, abductors, and adductors.
J. Muscles are named according to action, shape, origin and insertion, number of divisions, location, and direction of fibers.
K. The major symptoms of muscular disorders are paralysis, weakness, pain, atrophy, and cramps.
   1. A contracture is an abnormal muscle shortening.
   2. Paralysis is a loss of responsiveness.
   3. Atrophy—deterioration—results from inaction.
   4. Hypertrophy results from abnormal overexercise.
   5. Two serious muscle disorders are muscular dystrophy and myasthenia gravis.
L. Intramuscular injections avoid major vessels.
M. Aerobic exercise is performed within the range of the immediate ability of the heart and lungs to supply the body's demand for oxygen.
   1. A minimal program of exercise is 30 minutes of aerobic exercise three or four times per week.
      a. This provides 80 per cent of the benefits of exercise.

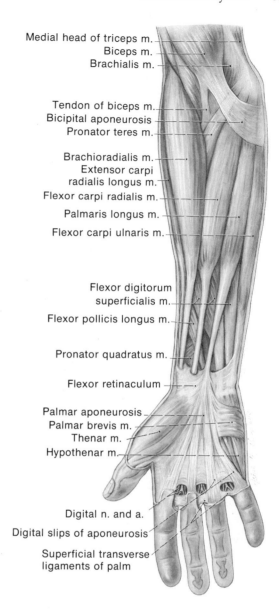

Figure 5-18 Muscles of the palmar aspect of the right hand and forearm.

Labels in figure:
Medial head of triceps m.
Biceps m.
Brachialis m.
Tendon of biceps m.
Bicipital aponeurosis
Pronator teres m.
Brachioradialis m.
Extensor carpi radialis longus m.
Flexor carpi radialis m.
Palmaris longus m.
Flexor carpi ulnaris m.
Flexor digitorum superficialis m.
Flexor pollicis longus m.
Pronator quadratus m.
Flexor retinaculum
Palmar aponeurosis
Palmar brevis m.
Thenar m.
Hypothenar m.
Digital n. and a.
Digital slips of aponeurosis
Superficial transverse ligaments of palm

      b. It improves your ability to handle both physical and emotional stress.
   2. Aerobic exercise is also defined as between 60 and 80 per cent of your maximum heart rate (MHR = 220 – your age; see box on page 97).

Text continues on page 97

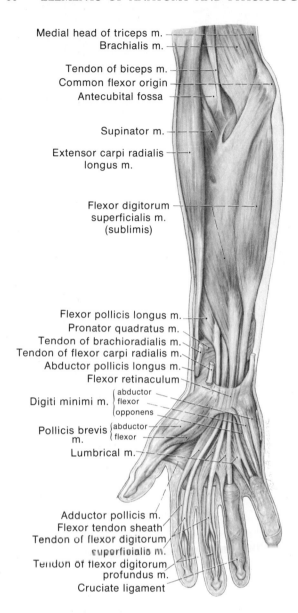

Medial head of triceps m.
Brachialis m.
Tendon of biceps m.
Common flexor origin
Antecubital fossa
Supinator m.
Extensor carpi radialis longus m.
Flexor digitorum superficialis m. (sublimis)
Flexor pollicis longus m.
Pronator quadratus m.
Tendon of brachioradialis m.
Tendon of flexor carpi radialis m.
Abductor pollicis longus m.
Flexor retinaculum
Digiti minimi m. { abductor / flexor / opponens
Pollicis brevis m. { abductor / flexor
Lumbrical m.
Adductor pollicis m.
Flexor tendon sheath
Tendon of flexor digitorum superficialis m.
Tendon of flexor digitorum profundus m.
Cruciate ligament

Figure 5–19 Second layer of muscles of the right hand and forearm, palmar aspect.

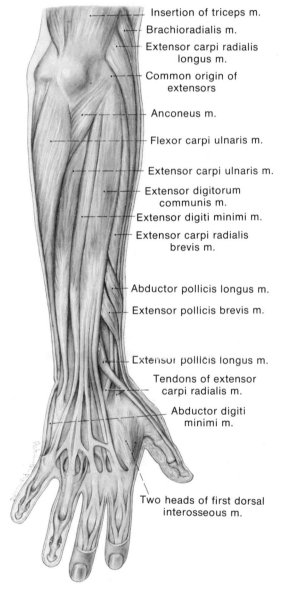

Insertion of triceps m.
Brachioradialis m.
Extensor carpi radialis longus m.
Common origin of extensors
Anconeus m.
Flexor carpi ulnaris m.
Extensor carpi ulnaris m.
Extensor digitorum communis m.
Extensor digiti minimi m.
Extensor carpi radialis brevis m.
Abductor pollicis longus m.
Extensor pollicis brevis m.
Extensor pollicis longus m.
Tendons of extensor carpi radialis m.
Abductor digiti minimi m.
Two heads of first dorsal interosseous m.

Figure 5–20 Posterior view of the right forearm and hand, showing the superficial muscles.

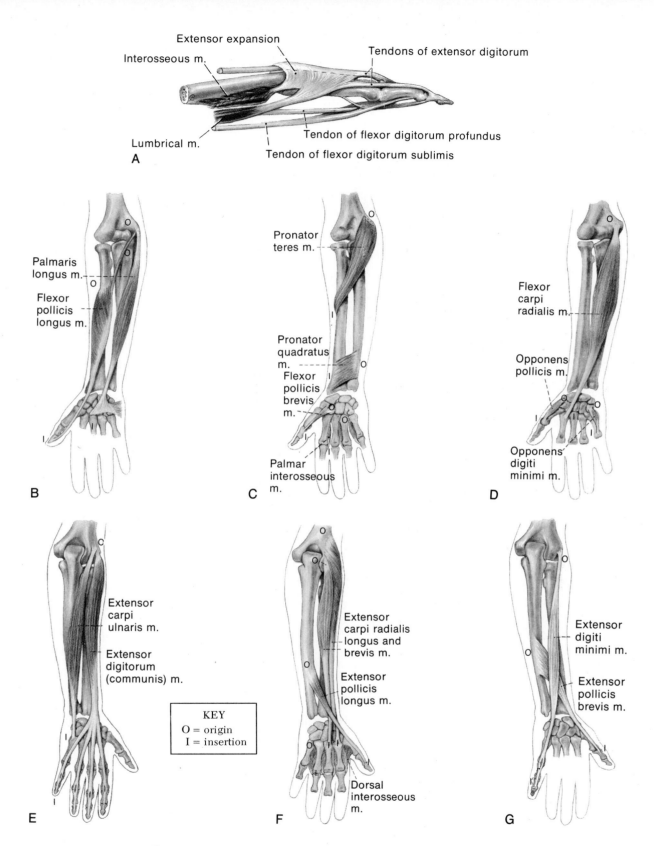

Figure 5-21 Muscles that move the thumb and fingers and the wrist.

Extensor expansion

Interosseous m.

Tendons of extensor digitorum

Lumbrical m.

Tendon of flexor digitorum profundus

Tendon of flexor digitorum sublimis

A

Palmaris longus m.

Flexor pollicis longus m.

B

Pronator teres m.

Pronator quadratus m.

Flexor pollicis brevis m.

Palmar interosseous m.

C

Flexor carpi radialis m.

Opponens pollicis m.

Opponens digiti minimi m.

D

Extensor carpi ulnaris m.

Extensor digitorum (communis) m.

KEY
O = origin
I = insertion

E

Extensor carpi radialis longus and brevis m.

Extensor pollicis longus m.

Dorsal interosseous m.

F

Extensor digiti minimi m.

Extensor pollicis brevis m.

G

87

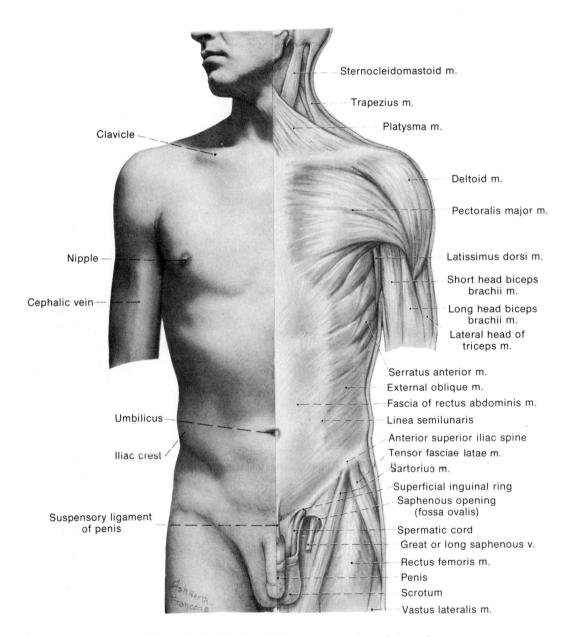

Sternocleidomastoid m.

Trapezius m.

Platysma m.

Clavicle

Deltoid m.

Pectoralis major m.

Latissimus dorsi m.

Nipple

Short head biceps
brachii m.

Cephalic vein

Long head biceps
brachii m.

Lateral head of
triceps m.

Serratus anterior m.

External oblique m.

Fascia of rectus abdominis m.

Linea semilunaris

Umbilicus

Anterior superior iliac spine

Tensor fasciae latae m.

Iliac crest

Sartorius m.

Superficial inguinal ring

Saphenous opening
(fossa ovalis)

Spermatic cord

Suspensory ligament
of penis

Great or long saphenous v.

Rectus femoris m.

Penis

Scrotum

Vastus lateralis m.

Figure 5–22 Muscles of the anterior surface of the male.

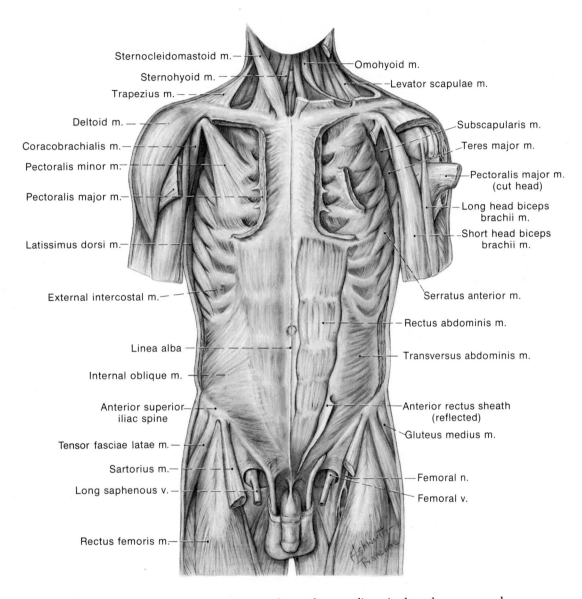

Sternocleidomastoid m.
Sternohyoid m.
Trapezius m.
Deltoid m.
Coracobrachialis m.
Pectoralis minor m.
Pectoralis major m.
Latissimus dorsi m.
External intercostal m.
Linea alba
Internal oblique m.
Anterior superior iliac spine
Tensor fasciae latae m.
Sartorius m.
Long saphenous v.
Rectus femoris m.

Omohyoid m.
Levator scapulae m.
Subscapularis m.
Teres major m.
Pectoralis major m. (cut head)
Long head biceps brachii m.
Short head biceps brachii m.
Serratus anterior m.
Rectus abdominis m.
Transversus abdominis m.
Anterior rectus sheath (reflected)
Gluteus medius m.
Femoral n.
Femoral v.

Figure 5-23 Superficial musculature; skin and pectoralis major have been removed.

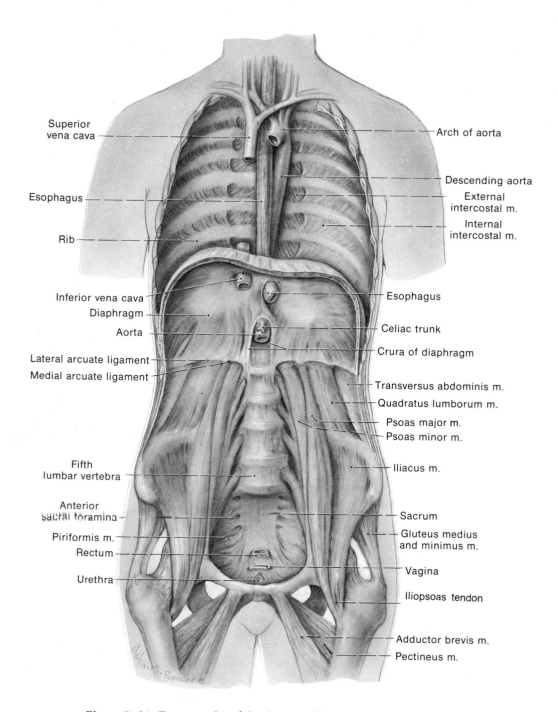

Superior vena cava
Arch of aorta
Descending aorta
External intercostal m.
Internal intercostal m.
Esophagus
Rib
Inferior vena cava
Esophagus
Diaphragm
Celiac trunk
Aorta
Crura of diaphragm
Lateral arcuate ligament
Medial arcuate ligament
Transversus abdominis m.
Quadratus lumborum m.
Psoas major m.
Psoas minor m.
Iliacus m.
Fifth lumbar vertebra
Anterior sacral foramina
Sacrum
Gluteus medius and minimus m.
Piriformis m.
Rectum
Vagina
Urethra
Iliopsoas tendon
Adductor brevis m.
Pectineus m.

Figure 5–24 Deep muscles of the thoracic, abdominal, and pelvic cavities.

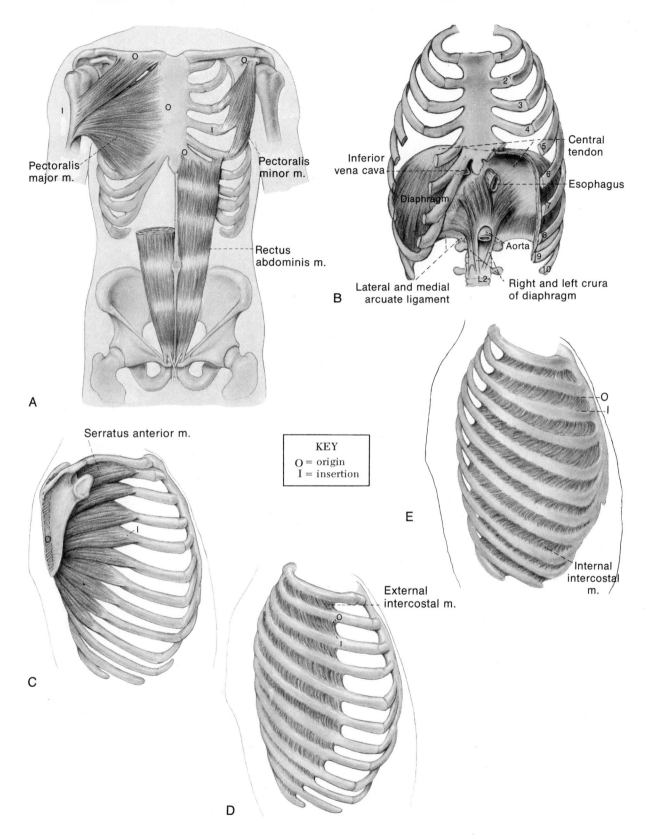

Figure 5-25 Muscles of respiration.

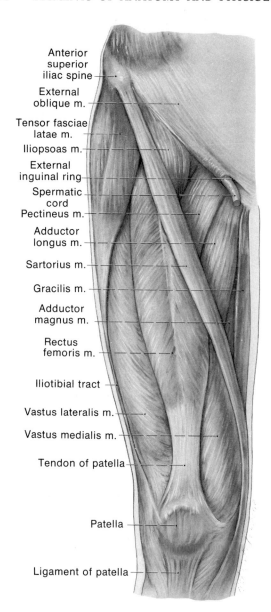

Anterior
superior
iliac spine

External
oblique m.

Tensor fasciae
latae m.

Iliopsoas m.

External
inguinal ring

Spermatic
cord

Pectineus m.

Adductor
longus m.

Sartorius m.

Gracilis m.

Adductor
magnus m.

Rectus
femoris m.

Iliotibial tract

Vastus lateralis m.

Vastus medialis m.

Tendon of patella

Patella

Ligament of patella

Figure 5–26 Superficial muscles of the right upper leg, anterior surface.

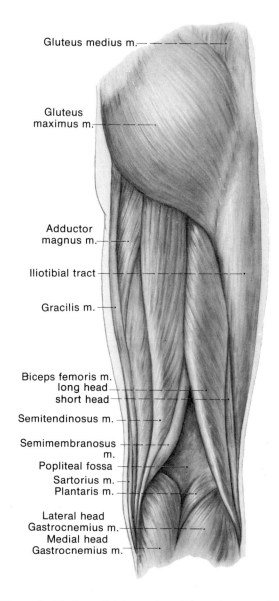

Gluteus medius m.

Gluteus
maximus m.

Adductor
magnus m.

Iliotibial tract

Gracilis m.

Biceps femoris m.
long head
short head

Semitendinosus m.

Semimembranosus
m.

Popliteal fossa

Sartorius m.

Plantaris m.

Lateral head
Gastrocnemius m.

Medial head
Gastrocnemius m.

Figure 5–27 Superficial muscles of the right upper leg, posterior surface.

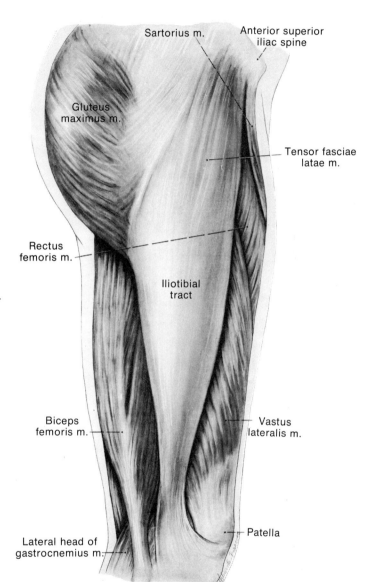

Sartorius m.

Anterior superior
iliac spine

Gluteus
maximus m.

Tensor fasciae
latae m.

Rectus
femoris m.

Iliotibial
tract

Biceps
femoris m.

Vastus
lateralis m.

Patella

Lateral head of
gastrocnemius m.

Figure 5–28   Lateral view of superficial muscles of the right upper leg.

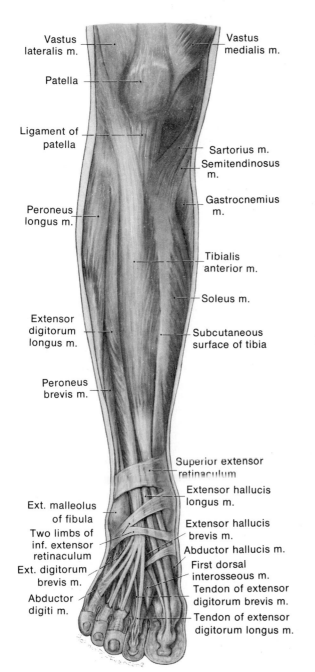

Vastus lateralis m.

Vastus medialis m.

Patella

Ligament of patella

Sartorius m.

Semitendinosus m.

Gastrocnemius m.

Peroneus longus m.

Tibialis anterior m.

Soleus m.

Extensor digitorum longus m.

Subcutaneous surface of tibia

Peroneus brevis m.

Superior extensor retinaculum

Extensor hallucis longus m.

Ext. malleolus of fibula

Two limbs of inf. extensor retinaculum

Ext. digitorum brevis m.

Abductor digiti m.

Extensor hallucis brevis m.

Abductor hallucis m.

First dorsal interosseous m.

Tendon of extensor digitorum brevis m.

Tendon of extensor digitorum longus m.

Figure 5–29 Superficial muscles of the right lower leg and foot, anterior surface.

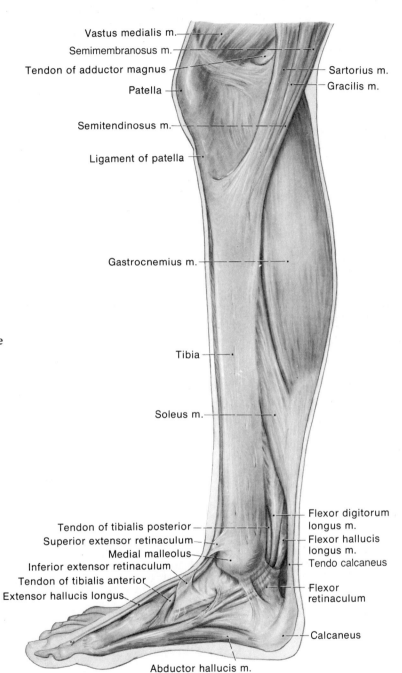

Vastus medialis m.
Semimembranosus m.
Tendon of adductor magnus
Patella
Semitendinosus m.
Ligament of patella

Sartorius m.
Gracilis m.

Gastrocnemius m.

Tibia

Soleus m.

Tendon of tibialis posterior
Superior extensor retinaculum
Medial malleolus
Inferior extensor retinaculum
Tendon of tibialis anterior
Extensor hallucis longus

Flexor digitorum longus m.
Flexor hallucis longus m.
Tendo calcaneus
Flexor retinaculum

Calcaneus

Abductor hallucis m.

Figure 5–30 Superficial muscles of the lower right leg and foot, medial view.

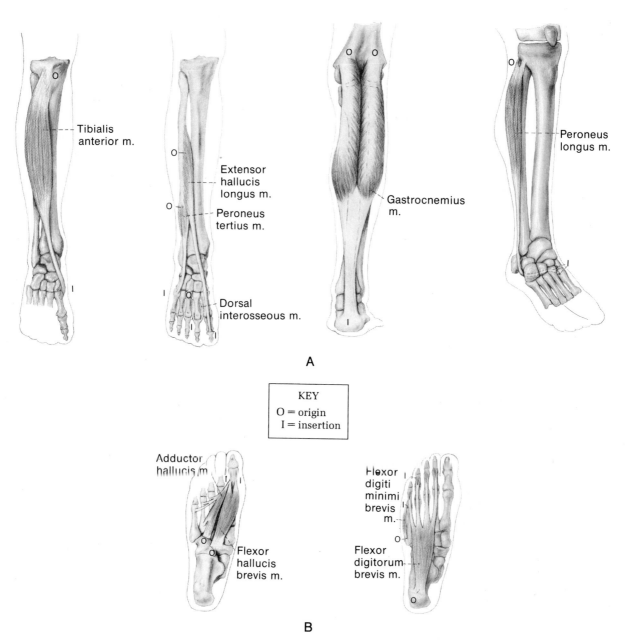

KEY
O = origin
I = insertion

Figure 5-31 Muscles that move the foot *(A)* and toes *(B)*.

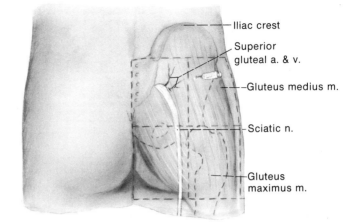

Figure 5-32 Intramuscular injection in the gluteal region should be in the upper outer quadrant.

Aerobic Exercise

The muscle tissues need regular exercise in order to function efficiently and effectively. A sedentary lifestyle leads to muscle degeneration and a decrease of the overall capacity of all organ systems. This is particularly true of the cardiovascular system.

Sports medicine and physical therapy research has determined that the body needs about 30 minutes of aerobic exercise three to four times per week in order to maintain the capacities of the cardiovascular system, skeletal muscles, and nervous system. Even with this minimal level of exercise, the body gains as much as 80 per cent of the benefits of more ambitious exercise programs.

Aerobic exercise is defined as exercise within the range of the immediate ability of the heart and lungs to supply the body's demand for oxygen. This is in contrast to anaerobic exercise that demands more oxygen than the heart and lungs can supply at the time of exercise. In anaerobic exercise, such as sprinting, an oxygen "debt" builds up, and the individual becomes out of breath.

Aerobic exercise has come to be more specifically defined as exercise within the range between 60 and 80 per cent of maximum heart rate. Maximum heart rate (MHR) is calculated by the formula:

$$220 - \text{Your Age} = \text{MHR}$$

The benefits of aerobic exercise include an increased ability to handle both physical and emotional stress. Cardiovascular fitness has been shown to enhance the use of oxygen by all organ systems.

The tremendous importance of exercise during a period of healing or recovery from illness has been demonstrated by recent physical therapy research. The old-fashioned prescription for bed rest as a response to disease is no longer widely recommended. Even this temporary lack of exercise can create problems as damaging in the long run as the direct effects of the original disease or injury. One consequence of this new thinking has been the recent growth in popularity of outpatient, or day, surgery, in which there is no overnight stay in the hospital.

Table 5-1   **MAJOR MUSCLES**

MUSCLE	ORIGIN	INSERTION	FUNCTION	INNERVATION
Head and Neck				
Frontalis	Galea aponeurotica	Frontal bone above supraorbital line	Elevates eyebrows and wrinkles skin of forehead	Facial
Zygomaticus major	Zygomatic bone	Orbicularis oris	Pulls angle of mouth upward and backward when laughing	Facial
Orbicularis oris	Muscle fibers surrounding the opening of the mouth	Angle of mouth	Closes lips	Facial
Masseter	Zygomatic process and adjacent portions of maxilla	Angle and lateral surface of ramus of mandible	Closes jaw	Trigeminal
Sternocleidomastoid (right and left)	Two heads from sternum and clavicle	Tendon into mastoid portion of temporal bone	Flexes vertebral column, rotates head	Spinal accessory
Trapezius	Occipital bone, seventh to twelfth thoracic vertebrae	Acromial process of clavicle and spine	Draws head to one side, rotates scapula	Spinal accessory
Shoulder and Trunk				
Pectoralis major	Anterior surface of sternal half of clavicle, sternum, six upper ribs	Crest and greater tubercle of humerus	Flexes, adducts, rotates arm	Anterior thoracic
Deltoid	Clavicle, scapula	Lateral surface of body of humerus	Abducts arm	Axillary
Latissimus dorsi	Vertebrae, ilium	Humerus	Extends, adducts, rotates arm medially; draws shoulder downward and backward	Thoracodorsal
Rectus abdominis	Crest of pubis and ligaments covering symphysis	Cartilages of fifth, sixth, and seventh ribs	Flexes vertebral column, assists in compressing abdominal wall	Branches of seventh to twelfth intercostal
External oblique	Lower eight ribs	Anterior half of outer lip of iliac crest; anterior rectus sheath	Compresses abdominal contents	Branches of eighth to twelfth intercostal; iliohypogastric

Table 5-1 MAJOR MUSCLES *Continued*				
MUSCLE	**ORIGIN**	**INSERTION**	**FUNCTION**	**INNERVATION**
		Shoulder and Trunk		
Diaphragm	Xiphoid process, costal cartilages, lumbar vertebrae	Central tendon	Pulls central tendon downward to increase vertical diameter of thorax	Phrenic
		Arm and Shoulder		
Flexor pollicis longus	Radius	Base of distal phalanx of thumb	Flexes second phalanx of thumb	Posterior interosseus
Biceps brachii	Scapula	Radius	Flexes lower arm, rotates hand	Musculo-cutaneous
Triceps brachii	Scapula and humerus	Ulna	Extends and adducts forearm	Radial
Brachioradialis	Humerus	Lower end of radius	Flexes forearm	Radial
Flexor carpi radialis	Humerus	Second and third metacarpals	Flexes, abducts wrist	Median
		Hip, Thigh, and Leg		
Iliopsoas, psoas major, psoas minor	Ilium, vertebrae, femur	Femur, ilium, vertebrae	Flexes and rotates thigh Flexes trunk	Second and third lumbar First lumbar
Gluteus maximus	Ilium, sacrum, coccyx	Femur	Extends thigh	Inferior gluteal
Gluteus medius	Ilium	Strong tendons that run into lateral surface	Abducts, rotates thigh medially	Superior gluteal
Quadriceps femoris group (rectus femoris, vastus lateralis, vastus medialis, vastus intermedius)	Ilium and femur	Patella and tibia	Extends leg, flexes thigh	Femoral
Gastrocnemius	Femur and capsule of knee	Tendon calcaneus (Achilles tendon or hamstring)	Points toes, flexes leg, supinates foot	Tibial
Tibialis anterior	Upper tibia	Undersurface of medial cuneiform and base of first metatarsal	Dorsally flexes foot	Deep peroneal
Abductor hallucis	Calcaneus	Proximal phalanx of great toe	Abducts, flexes great toe	Medial plantar

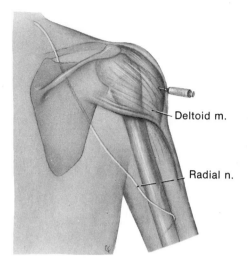

Deltoid m.

Radial n.

Figure 5–33 Intramuscular injection into the deltoid, two to three fingerbreadths below the acromion.

REVIEW QUESTIONS

1. Distinguish and describe the internal and external functions of the muscular system.

2. What is fascia?

3. Name the three types of muscle tissue and compare their characteristics.

4. How much longer than wide are striated muscle cells?

5. Which types of muscle are under voluntary control? Where are these types of muscle located? What are they called?

6. Identify several organs that are composed primarily of smooth muscle cells.

7. What characteristic of cardiac muscle allows it to perform the special needs of the regular pumping action of the heart?

8. Explain the difference between isotonic and isometric contraction.

9. What is muscle tone? What might level of muscle tone indicate about a person's health? How can you increase muscle tone?

10. What is the appropriate role of exercise in all convalescence?

11. Construct a diagram of the upper and lower arm and shoulder, labeling the origins and insertions of the biceps. Construct a similar diagram for the triceps. Based on these diagrams explain how skeletal muscles produce movement.

12. Define contracture. How is it treated?

13. What is paralysis and what is its invariable cause?

14. What are atrophy and hypertrophy?

15. Briefly characterize muscular dystrophy and myasthenia gravis.

16. In giving an intramuscular injection one always pulls back on the syringe plunger before injecting. What is the purpose of this procedure?

17. Distinguish aerobic and anaerobic exercise. Describe a minimal weekly aerobic exercise program. Discuss the benefits of a regular minimal aerobic exercise program.

S I X

The Nervous System

O B J E C T I V E S

The aim of this chapter is to enable the student to do the following:

- List the general functions of the nervous system.

- Explain the anatomic and functional divisions of the nervous system.

- Describe the structure of neurons and distinguish between the different types.

- Explain the distribution and function of myelin.

- Define reflex arc and list its elements.

- Describe the events that lead to the propagation of a nerve impulse and its transmission from one neuron to another.

- Describe the principal features and functions of the spinal cord.

- Construct one or more diagrams identifying the major regions of the cerebral hemispheres, brainstem, and cerebellum and list their functions.

- Describe the origin, function, and circulation of the cerebrospinal fluid.

- List the major types of brain activity recorded by the EEG.

- Describe the anatomy and distribution of the cranial and spinal nerves.

- Outline the anatomic and functional characteristics of the sympathetic and parasympathetic divisions of the autonomic nervous system.

- Construct a diagram identifying the structures of the eye and explain the functions of each.

- Explain the difference in rod and cone function.

- Describe and diagram image formation on the retina.

- Construct a diagram identifying the structures of the ear and explain the functions of each.

- Summarize the sequence of events in the production of sound.

- Construct a diagram identifying the structures underlying the senses of smell and taste and explain the functions of each.

- Identify and describe various disorders of the nervous system.

THE NERVOUS SYSTEM: AN OVERVIEW

What Does the Nervous System Do?

The nervous system, in association with the endocrine system (Chapter 7), controls and coordinates the workings of the component parts of the body. In its most simple conception, the nervous system is a communication network that transmits information by electrical signals throughout the body.

The nervous system accomplishes its function by means of a vast network of nerves that carry signals into and out of the central nervous system (the brain and spinal cord). The brain, and to a lesser extent the spinal cord, serves to interpret and process incoming signals in order to produce appropriate outgoing signals. The higher centers of the brain (the cerebrum) are generally recognized as being responsible for thought processes and conscious activities.

What Types of Cells Are Found in the Nervous System?

Two major kinds of cells make up the nervous system. The *neurons* (nerve cells) conduct and process electrical impulses (signals) from one area of the body to another. These are, therefore, the cells that perform the major work of the nervous system. The *neuroglia* (nu-rog'le-ah) are cells of a special kind of connective tissue. They do not transmit nerve impulses but serve to support, repair, and perhaps nourish the neurons. The neuroglia, or *glial* (gli'al) cells (from the Latin word for glue), differ in size and shape according to their particular function.

THE NEURON

What Does a Neuron Look Like? How Does It Work?

Neurons are usually considered to have three main parts: the axon fibers, the dendrite fibers, and the main cell body.

The axon fibers, or *axons*, normally conduct impulses away from the main cell body. The dendrite fibers, or *dendrites*, normally conduct impulses *toward* and into the main cell body. To remember which type of fiber conducts impulses which way, you should associate the "a" of an *axon* with *away* from.

These neuron fibers are actually part of the cell body, evidenced by the fact that they contain cyto-

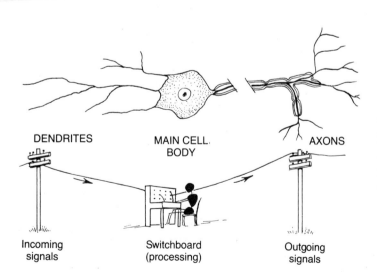

DENDRITES   MAIN CELL BODY   AXONS

Incoming signals   Switchboard (processing)   Outgoing signals

Figure 6-1 A typical neuron. Incoming signals travel along the dendrites, and outgoing signals travel along the axon. The main cell body processes the signals. The neuron is like a telephone communication system, except that in a neuron, signals normally travel in only one direction—in the dendrites and out the axon.

plasm, which is continuous with the cytoplasm of the main cell body. In other words, the axons and dendrites are actually extensions of the main cell body. The axons and dendrites are often extremely long—up to 2 feet or more for neurons serving the feet. Anatomists often refer to these fibers simply as *nerves.* And this has become the proper definition of the word "nerve": that is, it refers to one of the long fibers of a neuron.

The main cell body of a neuron contains the nucleus of the cell. Current theory holds that the main cell body functions to change the nature and direction of signals passing through it. However, the mechanisms and reasons for such changes are not well understood. The main cell body can be thought of as a telephone switchboard through which incoming signals are processed and directed to the appropriate outgoing fiber (Fig. 6–1).

How Are Nerve Fibers Insulated?

What Is the Function of Myelin?

Extending the comparison of the nervous system network to a telephone network, telephone wires are normally insulated (covered) with a nonconducting substance to prevent signals on one wire from interfering with signals on another. Similarly, nerves (long neuron fibers) are normally insulated with a nonconducting material called *myelin.* The myelin covering on nerves is made up of non-nervous Schwann cells, which wind around the nerve fibers, somewhat like several turns of thick tape around a telephone wire (Fig. 6–2).

Nerve cells, including their fiber extensions, all naturally appear gray. Schwann cells, however, appear distinctly white. As a result, some areas of the nervous system look gray and others white. Anatomists have come to refer to the different areas by use of the expressions *gray matter* and *white matter.*

The main cell bodies of the neurons are never covered with myelin; therefore, groups of main cell bodies are always gray matter. Furthermore, whenever gray matter is examined, it is most often composed of main cell bodies. White matter, on the other hand, is always made up of myelinated nerves (fibers).

What Do the Three Classes of Neurons Do?

There are actually three different classes, or categories, of neurons, distinguished on the basis of the duties they perform. *Sensory neurons* bring messages into the central nervous system. *Motor neurons* carry messages out of the central nervous system. *Interneurons* transmit messages between sensory and motor neurons, always within the confines of the central nervous system.

The sensory neurons carry all the sensory signals from all over the body into the central nervous system. These sensory signals inform the central nervous system of the internal workings of each part of the body *and* also of the external or environmental situation (as with the eyes and ears). We are only consciously aware of a small portion of these sensory signals as *sensations* or *perceptions.*

The motor neurons carry the signals that go out from the central nervous system to the various parts of the body. These motor signals activate or instruct each part of the body to accomplish its functions, either internal, such as digestion, or external, such as walking and talking.

The interneurons (sometimes called internuncial neurons) are located exclusively within the central nervous system. They carry messages between the sensory and motor neurons and are commonly connected to other interneurons. This network of interconnections of the interneurons in the central nervous system makes possible the coordination of complex behaviors.

What Is a Reflex Arc?

A *reflex arc* is a complete two-way communication unit. Since neurons carry messages in only one direction, a reflex arc must be made up of at least two neurons, one sensory and one motor. In fact, most reflex arcs also involve one or more interneurons as well (Figs. 6–2 and 6–3).

As a rule, reflex arcs (properly called) control only the simplest or most primitive and automatic behaviors of the particular parts of the body. An example of a simple reflex action is the contraction of the pupil of the eye when exposed to bright light; this primitive response serves to protect the sensi-

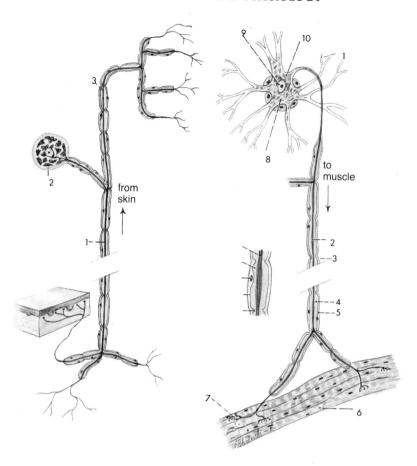

Figure 6-2 Motor and sensory neurons.

tive retina (back of the eye) from damage. The sensory neurons connected to the back of the eye bring the information that there is a bright light to the brain, and the motor neuron carries the activating signal back to the pupil, causing it to contract.

Most reflex behaviors that have been identified have a similar *primitive protective function*, and they are fairly *automatic*.

As behaviors or responses to stimuli become increasingly complex, they are most often processed through the brain centers. Most everyday actions involve a smooth, integrated combination of involuntary (automatic) reflex actions and consciously controlled actions (involving the brain centers).

How Are Signals Transmitted?

Neurons transmit impulses or signals by an electrical (or electrochemical) process. The process begins when the end of the dendrite is stimulated. The stimulus causes a rapid in and out exchange of sodium and potassium ions at the point of stimulation. This process is called "depolarization." It proceeds to adjacent areas of the dendrite fiber, and so on down the line, creating an electrical wave that sweeps along the length of the neuron, out to the tip of the axon (Fig. 6-4).

The rapid in and out exchange of ions takes only a small fraction of a second, but the fiber cannot be stimulated to start another impulse until the ions return to their normal or "ready" position. This "return to normal" process is called "repolarization."

The larger the nerve fiber and the thicker the myelin sheath, the more rapid the rate of conduction of an impulse down the length of the fiber. The range is from 100 meters per second for the largest nerve fibers to about 0.5 meter per second for the smallest.

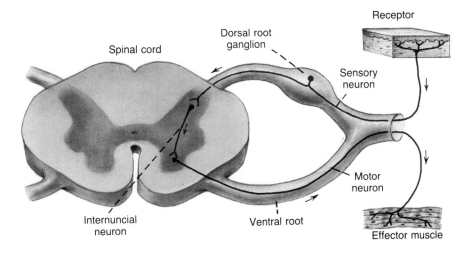

Figure 6-3 Simple reflex arc.

How Does an Impulse Get from One Neuron to Another?

The transmission of an impulse from one neuron to another occurs across a special neuron-to-neuron junction called the *neural synapse* (the point at which an impulse passes from one nerve cell to another) (Fig. 6–2).

Consider a sensory signal reaching the end of its axon in the central nervous system. What happens at that point is the impulse stimulates the release of a special chemical, called a neurotransmitter, stored at the tip of the fiber. The neurotransmitter is a chemical messenger, traveling across the synapse to the dendrite of the next cell. On reaching the connecting neuron, this chemical messenger stimulates the next cell to transmit an electrical impulse, which

Figure 6-4 Schematic representation of the events responsible for the resting membrane potential of a nerve fiber and the action potential. Sodium is actively pumped out of and potassium moves into the cell interior. Some inward diffusion of sodium and outward diffusion of potassium occur as a result of the concentration gradients created by the active transport mechanism. The more rapid outward diffusion of potassium gives rise to the negative resting potential. A stimulus opens the sodium channels, flooding the interior with sodium, reversing the membrane potential. Closing of the sodium channels is followed by opening of the potassium channels and a rapid outflow of potassium, which returns the membrane potential to negative. This transitory reversal of potential, called the action potential or nerve impulse, is propagated along the membrane.

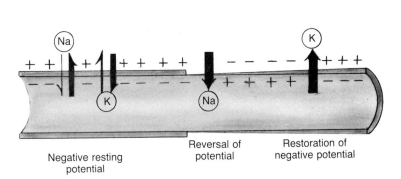

then travels the length of that cell by the electrical process.

In a reflex arc, for example, the impulse begins in a sensory neuron and is transmitted electrically along the cell to the synapse. Here the chemical messenger is released and quickly (almost instantaneously) crosses the junction, contacting the next neuron (either a motor neuron or interneuron). This contact stimulates a new (continued) electrical impulse in the contacted neuron and so on.

Since the neurotransmitters are stored only at the ends of the axon fibers, the synapse is only a *one way junction.* This synaptic property is the real reason why nerve impulses normally travel in only one direction through a nerve cell. Although the nerve fibers are *able* to carry impulses in a reverse direction, this does not normally occur, since reverse impulses can never cross a synapse and, therefore, simply die out whenever they occur.

How Do Signals Start and Stop?

A normal sensory impulse, once started, does not necessarily lead to the production of a motor signal. Interneurons often stop the impulse. In a simple, direct, sensory-to-motor reflex arc, however, a sensory impulse will almost always lead to a motor signal activating the appropriate response; that is, the response to the stimulus is automatic.

At the end of each dendrite of a sensory neuron is a specialized microscopic ending called a *sensory receptor.* These receptors are sensitive to different types of stimuli. For instance, some are stimulated by cold and some by heat, some by light, and some by sound; others are sensitive to specific concentrations of chemicals in the blood. One rather interesting type of sensory receptor is the *baroreceptor,* which is sensitive to the stretching of the walls of arteries caused by increased blood pressure. A sensory neuron transmits a signal when its sensory receptors are stimulated by their characteristic stimulus.

At the end of each axon of a motor neuron is a specialized microscopic ending called an *effector* (or effector ending). When an electrical motor impulse reaches these miniature organs, they release a special chemical, which activates or deactivates the particular part of the body being served; for example, a muscle or digestive organ.

What Is the Language of the Nervous System?

For a long time scientists believed that neurons could each carry many types of messages, depending on how they were stimulated. Experiments have shown, however, that in most instances each neuron transmits only one type of signal. In this sense, neurons are unlike telephone lines. For instance, each sensory neuron or, more accurately, each sensory receptor is sensitive to only one type of stimulus, not several. Similarly, each motor neuron activates only one part and in only one way, not several; for instance, one part of one muscle at one strength.

As a result of this fact, numerous neurons must be present in each area of sensitivity in order for the nervous system to be able to sense a variety of stimuli. And similarly, many different motor neurons must serve each area or organ in order for there to be a variety of possible motor responses for each component.

To take an example, one sensory neuron is needed in each area of the skin to transmit the message "cold" (another is needed for heat, another for pressure, and so on) and a different sensory neuron is needed to transmit the message "very cold." With motor neurons the situation is similar; each motor neuron serves a limited function, so that in many cases one motor neuron is needed to turn some part on and another is needed to turn it off (see Autonomic Nervous System later on).

In other words, each neuron transmits only *one message.* So when it is cold, but not very cold, the first neuron, above, will fire but not the second. Each sensory neuron then has its own particular (characteristic) stimulus, by virtue of the type of sensory receptor endings it has. If that stimulus is present, the neuron will be triggered; if that stimulus is not present, it will not fire.

Neurons cannot be stimulated partially or in degrees; they either fire and transmit their signal, or they don't fire at all and no signal is sent. They do not carry weaker or stronger signals — just one signal, just one message. This is known as the *all-or-none rule* governing the behavior of neurons. It might be remembered as the basic grammatical rule of the language of the nervous system.

These facts about the nature of neurons —

about their language—help us to understand the basis for the organization of the network of millions of nerves throughout the body.

What Are the Two Main Divisions of the Nervous System?

The nervous system is structurally divided into two main parts: the *central nervous system* (CNS) (Fig. 6–5), which is composed of the spinal cord and brain, and the *peripheral nervous system* (PNS), which involves all the nerves and nerve centers of the outlying or peripheral parts of the body.

THE CENTRAL NERVOUS SYSTEM

What Does the Spinal Cord Look Like?

The spinal cord is enclosed in the bony *vertebral column* and extends from the lower brain and down the midline of the back to the pelvic region. Inside

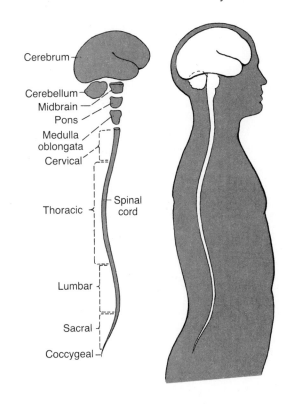

Figure 6–5 Diagram showing major anatomic divisions of the central nervous system.

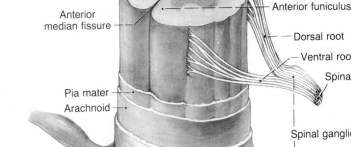

Figure 6–6 Section of spinal cord illustrating formation of a spinal nerve and layers of meninges.

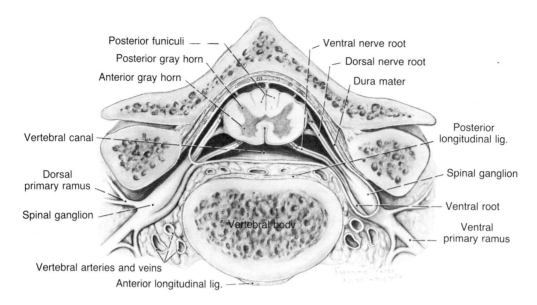

Figure 6-7   Relation of spinal cord and nerves to vertebra.

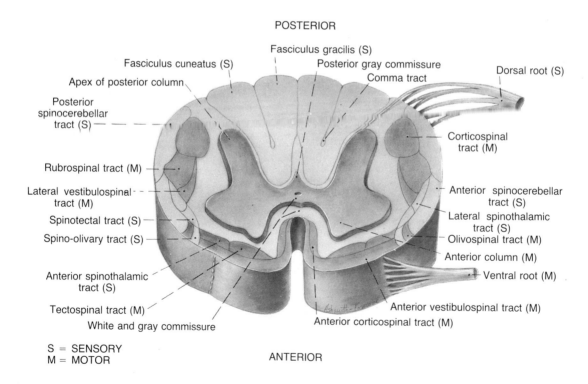

Figure 6-8   Major ascending and descending tracts of the spinal cord.

the vertebral column the spinal cord is covered by three protective membranes called the *meninges* (me-nin'jez). The three layers of the meninges are the *dura mater* (lines the vertebrae), the *pia mater* (covers the cord), and the *arachnoid* (ah-rak'noid) *membrane,* which lies between them (Fig. 6–6). This middle layer is composed of a network of spaces filled with a specialized fluid called the *cerebrospinal fluid.* The composition of the cerebrospinal fluid is very similar to that of the plasma portion of blood, but its function seems to be only protective, since no evidence exists that it participates in the operation of the nervous system. This fluid also surrounds and circulates through the hollows (ventricles) of the brain (see Fig. 6–10).

A cross section of the spinal cord shows an inner region of gray matter in the shape of an H, which is surrounded by a region of white matter. The inner, gray-matter region is composed mainly of cell bodies of neurons. The outer, white-matter region is made up of bundles of myelinated axons known as *tracts,* which transmit impulses between the brain and the lower areas of the body (Figs. 6–7 and 6–8).

What Are the Two Functions of the Spinal Cord?

The activity of the spinal cord can best be understood by dividing it into two functions: the *reflex function* and the *brain communication* function. When a specific sensory impulse enters the spinal cord, either it can be switched directly (or through an interneuron) to an outgoing motorneuron making a reflex arc, or it can be switched to travel up the (white matter) nerve fiber tracts of the spinal cord to the brain. The *spinal cord reflexes* (primitive protective reflex behaviors below the head) result from the direct switching that is independent of the brain centers (see Fig. 6–3).

The *brain communication* function of the spinal cord is performed by the long nerve fiber tracts (white matter) that run the length of the cord, linking the brain centers with various parts of the body. The nerve tracts, which are from both sensory and motor neurons, transmit impulses directly to and from the brain and the sensory receptor and motor-effector sites (Fig. 6–9). In the later discussion of the

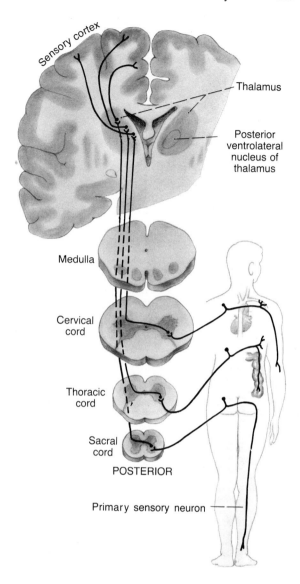

Figure 6–9 Lateral spinothalamic tract (pathway for pain and temperature.)

peripheral nervous system we will talk about these nerve fibers as they enter (sensory) and leave (motor) the central nervous system to connect with the various receptors and effectors throughout the body. The nerve fibers entering and leaving the cranial area are referred to as *cranial nerves,* and those to and from the spinal cord are referred to as *spinal nerves.*

These two functions of the spinal cord—reflex and brain communication— are easily seen to be distinct when an injury cuts the spinal cord all the way through. In such cases, the brain communication function *below the point of injury* is lost completely, resulting in a loss of sensation (anesthesia) and a loss of motor influence (paralysis). This is because the tracts—the direct communication lines—have been severed. However, the spinal cord reflexes continue to operate, so that all behaviors and responses controlled by spinal reflex arcs will persist. This occurs because the entire reflex arc (main cell bodies and nerve fibers) is located below the injury and *can* operate independently of the brain centers.

What Does the Brain Look Like?

As in the spinal cord, the brain is covered by a meninx, which is in fact continuous with the

meninges of the spinal cord. The cerebrospinal fluid fills the spaces of the arachnoid layer of the meningeal covering and also circulates through internal hollows or *ventricles* that lie deep inside the brain. These ventricles are connected by the *cerebral aqueduct* to the spinal cavity, which contains the spinal cord. The cerebrospinal fluid is continually being formed and reabsorbed by a sort of osmotic filtration process between the cavities and capillaries (Figs. 6–10 to 6–12). *Hydrocephalus*, or "water on the brain," results from blockages of this circulation caused by such disorders as congenital (present at birth) abnormalities or tumors.

The brain itself can be structurally and functionally divided into several main parts, as follows (Figs. 6–11 and 6–12):

1. *The hindbrain* includes the pons, medulla and cerebellum.

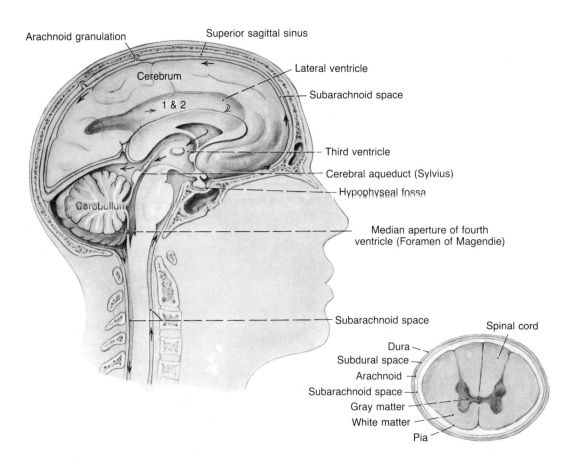

Figure 6–10 Circulation of cerebrospinal fluid in brain and spinal cord.

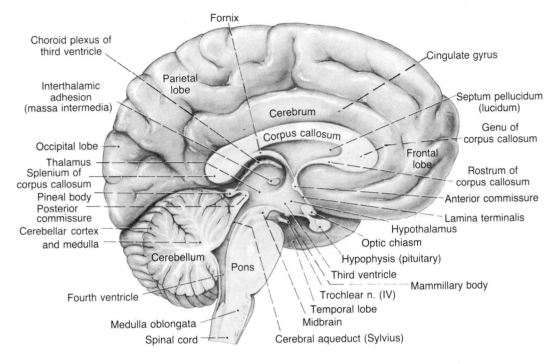

Figure 6–11 Sagittal view of the left half of the brain and spinal cord.

2. *The midbrain and interbrain* includes the thalamus, hypothalamus, and important motor centers.
3. *The forebrain,* the largest portion, is also referred to as the cerebrum.

What Are the Structures and Functions of the Hindbrain?

Moving up the spinal cord to the hindbrain, one first encounters the *medulla* (medulla oblongata), which is continuous with the spinal cord. The medulla is very similar in many ways to the spinal cord and has been called the bulb of the spinal cord. Internally, it contains several separate collections of the nerve cell bodies (gray matter), which are called *centers.* The outer portion of the medulla is made up of the continuation of the numerous myelinated (white matter) nerve fibers (both sensory and motor) that directly link the higher brain centers (through the spinal cord) to the various parts of the body.

The internal, gray-matter portions of the me-

dulla contain several important reflex centers. Among these are the reflex centers controlling three vital functions. The *respiratory reflex center* controls the muscles of respiration in response to chemical and other stimuli. The *cardiac reflex center* has a role in controlling the rate of heartbeat. And the *vasomotor reflex center* (*vas* is Latin for vessel) activates constriction of the blood vessels and hence aids in maintaining proper blood pressure.

The *pons* is a bridgelike structure continuous with the medulla and lying anterior to the cerebellum. It is almost entirely composed of white matter linking the various parts of the brain to each other. The pons serves as a relay station from the medulla to the higher centers of the brain. In addition, several important reflex centers for cranial nerves are located in this area.

The *cerebellum* is a large, gray, oval body located posterior to the medulla and pons. The internal portion, called the *vermis,* is made up of white matter and is surrounded by two lateral *hemispheres* of gray matter; note that the medulla and spinal cord are of the opposite make-up—internal gray matter and external white matter. The determina-

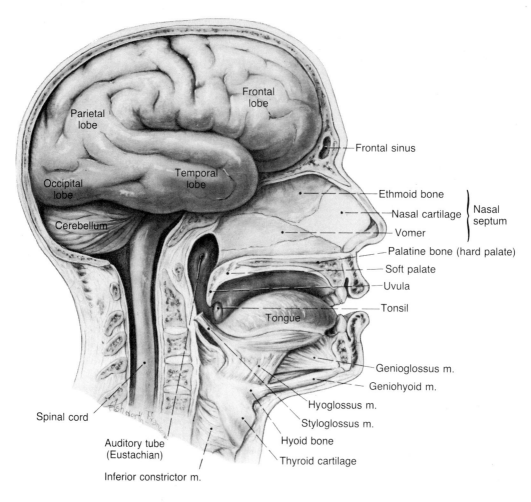

Figure 6-12 Sagittal section through the head (brain intact).

tion of the functions of the cerebellum has come primarily from observing the problems that arise in patients with cerebellar injuries and in experimental animals with all or part of the cerebellum removed. From these observations and studies it has been determined that the cerebellum functions in coordinating movements, such as in walking or more strenuous activity; in sustaining posture by maintaining muscle tone; and in controlling the balance and spatial orientation of the individual. A patient with cerebellar damage displays jerkiness of movement, lack of coordination, and deterioration of muscle tone and posture and has difficulty in maintaining balance.

Scattered throughout the area of the midbrain, pons, and medulla are numerous large and small neurons that are related to each other by small processes (cellular extensions). These neurons and their fibers constitute the *reticular formation*, or the *reticular activating system* (RAS), which controls the overall degree of central nervous system activity, including the control of wakefulness and sleep, and at least part of our ability to direct our attention.

What Are the Structures and Functions of the Midbrain and Interbrain?

The area just above and forward of the pons is referred to as the *midbrain*. It is composed of several nuclear masses that are of great importance in motor coordination—relating and integrating motor signals from several parts of the brain. Of particular interest are three of these mass centers: the *superior colliculi* (ko-lik'u-li), which are involved in visual reflexes; and two posterior mass centers, the *inferior colliculi*, which are associated with hearing. When the superior part of the midbrain is injured or diseased, an abnormality of eye movements results, particularly a paralysis of upward gaze. The midbrain, pons, and medulla together are commonly referred to as the *brainstem*.

The *interbrain*, also referred to as the diencephalon, is located anterior to the midbrain. It is composed of two important structures, the thalamus and the hypothalamus. The *thalamus* (thal'ah-mus) is a relatively large mass of gray matter located in the medioposterior portion of each cerebral hemisphere. It operates to integrate and process sensory stimuli, suppressing some and magnifying others. The *hypothalamus*, a much smaller structure, is located in the midline area below the thalamus. For its size, the hypothalamus is perhaps the most significant single structure so far considered. It has been found to be of central importance in a wide variety of functions, including control of the chief endocrine gland (the pituitary), which influences almost all secretions of the endocrine system; control of

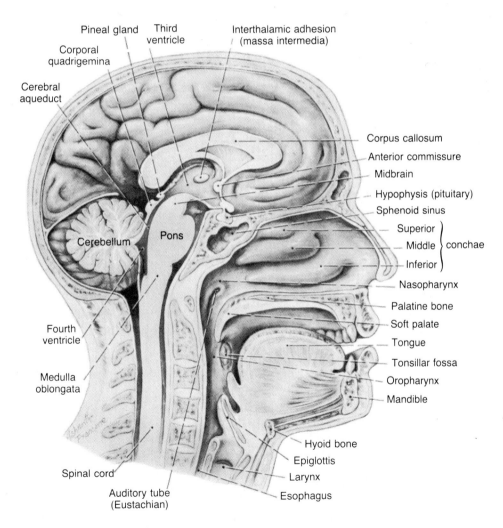

Figure 6–13 Sagittal section through the head showing relationship of cerebellum, cerebrum, and spinal cord to other parts of the head and neck.

appetite, sleep, and some emotions (such as fear and pleasure); and control of much of the activity of the autonomic (unconscious) nervous system, which activates and regulates the functioning of almost all of the internal (visceral) organs.

What Are the Structures and Functions of the Forebrain?

The forebrain, or *cerebrum*, is the largest part of the brain, and it controls all the "higher" functions and activities of the human body. It is divided into two hemispheres by the *longitudinal fissure.* These hemispheres are connected only in their lower middle portion, referred to as the *corpus callosum* (kahlo'sum). The outer layer of the cerebral hemispheres, called the *cerebral cortex,* is composed of gray matter. The internal portion, called the *cerebral medulla,* is composed of white matter.

The nerve fibers (tracts) of the neurons contained in the cerebrum that communicate with the lower parts of the body "cross over" in the area of the medulla. As a result, the left hemisphere serves the right side of the body and the right hemisphere serves the left side.

The cerebral cortex of each hemisphere is divided into four *lobes.* Each lobe has been found to control certain categories of functions (Figs. 6–13 and 6–14):

1. The *frontal lobe* contains the motor cortex, which controls the voluntary movements of all the muscles of the body. Also located in the frontal lobe are the *verbal speech* and *written speech* centers, which control the muscles of the tongue, soft palate, and larynx and the muscles of the hand and arms, respectively.
2. The *parietal lobe* contains the sensory reception area and enables awareness of pain, touch, and temperature as well as judgments of distances, sizes, and shapes.
3. The *temporal lobe* contains the auditory center, which enables awareness of distinct sounds, and

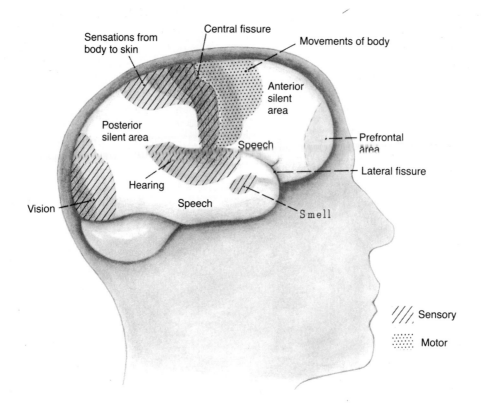

Figure 6-14 Projection areas of the cerebral cortex.

also the auditory speech center, which functions in the understanding of spoken language.

4.   The *occipital* (ok-sip'i-tal) *lobe* contains the visual center, enabling awareness of distinct visual phenomena, and also the visual speech center, which functions in the understanding of written language (reading). The olfactory (smell) center is located in the cerebral core.

More generally, the cerebrum controls conscious mental processes, sensations, emotions, and voluntary movements.

THE PERIPHERAL NERVOUS SYSTEM

What Are the Two Main Subdivisions of the Peripheral Nervous System?

The peripheral nervous system is made up of all the nerves and nerve centers of the outlying or peripheral parts of the body. Any part of the nervous system not contained in the central nervous system is a component of the peripheral nervous system. The two main subdivisions are the *cranial nerves* and the *spinal nerves.*

What Are the Cranial Nerves?

The cranial or cerebral nerves consist of 12 pairs of symmetrically arranged nerves attached to the brain (Figs. 6–16 and 6–17). Each leaves the skull through a foramen (small opening in the bone) at its base. The site where the fibers composing the nerve enter or leave the brain surface is usually termed the superficial origin of the nerve; and the more deeply placed group of neurons from which the fibers arise (motor) or around which they terminate (sensory) is called the nucleus of origin or *deep origin* of the nerve (Table 6–1). The sensory cranial nerve fibers bring in sensory impulses of special senses (such as smell, vision, and hearing) and general senses (such as pain, touch, temperature, deep muscle sense,

---

What Is an Electroencephalogram (EEG)?

Human brain cells generate electrical potentials that can be measured through the skull and are the basis of electroencephalography, a clinical diagnostic procedure used as an aid in diagnosis of epilepsy, brain tumor, hemorrhage, and other disorders. The electroencephalogram (elek"tro-en-sef'ah-lo-gram") (EEG) is recorded by placing electrodes on the individual's head. The EEG varies from the nonrhythmic, high frequency, low voltage waves of the mentally active state (beta waves; 15 to 60 cycles/second, 5 to 10 microvolts), through the more rhythmic, lower frequency, higher voltage activity of the relaxed state (alpha waves; 8 to 10 cycles/second, about 50 microvolts), to the highly rhythmic, slow, large waves of deep sleep producing synchronous cortical activity (delta waves; 1 to 5 cycles/second, 20 to 200 microvolts). (Alpha, beta, and delta waves are illustrated in Fig. 6–15.)

The alpha rhythm of the inattentive brain, usually recorded with the eyes closed, will be replaced by the beta activity by simply opening the eyes in bright light. Slow, large waves are seen in the awake state only in early childhood. Their occurrence in adults other than during sleep is an indication of some brain disorder.

In the course of a night's sleep, episodes occur during which the eyes dart back and forth (although the muscles are in general relaxed), dreaming occurs, and the EEG shows characteristics of the awake states (beta-type activity).

---

pressure, and vibration). The motor cranial nerve fibers carry outgoing motor signals activating voluntary and involuntary muscles, organs, and glands. Figures 6–18 to 6–23 detail several of the cranial nerves.

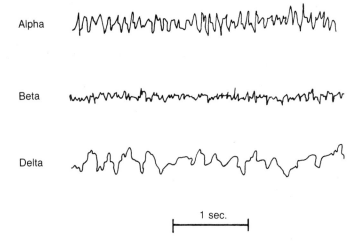

Alpha

Beta

Delta

1 sec.

Figure 6–15   Principal types of normal EEG waves.

What Are the Spinal Nerves?

There are 31 pairs of nerves emerging from the spinal cord along almost its entire length (Fig. 6–24). Each pair is made up of a *dorsal root* and a *ventral root*. The ventral root nerve carries motor signals, and the dorsal root nerve carries sensory signals. Along each dorsal root are found concentrations of sensory nerve cell main bodies; these collections are called dorsal root ganglia. The ganglia are gray matter, since main cell bodies are never covered by myelin, even when located outside the central nervous system. The main cell bodies for the ventral (motor) roots are located inside the spinal column, forming the internal gray matter of the spinal cord (Fig. 6–25).

Each spinal nerve branches into a small, posterior division and a larger, anterior division a short distance after emerging from the spine. The anterior branches interlace to form networks called *plexuses* (plek'sus-eez), from which branches then reemerge to innervate the motor effector organs (Figs. 6–26 to 6–28).

What Is the Autonomic Nervous System?

The autonomic nervous system is a functionally specialized subsystem of the total nervous system. The overall function of the autonomic nervous sys-tem seems to be to maintain homeostasis (since it controls the most important homeostatic effector organs) of the internal environment, particularly with respect to temperature and composition. It generally controls body functions that are considered to be involuntary, acting on the internal (visceral) *effectors* such as smooth and cardiac muscle, exocrine glands (sweat and salivary), and some endocrine glands (Fig. 6–29).

The autonomic nervous system is strictly a motor system (Table 6–2). Anatomically and functionally, it is the motor pathway linking the control centers of the brain with the internal organs and secretory cells. The corresponding sensory portion of the nervous system serving these areas is not considered to be part of the autonomic system.

Unlike the motor portion of the voluntary (somatic) division of the nervous system, the autonomic system displays in part an organizational network of motor ganglia. These *ganglia* are synaptic junctions and relay centers in the divided motor signal transmission system of the autonomic system. On the spinal side there are motor neurons with their main bodies inside the spinal cord (as with the voluntary system), and these are called preganglionic neurons. However, unlike the voluntary system, these preganglionic neurons do not reach the effectors; instead, they synapse (connect) with the postganglionic neurons, whose main cell bodies go to make up the bulk of the ganglion. It is the postganglionic neuron nerve fiber that finally carries the motor signal from the ganglion to the

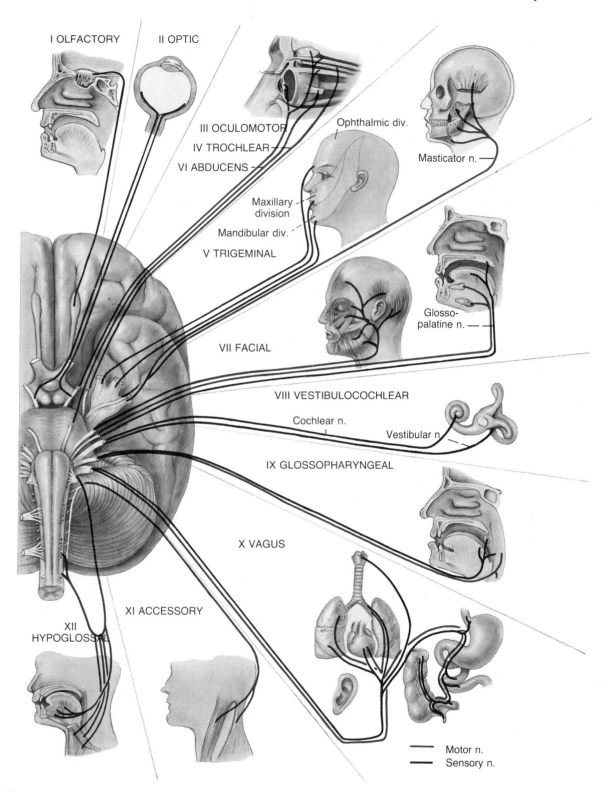

I OLFACTORY

II OPTIC

III OCULOMOTOR

IV TROCHLEAR

VI ABDUCENS

Ophthalmic div.

Masticator n.

Maxillary
division

Mandibular div.

V TRIGEMINAL

VII FACIAL

Glosso-
palatine n.

VIII VESTIBULOCOCHLEAR

Cochlear n.

Vestibular n

IX GLOSSOPHARYNGEAL

X VAGUS

XI ACCESSORY

XII
HYPOGLOSSAL

Motor n.
Sensory n.

Figure 6–16 Distribution of cranial nerves. (After Netter.)

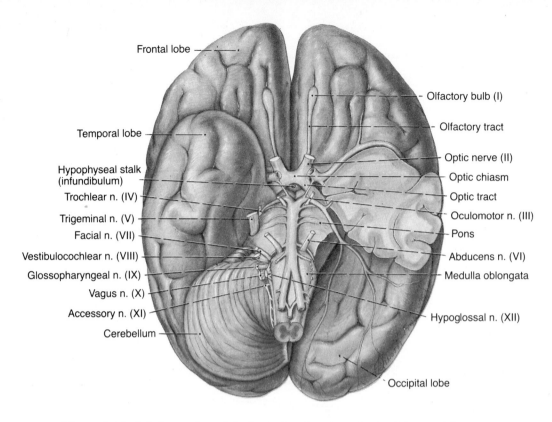

Figure 6–17 Inferior surface of the brain showing sites of exit of the cranial nerves.

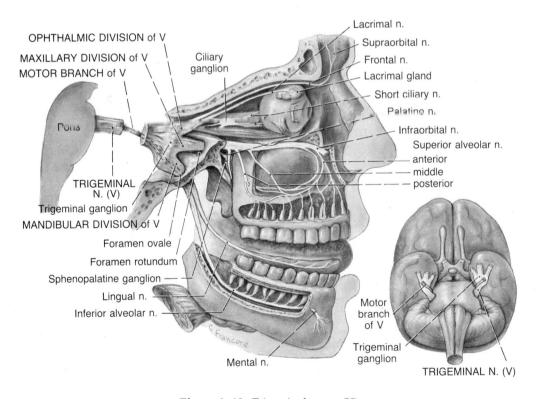

Figure 6–18 Trigeminal nerve (V).

118

Table 6–1   CRANIAL NERVES

NUMBER	NAME	ORIGIN	EXIT FROM SKULL	FUNCTION
I	Olfactory	Cells of nasal mucosa	Cribriform plate of ethmoid	Sensory: olfactory (smell)
II	Optic	Ganglion cells in retina	Optic foramen	Sensory: vision
III	Oculomotor	Midbrain	Superior orbital fissure	Motor: external muscles of eyes except lateral rectus and superior oblique; levator palpebrae superioris Parasympathetic: sphincter of pupil and ciliary muscle of lens
IV	Trochlear	Roof of midbrain	Superior orbital fissure	Motor: superior oblique muscle
V	Trigeminal	Lateral aspect of pons		
	Ophthalmic branch	Semilunar ganglion	Superior orbital fissure	Sensory: cornea; nasal mucous membrane; skin of face
	Maxillary branch	Semilunar ganglion	Foramen rotundum	Sensory: skin of face; oral cavity; anterior two thirds of tongue; teeth
	Mandibular branch	Semilunar ganglion	Foramen ovale	Motor: muscles of mastication Sensory: skin of face
VI	Abducens	Lower margin of pons	Superior orbital fissure	Motor: lateral rectus muscle
VII	Facial	Lower margin of pons	Stylomastoid foramen	Parasympathetic: lacrimal, submandibular, and sublingual glands Motor: muscles of facial expression Sensory: taste, anterior two thirds of tongue
VIII	Vestibulocochlear			
	Vestibular	Lower border of pons	Internal auditory meatus	Sensory: equilibrium
	Cochlear	Lower border of pons	Internal auditory meatus	Sensory: hearing
IX	Glossopharyngeal	Medulla oblongata	Jugular foramen	Motor: stylopharyngeus muscle Sensory: tongue (posterior one third), taste, pharynx Branch to the carotid sinus
X	Vagus	Medulla oblongata	Jugular foramen	Sensory: external meatus, pharynx, and larynx Motor: pharynx and larynx Parasympathetic: thoracic and abdominal viscera
XI	Accessory	Medulla oblongata	Jugular foramen	Motor: trapezius and sternocleidomastoid muscles
XII	Hypoglossal	Anterior lateral sulcus between olive and pyramid	Hypoglossal canal	Motor: muscles of tongue

effector organ. Recall that in the somatic (voluntary) nervous system the motor neuron cell bodies are located inside the spinal cord, with fibers extending directly out to the effector (such as skeletal muscles).

The autonomic nervous system can be further divided into the sympathetic and parasympathetic nervous systems. These two systems both operate in the organs controlled by the autonomic system. The two sets of nerves from these subsystems have opposing functions — one stimulates and the other inhibits the activity of a given organ. Thus, the heart rate is slowed by the parasympathetic and accelerated by the sympathetic division. In general, the parasympathetic system is concerned with restora-

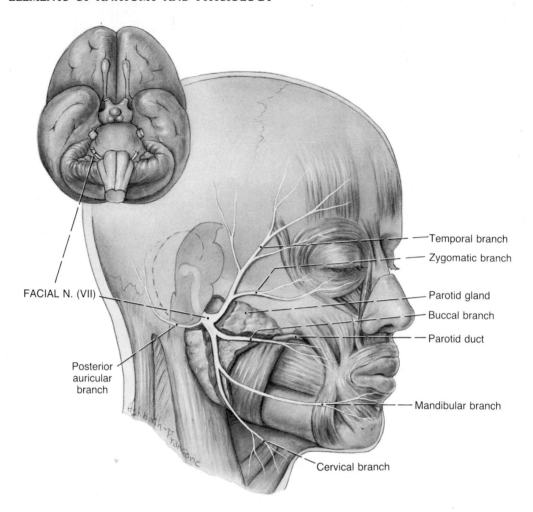

FACIAL N. (VII)

Temporal branch

Zygomatic branch

Parotid gland

Buccal branch

Parotid duct

Posterior
auricular
branch

Mandibular branch

Cervical branch

Figure 6–19   Facial nerve (VII).

tive processes, and the sympathetic, with processes involving energy expenditure. The sympathetic system is sometimes called the "fight or flight" system, since stimulation through the sympathetic division alone does those things that would prepare one to either fight or flee.

The sympathetic nerves arise from all the thoracic segments and from the first few lumbar segments of the spinal cord. The parasympathetic nerves arise from the third, seventh, ninth, and tenth cranial nerves and from the second, third, and fourth sacral segments of the spinal cord.

SPECIAL SENSES

How Are the Sensory Receptors Organized?

At the beginnings of the dendrites of the sensory neurons are specialized receptors, microscopic sense organs. Literally millions of these sensory receptors are scattered in almost every part of the body. Some receptors are designed to respond to

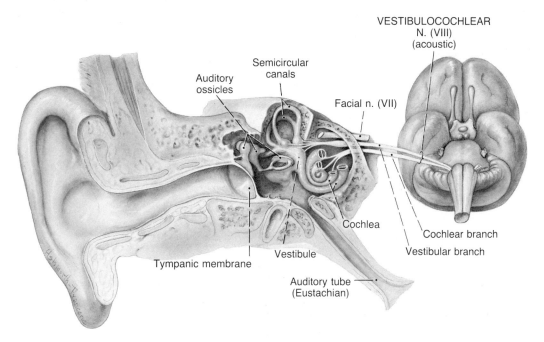

Figure 6–20 Vestibulocochlear nerve (VIII).

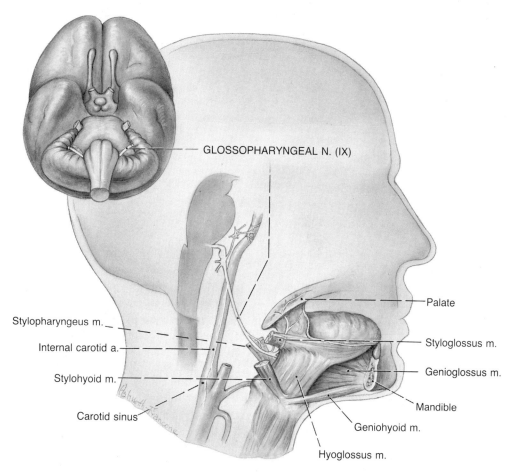

Figure 6–21 Glossopharyngeal nerve (IX).

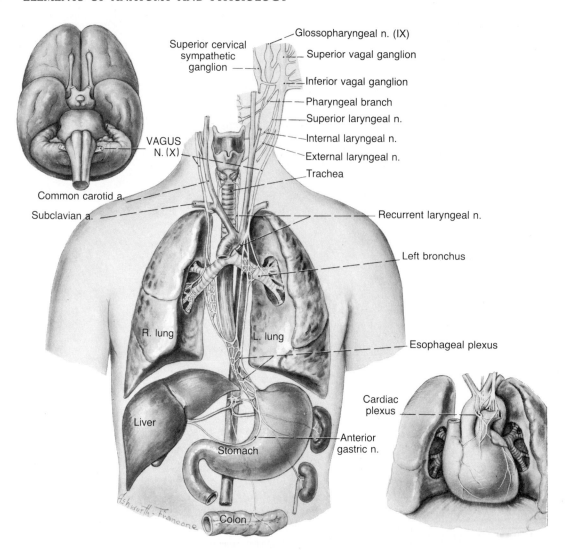

Figure 6-22   Vagus nerve (X).

special types of external stimuli in a limited area; examples are the receptors for vision, hearing, taste, and smell. Other receptors, such as those sensitive to touch, pressure, temperature, and positions of the body, are more generally distributed. When stimulated, a receptor organ produces impulses in the sensory neuron, which transmits the impulses to the spinal cord or brain.

The sensation of pain seems to arise not from special receptor organs, but rather from *free nerve endings*; that is, branchings of the dendrite fibers without any specialized end organs. These pain

sensation endings are the most widely distributed of any type of sensory receptor. They are found in the skin, muscles, and joints, and, to a lesser extent, in most internal organs (including the blood vessels and viscera).

Internal sensations such as hunger and thirst seem to be more complex, arising from a variety of conditions that stimulate receptors in the stomach, intestines, and throat as well as receptors that monitor the level of various nutrients in the blood. Hunger, in particular, involves several types of sensory stimulation, taken individually or together.

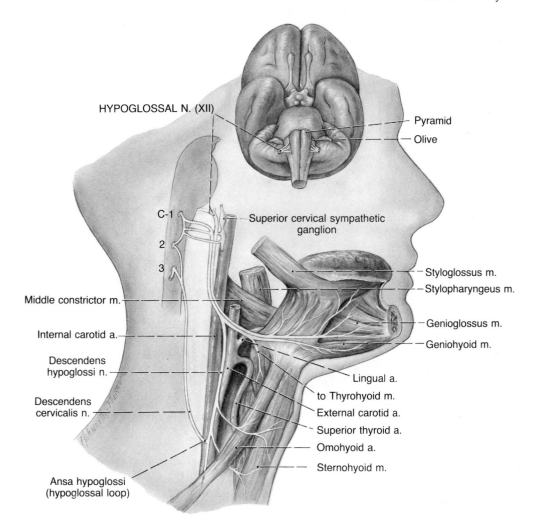

HYPOGLOSSAL N. (XII)

Pyramid

Olive

C-1

2

3

Superior cervical sympathetic ganglion

Styloglossus m.

Stylopharyngeus m.

Genioglossus m.

Geniohyoid m.

Middle constrictor m.

Internal carotid a.

Descendens hypoglossi n.

Descendens cervicalis n.

Lingual a.

to Thyrohyoid m.

External carotid a.

Superior thyroid a.

Omohyoid a.

Sternohyoid m.

Ansa hypoglossi (hypoglossal loop)

Figure 6-23   Hypoglossal nerve (XII).

The two major receptor structures considered next operate in conjunction with the functioning of gross anatomic sensory organs that aid in gathering sensory information from the environment as the attention directs.

What Does the Eye Look Like? How Does It Work?

The lining of the eyeball is made up of three partially specialized membrane layers: the sclera, the choroid, and the retina. The *sclera* (skle′rah) is the tough outer layer composed of connective tissue. What is commonly referred to as the "white" of the eye is part of the frontal portion of the sclera (Fig. 6–30). In the center of the frontal surface of the sclera is a specialized transparent area known as the *cornea.* Lying over the cornea is a limited protective mucous membrane referred to as the *conjunctiva* (kon″junk-ti′vah), which aids in keeping particles from irritating the corneal surface.

The *choroid* layer is also specialized in the frontal area of the eyeball, being made up of two involuntary muscles, the iris and the ciliary muscle. The *iris* is a colored, doughnut-shaped muscle. The open area in the middle of the iris is called the *pupil* (Figs.

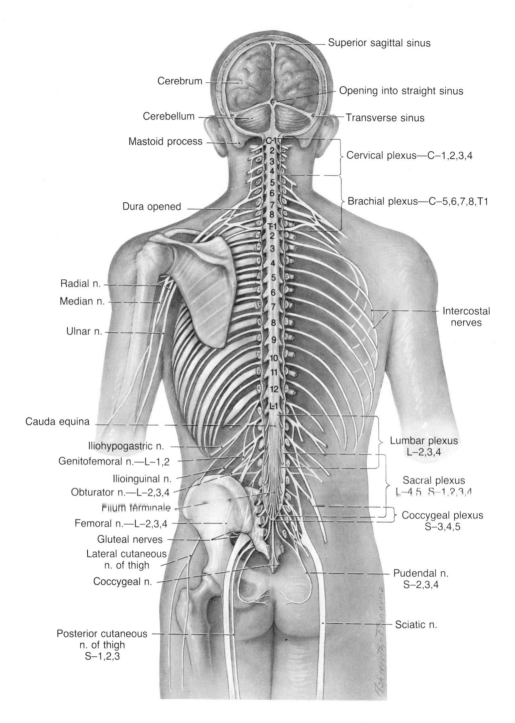

Superior sagittal sinus

Cerebrum

Opening into straight sinus

Cerebellum

Transverse sinus

Mastoid process

Cervical plexus—C–1,2,3,4

Brachial plexus—C–5,6,7,8,T1

Dura opened

Radial n.

Median n.

Intercostal nerves

Ulnar n.

Cauda equina

Iliohypogastric n.

Lumbar plexus L–2,3,4

Genitofemoral n.—L–1,2

Ilioinguinal n.

Sacral plexus L–4,5 S–1,2,3,4

Obturator n.—L–2,3,4

Filum terminale

Coccygeal plexus S–3,4,5

Femoral n.—L–2,3,4

Gluteal nerves

Lateral cutaneous n. of thigh

Pudendal n. S–2,3,4

Coccygeal n.

Sciatic n.

Posterior cutaneous n. of thigh S–1,2,3

Figure 6-24 Spinal cord and nerves emerging from it.

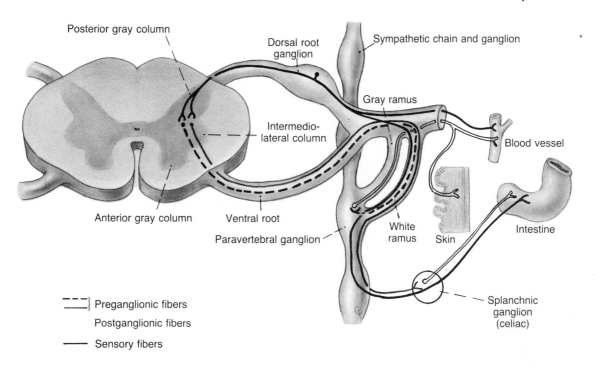

Figure 6-25 Pathways for distribution of sympathetic fibers.

6-31 and 6-32). In normal bright daylight the iris is relaxed, and the pupil opening is small. In dim light the spokelike muscle fibers of the iris contract, widening the pupil opening and thus allowing more light to enter the interior of the eyeball.

The *ciliary muscle* is attached to the *lens* of the eye; both of these structures lie behind the iris and pupil opening. The lens is held in place by a ligament attached to the ciliary muscle. When one focuses on distant objects, the ciliary muscle relaxes, and the curve of the lens is flattened. When one is looking at close objects, as when reading, the ciliary muscle contracts, causing the lens to bulge into a more pronounced curvature. These changes in the curvature of the lens operate to focus light images on the internal surface (retina) of the back of the eyeball.

The interior lining of the eyeball is referred to as the *retina*. The portion of the retina directly across the chamber behind the lens is the only area sensitive to light. This light-sensitive area contains two types of microscopic light receptors, the rods and the cones, which derive their names from their shapes. The *cones* are stimulated by fairly bright light and are of central importance in daylight and in most color vision. The *rods* operate in dim light and are necessary for good night vision. The rods tend to be located away from the point of central focus. This is demonstrated by the fact that if one looks slightly away from a dimly lit object or a dim light source (such as a star at night), the object is seen more clearly. Figures 6-33 to 6-35 show some common abnormalities in vision and how they are corrected.

What Does the Ear Look Like? How Does It Work?

The ear consists of three portions: an external, a middle, and an inner ear. The external ear has two parts, the ear flap (auricle or pinna) and the ear canal (external acoustic meatus). The ear flap functions to collect sounds, which then travel along the ear canal to the eardrum (Figs. 6-36 and 6-37).

The *middle ear* (tympanic cavity) is a tiny hollow in the temporal bone. The tympanic membrane, or

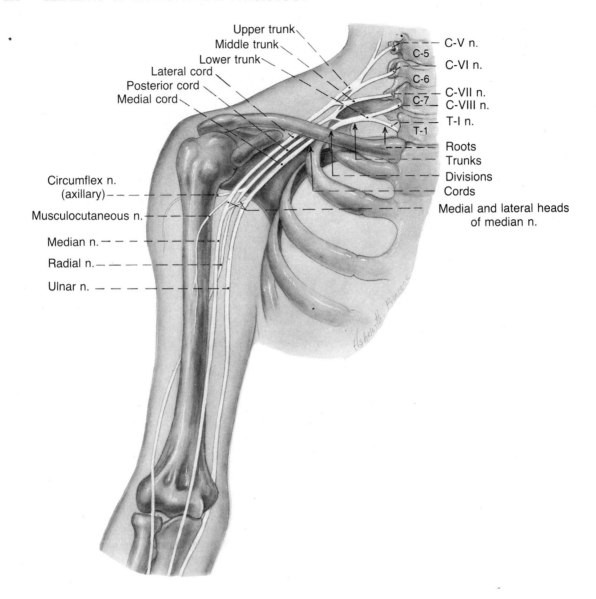

Upper trunk
Middle trunk
Lower trunk
Lateral cord
Posterior cord
Medial cord

C-V n.
C-5
C-VI n.
C-6
C-VII n.
C-7
C-VIII n.
T-I n.
T-1
Roots
Trunks
Divisions
Cords
Medial and lateral heads
of median n.

Circumflex n.
(axillary)

Musculocutaneous n.

Median n.

Radial n.

Ulnar n.

Figure 6–26 Brachial plexus and its skeletal relations.

eardrum, separates the middle ear from the external ear canal. Within the middle ear cavity are three very small bones: the malleus (hammer), the incus (anvil), and the stapes (stirrup). The malleus (mal'-e-us) is attached to the eardrum and to the incus. In sequence, the other end of the incus is connected to one end of the stapes, and the stapes then terminates at the oval window (the opening to the inner ear). Sound vibrations striking the eardrum are

translated to the inner ear by the mechanical movement of the three small bones of the middle ear.

The middle ear cavity has multiple openings: the opening covered by the tympanic membrane; the auditory, or eustachian, tube (connecting with the throat); the openings into the mastoid cavity (sinuses); and the openings into the inner ear. The eustachian tube is frequently the pathway for the spread of infections, which may begin with a sore

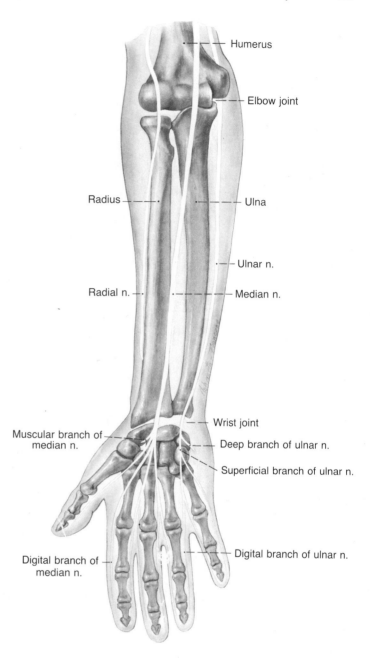

Humerus

Elbow joint

Radius

Ulna

Ulnar n.

Radial n.

Median n.

Wrist joint

Muscular branch of median n.

Deep branch of ulnar n.

Superficial branch of ulnar n.

Digital branch of median n.

Digital branch of ulnar n.

Figure 6–27 Nerves of right forearm and hand (palmar view).

throat and lead to middle ear infection (otitis media) or infection of the mastoid spaces (mastoiditis).

The *inner ear* consists of bony and membranous labyrinths. The bony labyrinth, composed of a series of canals hollowed out of the temporal bone, is filled with a fluid called perilymph. The membranous labyrinth lies within the bony labyrinth and is filled with a fluid called endolymph. Each labyrinth has three parts: the *vestibule* and *semicircular canals*, which contain the sensory receptors for balance, and the *cochlea* (kok'le-ah) (like a snail shell), which contains the sensory receptors for hearing. The portion of the cochlea that contains the hearing receptors is referred to as the organ of Corti.

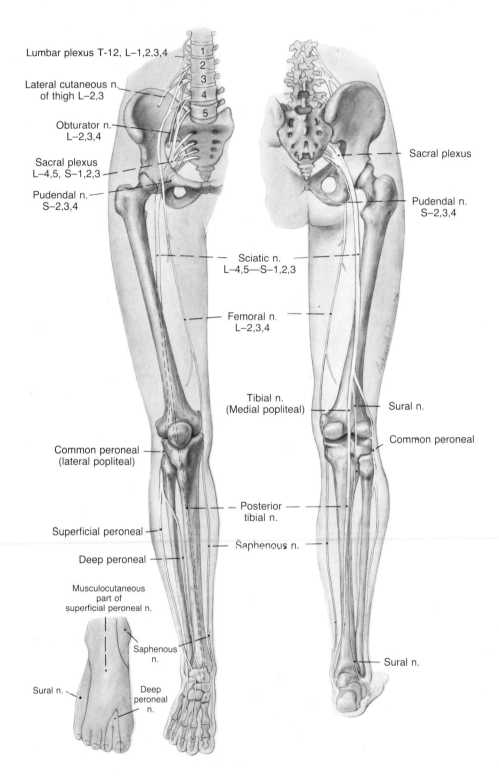

Figure 6-28 Anterior and posterior views of the right leg and foot, showing lumbar and sacral plexuses and the regions supplied. Inset shows areas of the foot supplied by the nerves.

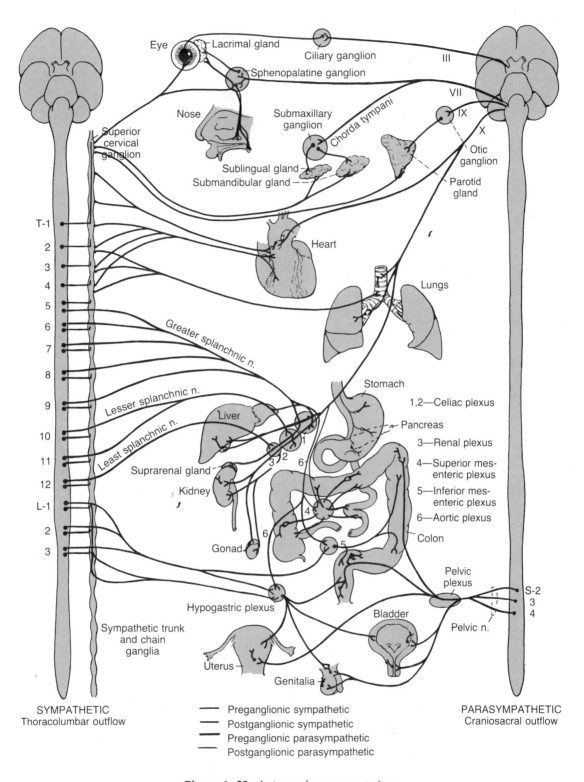

Figure 6–29 Autonomic nervous system.

Table 6-2   FUNCTIONS OF THE AUTONOMIC NERVOUS SYSTEM

ORGAN	SYMPATHETIC STIMULATION	PARASYMPATHETIC STIMULATION
Eye		
Iris	Accommodates for far vision	Accommodates for near vision
Ciliary muscle	Dilates pupil	Constricts pupil
	Lens flattens (inhibits)	Lens bulges (stimulates)
Glands		
Lacrimal	Vasoconstriction	Stimulation of secretion high in enzyme content
Sweat	Copious sweating	Secretion of tears
Heart		
Sinoatrial node	Increases rate	Decreases rate
Muscle	Increases force of contraction	
Lungs		
Bronchi	Dilation	Constriction
Stomach		
Sphincter	Contraction	Inhibition
Glands	Inhibition	Secretion
Intestine		
Wall	Inhibition	Increases tone of musculature
Anal sphincter	Contraction	Decreases tone of musculature
Pancreas	Diminishes enzyme secretion	Stimulates secretion of pancreatic enzymes
Suprarenal gland		
Medulla	Secretion	No known effect
Kidney	Decreases output	No known effect
Urinary bladder		
Detrusor	Inhibition	Excitation
Trigone (sphincter)	Excitation	Inhibition
Penis	Ejaculation	Erection
Arterioles in abdomen and skin	Constriction	
Arrector muscles of hair follicles	Contraction	

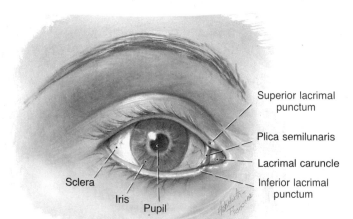

Superior lacrimal punctum

Plica semilunaris

Lacrimal caruncle

Inferior lacrimal punctum

Sclera

Iris

Pupil

Figure 6-30 External appearance of the eye and surrounding structures.

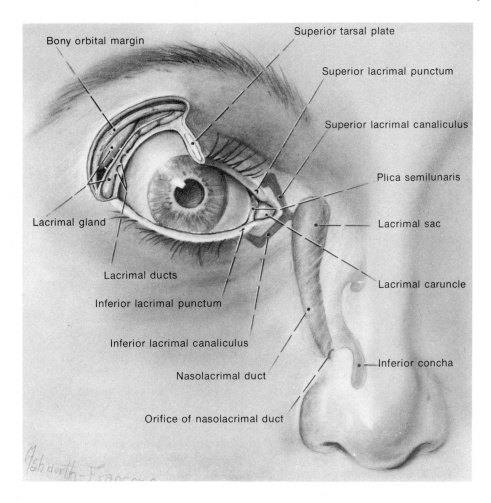

Bony orbital margin

Superior tarsal plate

Superior lacrimal punctum

Superior lacrimal canaliculus

Plica semilunaris

Lacrimal gland

Lacrimal sac

Lacrimal ducts

Lacrimal caruncle

Inferior lacrimal punctum

Inferior lacrimal canaliculus

Inferior concha

Nasolacrimal duct

Orifice of nasolacrimal duct

Figure 6–31 Lacrimal apparatus in relation to the eye.

Summary When sound is produced, the atmosphere is disturbed by sound waves radiating from the source. As sound waves impinge on the eardrum, the membrane vibrates at the same frequency as the source creating the sound. Sound vibrations are carried from the tympanic membrane by the small bones of the middle ear to the inner ear to be transformed into nerve impulses.

THE SENSE OF SMELL

How Does the Sense of Smell Work?

The thousands of receptors for smell are found in an area about 2.5 cm square in the roof of each nasal cavity. These *olfactory receptor cells* are neurons. At the mucosal surface they divide into many fine hairlike cilia (Fig. 6–38). Nowhere else in the body are nerve endings so exposed. The axons from these olfactory neurons pass through the cribriform plate of the ethmoid bone as olfactory nerves to the *olfactory bulb* just above each nasal cavity (Fig. 6–39).

Less is known about the physiology of the sense of smell than about any of the other special senses. In order for a substance to arouse the sensation of smell it must first be volatile so that it can be carried by air currents to the olfactory receptors. That portion of the nasal cavity containing the olfactory receptors is poorly ventilated. The amount of air reaching the region is greatly increased by *sniffing*, thereby increasing the intensity of the odor.

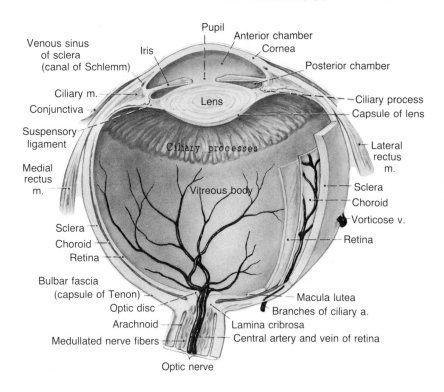

Figure 6–32 Midsagittal section through the eyeball showing layers of retina and blood supply. (After Lederle.)

Humans can distinguish between 2000 and 4000 different odors. And the direction from which the odor comes can often be detected by the difference in arrival time between the two nostrils.

Receptors for smell adapt quickly, so that after about a minute or more of continuous stimulation by a specific odor, the ability to recognize that odor is lost. However, if another odor is immediately smelled, adaptation to the first in no way seems to impair the sensing of the second.

THE SENSE OF TASTE

How Does the Sense of Taste Work?

Like the sense of smell, the sense of taste provides a chemical sensitivity enabling an organism to decide whether something should be ingested or rejected. The specialized structures for the reception of taste are the *taste buds*. Approximately 9000 of these structures are found on the tongue.

Taste buds are onion-shaped receptors containing a tiny pore opening onto the surface of the tongue. They measure 50 to 70 micrometers in diameter and consist of supporting cells and 5 to 18 gustatory receptors, or hair cells. The hairs project into the taste pore. The buds are found in numerous small projections on the tongue, referred to as papillae (pah-pil'e) (Fig. 6–40). The large papillae, located in a V-line on the posterior portion of the tongue, are *vallate papillae*. The *fungiform papillae* are smaller and more numerous and are located chiefly on the tip and sides of the tongue.

Only when a substance is in solution can it stimulate the gustatory hairs. Substances arousing taste sensations are believed to alter in some way the ionic permeability of the hair membranes, thereby evoking a change in the electrical potential of the gustatory cells.

Taste buds show sensitivity to combinations of four primary taste sensations: sweet, salty, sour, and bitter. Their distribution on the tongue gives rise to maximum sensitivity to sweet taste at the tip, salty taste at the tip and sides, sourness at the sides, and bitterness at the back (Fig. 6–41).

Acids taste sour, the sourness being generally

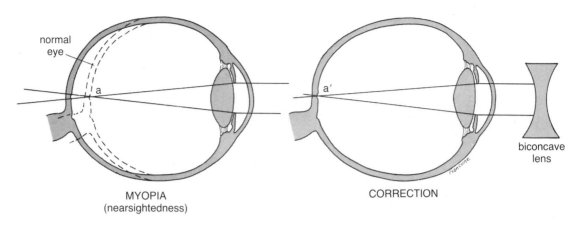

MYOPIA
(nearsightedness)

CORRECTION

Figure 6-33 Myopia, or nearsightedness; note how the image focuses in front of the retina. A biconcave lens is used as a corrective device for this condition—*a* indicates incorrect point of focus; *a'* indicates focus after correction.

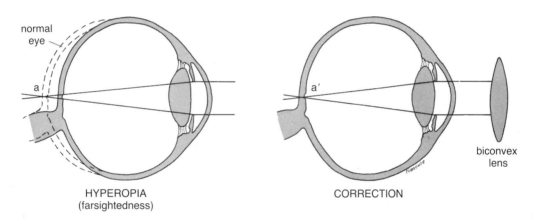

HYPEROPIA
(farsightedness)

CORRECTION

Figure 6-34 Hyperopia, or farsightedness; note how the image focuses behind the retina. A biconvex lens is used as a corrective device for this condition—*a* indicates incorrect point of focus; *a'* indicates focus after correction.

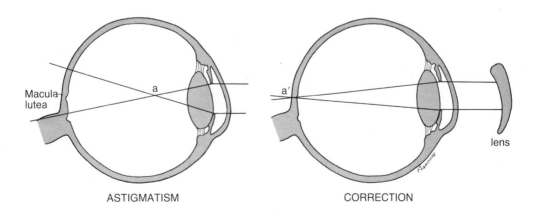

ASTIGMATISM

CORRECTION

Figure 6-35 Astigmatism: uneven focusing of the image resulting from distortion of the curvature of the lens or cornea—*a* indicates incorrect point of focus; *a'* indicates focus after correction.

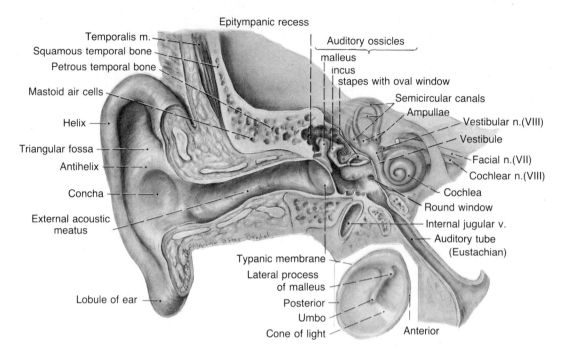

Figure 6-36   Frontal section through the outer, middle, and internal ear.

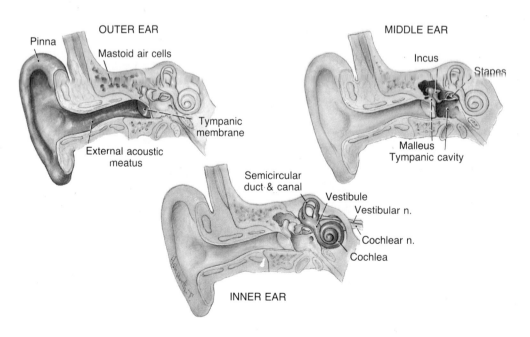

Figure 6-37   Three divisions of the ear.

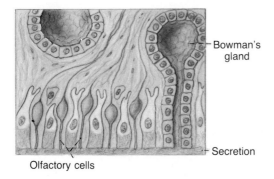

Figure 6-38 Olfactory epithelium showing supporting cells and olfactory cells.

proportional to the hydrogen ion concentration. Sweet substances are usually organic and include sugars and alcohols. Bitter-tasting substances are frequently organic also and include chemicals classified as alkaloids, such as quinine, caffeine, and nicotine.

Flavor is the result of a variety of tastes synthesized from the four basic taste components. Many substances are identified by combinations of gustatory and olfactory sensations aided by touch, pressure, temperature, and pain sensations.

CLINICAL CONSIDERATIONS

What Are the Results of Injury to the Spinal Cord?

The spinal cord either may be partially injured (as by blunt trauma) or may be severed completely (cut through). *Partial injuries* produce weakness, abnormal sensations, and decreased ability to sense pain and temperature. If the spinal cord is *severed completely*, communication between the higher centers and the sensory and motor neurons is lost

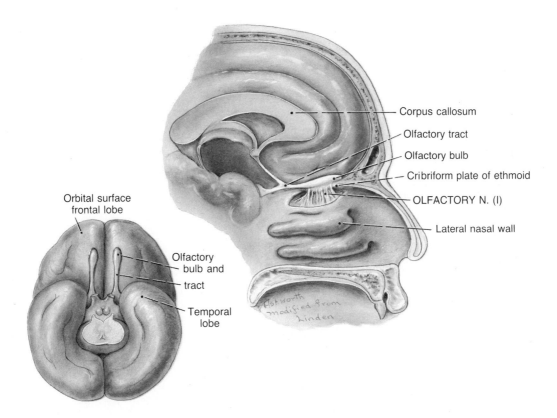

Figure 6-39 Olfactory nerve (I).

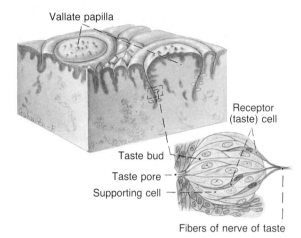

Figure 6-40 Taste bud and section from tongue showing where it is found.

below the point of transection. This results in a total loss of sensation and a loss of conscious motor control (paralysis) below the point of transection.

What Is Multiple Sclerosis?

Multiple sclerosis (skle-ro'sis) is a disease of the central nervous system that is characterized by a patchy demyelinization (loss of the myelin covering) in many (multiple) areas, resulting in a variety of symptoms involving both sensory and motor systems. These symptoms include virtually all the dysfunctions (abnormal functionings) of the nervous system. Multiple sclerosis is a chronic disease, and the symptoms will sometimes disappear for months or years at a time.

What Is Hydrocephalus?

Hydrocephalus, or "water on the brain," is a condition that occurs when blockage of circulation of cerebrospinal fluid increases the pressure on the brain and spinal cord. The signs and symptoms of hydrocephalus may be evident at the time of birth. The head enlarges, and the veins of the scalp dilate and become prominent (Fig. 6-42).

Surgical treatment consists of diverting the cerebrospinal fluid from one compartment into another in the normal fluid pathways, or from the cerebrospinal fluid compartments to some other area of the body, where it can be absorbed. One diverting technique is described in Figure 6-43.

What Is Meningitis?

Meningitis (men"in-ji'tis) is an infection of the meninges. The diagnosis depends on the history of the infection, the so-called meningeal signs (such as stiffness of the neck), and any abnormalities of the spinal fluid. In the small infants, manifestations of mild meningitis are sometimes masked for days, with the symptoms suggesting a cold (upper respiratory infection).

What Are Convulsive Seizures?

Convulsive disorders are more commonly known as *epilepsy.* An attack characterized by only momentary suspension of consciousness is called *petit mal* (French for "little illness"). An attack in which immediate loss of consciousness and a violent generalized convulsion occur is called *grand mal.*

What Is a Concussion?

Concussion is defined as a temporary loss of consciousness or paralysis of nervous function as a

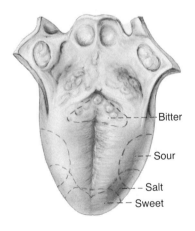

Figure 6-41 Taste areas of the tongue.

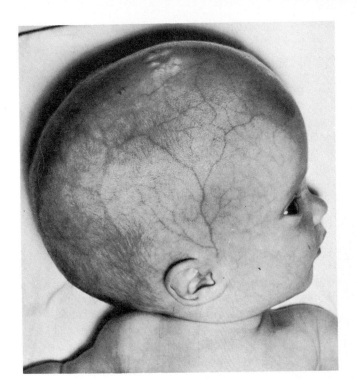

Figure 6–42 Child, age 4 months, with hydrocephalus.

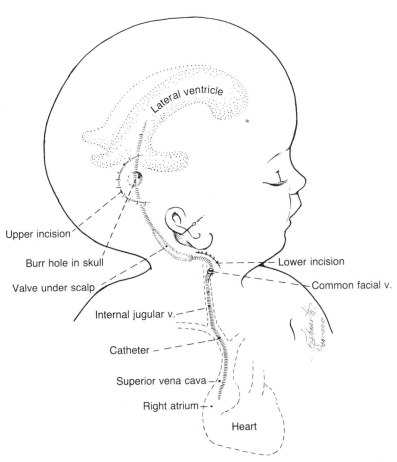

Upper incision

Burr hole in skull

Valve under scalp

Internal jugular v.

Catheter

Superior vena cava

Right atrium

Heart

Lateral ventricle

Lower incision

Common facial v.

Figure 6–43 Operative procedure for hydrocephalus in which a catheter drains the ventricular system into the right atrium.

137

result of a violent blow or shock. Even when consciousness is not lost, in a few days symptoms may arise including headache, dizziness, loss of self-confidence, nervousness, fatigue, inability to sleep, and depression. No account has been given of the mechanism of these symptoms.

Other symptoms may occur that are an indication of some process in addition to concussion. Symptoms include delayed traumatic collapse, epilepsy, coma, or acute drowsiness, confusion, or headaches. The basis of such symptoms can vary, ranging from contusion (a bruising) to laceration (a tearing wound), to subdural hemorrhage (bleeding beneath the dura).

Interestingly, many patients who suffer actual skull fractures do not have serious or prolonged disorders of cerebral function. On the other hand, autopsy in fatal head injuries may reveal an intact skull in 20 to 30 per cent of cases.

What Is Parkinson's Disease?

Parkinson's disease is characterized by involuntary tremors (shaking), decreased strength in movement, and rigidity; intellectual capabilities are not affected. Because of the characteristic shaking or tremors, it is commonly referred to as "shaking palsy."

What Is a Stroke?

Strokes, more formally referred to as cerebral vascular accidents, are specific disorders caused by a disease process in a blood vessel in the brain, most commonly either a blood clot or hemorrhage. In most cases the onset is abrupt and the development rapid, and symptoms reach a peak within seconds, minutes, or hours.

The specific symptoms of the resulting disorders vary depending on the part of the brain affected. Symptoms may be few and relatively unimportant or numerous and eventually fatal. Frequently, symptoms include paralysis, difficulty in speaking, and inability to write. Partial or complete recovery may occur over a period of hours to months.

SUMMARY

A. The nervous system, along with the endocrine system, controls and coordinates the component parts of the body.
   1. A vast network of nerves carries signals into and out of the central nervous system.
   2. The brain and spinal cord process incoming signals and produce outgoing signals.
   3. The higher centers of the brain are responsible for conscious thought and activities.
B. The nervous system is composed of neurons and glial cells.
   1. Glial cells support, repair, and nourish the neurons.
   2. Neurons conduct and process electrical impulses from one part of the body to another.
C. Neurons are composed of axon fibers, dendrite fibers, and the main cell body.
   1. The long axon and dendrite fibers are referred to as nerves.
   2. Axons conduct impulses away from, and dendrites toward, the main cell body.
   3. The main cell body functions to change the nature and direction of signals passing through it.
D. Nerves are normally insulated with a nonconducting material called myelin.
   1. The myelin covering is made up of Schwann cells.
   2. The Schwann cells wind around the nerve fibers.
   3. The main neuron bodies are never covered with myelin.
   4. Myelin-covered nerves appear white (white matter); uncovered main neuron bodies appear gray (gray matter).
E. There are three classes of neurons based on their functions.
   1. Sensory neurons bring messages into the central nervous system.
   2. Motor neurons carry messages out of the central nervous system.
   3. Interneurons transmit messages between sensory and motor neurons, always within the central nervous system.
F. A reflex arc is a complete two-way communication unit.
   1. The arc must be made of at least two

neurons, one sensory and one motor, and also typically an interneuron.

2. Reflex arcs control only the simplest or most primitive and automatic behaviors.

G. Neurons transmit signals by an electrochemical process.
1. The process begins with stimulation of the end of the dendrite.
2. A rapid in and out exchange of sodium and potassium ions, called depolarization, occurs at the point of stimulation.
3. Depolarization spreads to adjacent areas, creating an electrical wave that sweeps along the length of the neuron.
4. The nerve cannot be restimulated for a small fraction of a second until the fiber repolarizes.
5. Transmission is more rapid in larger nerves.

H. Neuron-to-neuron transmission occurs across a one-way junction called the neural synapse.
1. When the impulse reaches the end of the axon fiber, a special chemical stored at the tip is released.
2. The chemical travels rapidly across the synapse to stimulate the dendrite of the next cell.

I. At the end of each axon of a motor neuron is a specialized ending called an effector.
1. When the impulse reaches the effector, it releases a special chemical.
2. The special chemical activates or deactivates the part of the body being served.
3. Each motor neuron activates only one part in one way.

J. Sensory receptors at the ends of the dendrites are sensitive to different stimuli, but each is sensitive to only one type.
1. A sensory neuron transmits only when its sensory receptors are stimulated by their characteristic stimulus.
2. A sensory impulse may be stopped by an interneuron.
3. According to the all-or-none principle, neurons either fire completely and transmit or do not fire and do not transmit.

K. The nervous system is structurally divided into the central nervous system (CNS) and the peripheral nervous system.
1. The CNS is composed of the spinal cord and brain.
2. The peripheral nervous system involves all the nerves and nerve centers of the outlying parts of the body.

L. The spinal cord is enclosed in the bony vertebral column.
1. The spinal cord is covered by three protective membranes called the meninges.
   a. The three layers are called the dura mater, the pia mater (covering the cord), and the arachnoid (middle layer).
   b. The middle layer is a network of spaces filled with a cerebrospinal fluid that is much like plasma.
      i. The cerebrospinal fluid also circulates through hollow ventricles inside the brain.
      ii. The cerebral aqueduct connects the spinal cavity to the ventricles.
      iii. The fluid is continually being formed and reabsorbed by an osmotic filtration process.
2. A cross section of the spinal cord shows an inner region of gray matter surrounded by a region of white matter.
   a. The inner, gray matter is composed mainly of neuron cell bodies.
   b. The surrounding white matter is made up of bundles of myelinated axons known as tracts.
3. The activities of the spinal cord are divided into reflex functions and brain communication functions.
   a. Sensory impulses either enter a reflex arc or are switched to travel up the cord to the brain.
   b. The spinal cord reflexes (below the head) are primitive and protective.
   c. Communication between the brain and the lower areas of the body occurs by way of the long axon tracts (both sensory and motor).

M. The brain can be divided into three main functional areas.
1. The hindbrain is composed of the medulla, pons, and cerebellum.
   a. The medulla (oblongata), continuous with the spinal cord, contains reflex centers controlling respiration, heart rate, and blood vessel constriction.
   b. The pons is primarily a relay center and is composed entirely of white matter.

c. The cerebellum, gray matter surrounding white, is located posterior to the pons.
   i. It functions in coordinating movements, posture, balance, and spatial orientation.
   ii. The reticular activating system (RAS) controls wakefulness and ability to direct attention.

2. The midbrain and interbrain are composed of the colliculi, thalamus, and hypothalamus.
   a. The midbrain contains the superior and inferior colliculi and controls visual reflexes.
   b. The thalamus processes sensory stimuli, suppressing some and magnifying others.
   c. The hypothalamus is very important to a variety of functions, including control of the pituitary.

3. The forebrain, or cerebrum, is the largest part of the brain and controls "higher" level functions.
   a. Its two hemispheres, divided by the longitudinal fissure, are connected only at the corpus callosum.
   b. The outer cerebral cortex is gray matter.
   c. The inner cerebral medulla is white matter.
   d. The left hemisphere serves the right side of the body, and the right hemisphere serves the left side. This is known as "cross-over."
   e. The cerebral cortex of each hemisphere is divided into four lobes.
      i. The frontal lobe controls voluntary muscle movements and speech centers.
      ii. The parietal lobe contains the sensory reception area.
      iii. The temporal lobe contains the auditory center.
      iv. The occipital lobe contains the visual center.

N. The electroencephalogram records the electrical activity of the brain.
   1. The rapid beta waves reflect the active waking state.
   2. Alpha waves are associated with the awake but inattentive brain.
   3. Delta waves are the highly rhythmic, slow, large waves common to deep sleep.

O. The peripheral nervous system is divided into the cranial nerves and the spinal nerves.
   1. There are 12 symmetrical pairs of cranial nerves.
      a. Each nerve leaves the skull through a foramen.
      b. The superficial origin is where the nerve fiber leaves the surface of the brain.
      c. The deep origin is the location of the main cell bodies of the neurons.
   2. There are 31 pairs of nerves emerging from the spinal cord.
      a. Each nerve has a dorsal and a ventral root.
         i. The ventral root nerve carries motor signals.
         ii. The dorsal root nerve carries sensory signals.
      b. The main cell bodies of the ventral (motor) root nerves are the gray matter inside the spinal cord.
      c. The dorsal root ganglia (gray matter) are the main cell bodies of the sensory nerves.
      d. Spinal nerves form anterior and posterior branches soon after leaving the spine.
         i. Anterior branches interlace to form plexuses.
         ii. Branches reemerge from the plexuses to innervate the motor effector organs.

P. The autonomic nervous system (ANS) is a specialized subsystem of the overall nervous system.
   1. It generally controls bodily functions considered to be involuntary.
      a. The ANS links control centers of the brain with the internal organs and secretory cells.
      b. The ANS is strictly a motor system; the corresponding sensory systems are not part of the ANS.
   2. Unlike the somatic (voluntary) system, the ANS displays a divided motor signal transmission system.
      a. The motor ganglia are the synaptic junctions.
      b. Preganglionic neurons do not reach the

effectors (as they would in the somatic system).

    c. Postganglionic neuron fibers finally carry the motor signal from the ganglion to the effector.

  3. The ANS functions to maintain homeostasis, particularly temperature and body composition.

  4. The ANS can be further divided into two subsystems with opposing functions.

    a. The sympathetic is the "fight or flight" system, concerned with processes involving energy expenditure.

    b. The parasympathetic system inhibits activity and is concerned with restorative processes.

Q. At the beginnings of the dendrites of the sensory neurons are specialized receptors—microscopic sense organs.

  1. When stimulated, a receptor organ produces an impulse in the sensory neuron.

    a. Some localized receptors respond to special types of external stimuli: vision, hearing, taste, and smell.

    b. Others, more generally distributed, are sensitive to touch, pressure, temperature, and body positions.

  2. Pain arises from free nerve endings, without specialized sense organs. These are the most common and widely distributed nerve endings.

  3. Internal sensations like hunger and thirst are complex and involve a variety of receptors in several organ systems.

R. The functional lining of the eyeball is composed of three partially specialized membrane layers.

  1. The sclera is the tough outer layer of connective tissue.

    a. The "white" of the eye is the frontal sclera.

    b. In the frontal center is the specialized, transparent cornea.

    c. Lying over the cornea is the protective mucous membrane referred to as the conjunctiva.

  2. The choroid layer also consists of two specialized involuntary muscles.

    a. The iris is a colored, doughnut-shaped muscle.

      i. The pupil is the open area in the middle.

      ii. The pupil contracts (small opening) in bright light and relaxes (wide opening) in dim light.

    b. The lens is held in place by a ligament attached to the ciliary muscle (behind the iris/pupil opening).

      i. Focusing on distant objects relaxes the ciliary muscle and flattens the lens.

      ii. Focusing on near objects contracts the ciliary muscle and bulges the lens.

  3. The interior lining of the eyeball is referred to as the retina.

    a. Only the area directly across from the lens is sensitive to light.

    b. The central cones are stimulated by bright light and, in most persons, color.

    c. The rods, located away from the central focus, operate in dim light.

S. The ear consists of three portions: the external, middle, and inner ear.

  1. The external ear is composed of the ear flap and the ear canal and functions to collect sounds.

  2. The middle ear is a tiny hollow in the temporal bone.

    a. The tympanic membrane, or eardrum, separates the middle ear from the external ear canal.

    b. Three bones mechanically translate vibrations of the eardrum to the inner ear.

      i. The malleus (hammer) is attached to the eardrum and the incus (anvil).

      ii. The other end of the incus is connected to one end of the stapes (stirrup).

      iii. The stapes terminates at the oval window.

  3. The inner ear consists of bony and membranous labyrinths.

    a. The bony labyrinths, canals hollowed out of the temporal bone, are filled with perilymph.

    b. The membranous labyrinth lies within the bony labyrinth and is filled with endolymph.

    c. Each labyrinth has three parts: the vestibule, semicircular canals, and cochlea.

i. The vestibule and semicircular canals are the sensory receptors for balance.

ii. The cochlea (like a snail shell) contains the sensory receptors for hearing.

T. The receptors for the sense of smell are located in the roof of each nasal cavity.

1. The olfactory neurons divide into many cilia at the surface.

2. The axons pass through the ethmoid bone to the olfactory bulb.

3. Substances must be volatile to be smelled.

4. Sniffing improves the supply of air to the olfactory cells and increases the intensity of an odor.

5. Humans can distinguish between 2000 and 4000 odors.

U. The taste buds, located on the tongue, are the specialized structures for the reception of taste.

1. Taste buds are onion-shaped receptors with a tiny pore opening to the surface of the tongue.

2. There are about 9000 taste buds on the tongue, which are located on numerous small projections called papillae.

3. Only substances in solution stimulate taste.

4. Taste buds are sensitive to four primary tastes: sweet, salty, sour, and bitter.

V. There are a number of disorders of the nervous system.

1. If the spinal cord is severed, paralysis results below the point of transection.

2. Multiple sclerosis is characterized by patchy demyelinization, resulting in a range of motor and sensory dysfunctions.

3. Hydrocephalus ("water on the brain") results from blockage of circulation of the cerebrospinal fluid.

4. Meningitis is an inflammation of the meninges, usually due to infection.

5. Epilepsy is the general name for convulsive disorders or seizures.

6. Concussion is defined as a temporary loss of consciousness or paralysis of nervous function as a result of a violent blow or shock.

a. A contusion involves a bruising.

b. A laceration involves a tearing wound.

c. A subdural hemorrhage involves bleeding beneath the dura.

7. Parkinson's disease is characterized by involuntary tremors (shaking), decreased strength in movement, and rigidity in the presence of normal intelligence.

8. A stroke, or cerebral vascular accident, is caused by either a blood clot or hemorrhage.

REVIEW QUESTIONS

1. Besides the nervous system, which other bodily system also functions primarily in control and coordination?

2. List the major divisions of the nervous system and the subdivisions of each.

3. What are the main structures of the central nervous system and the peripheral nervous system?

4. The nervous system is made up of neurons and neuroglia. What is the primary function of each? What is myelin?

5. Draw a diagram of a neuron, identifying the cell body, dendrites, and axons. What is the function of each part?

6. What is the basis of the functional classification of the neurons?

7. What is a reflex arc? What are the minimum number of components?

8. Explain the all-or-none principle. Why does nerve conduction occur in only one direction at synapses?

9. Describe the sensory receptor for pain. What is the most prevalent type of dendrite nerve ending?

10. What are the two functions of the spinal cord? Describe the cross section of the spinal cord.

11. Why is the medulla the most vital part of the brain?

12. How does the arrangement of gray matter and white matter in the spinal cord differ from that in the brain?

13. What are the functions of the thalamus and hypothalamus? the cerebellum?

14. Describe the location, structure, and function of the reticular activating system (RAS).

15. What is meant when we say that most cerebral hemisphere pathways are "crossed pathways?"

16. What are the three main types of electrical brain activity recorded by an EEG?

17. List the 12 pairs of cranial nerves and give the principal function of each. Which are purely sensory?

18. Distinguish between the dorsal root and the ventral root of the spinal nerves. How many pairs of spinal nerves are there?

19. What are the main differences in structure and function between the autonomic and somatic nervous systems?

20. What is the functional relationship between the sympathetic and parasympathetic divisions of the autonomic nervous system?

21. Identify the three specialized features of the sclera in the front of the eyeball.

22. Using a diagram, explain how the lens is distorted by the ciliary muscle to produce a focused image (1) of distant objects and (2) of near objects.

23. Explain how the iris and the rods each operate to enhance night vision.

24. How are the sound vibrations of the air transmitted by the outer and middle ear to the inner ear?

25. What are the two types of sensory receptors found in the inner ear? What is the structural location of each?

26. Referring to the anatomy of the nose, explain why sniffing enhances the ability to identify and distinguish odors.

27. Identify the tastes that combine to make up the flavors of a cup of tea with lemon and a doughnut.

28. Define and characterize five common disorders of the nervous system.

S E V E N

The Endocrine System

The aim of this chapter is to enable the student to do the following:

- Explain the difference between endocrine and exocrine glands.

- Locate and describe each endocrine gland.

- Summarize the actions of the hormones secreted by each endocrine gland.

- Explain negative feedback and its role in regulating blood levels of the various hormones.

- Explain how various endocrine glands are stimulated to release their hormonal products.

- Describe the anatomic and physiologic relationship between the hypothalamus and the pituitary.

- Describe the major pathologic consequences of hypersecretion and hyposecretion of the endocrine hormones.

- Explain the physiologic functions of prostaglandins.

THE ENDOCRINE SYSTEM: AN OVERVIEW

What Does the Endocrine System Do?

There are actually two general systems in the body performing the overall functions of *control* and *communication.* The nervous system is responsible for rapid, short-interval control and accomplishes this through the use of fast-traveling nerve impulses. The *endocrine* (en'do-krin) *system*, on the other hand, is responsible for more general and longer-lasting control of bodily states. It accomplishes this by the use of *hormones* (chemical stimulants), which are secreted into and circulated by the blood stream. Nervous system controls act over seconds or fractions of seconds; endocrine system controls act over minutes, hours, and days.

In comparing the two systems, we find that the nervous system is responsible for the moment-to-moment control and coordination of skeletal muscles in the performance of movements, and the glands of the endocrine system secrete the hormones that control growth and stimulate sexual development during puberty. The endocrine glands also secrete hormones that regulate the amount of glucose in the blood and hormones that will excite the whole body, as when one is preparing to fight or flee in some situation.

What Structures Make Up the Endocrine System?

The endocrine system is made up of *eight endocrine glands*. A gland is any organ that produces and secretes special substances. Endocrine glands are those that secrete hormones directly into the blood. Another class of glands, the exocrine, discharge their secretions (usually enzymes) by means of ducts, and are not part of the endocrine system. The glands of the digestive system and the skin are ex-amples of *exocrine glands*. A few glandular organs, such as the pancreas, are made up of both types of glands operating independently. (The term endocrine is from the Greek *endo*, within, + *krine*, to separate or secrete. The term exocrine is similar: *exo*, outside, + *krine*, to secrete).

As can be seen in Figure 7–1, the glands of the endocrine system are located throughout the body. They are considered to make up *one system*, not only because of their similar type of function and similar means of active influence but also because of the many important interrelationships. These interrelationships will become apparent as we proceed.

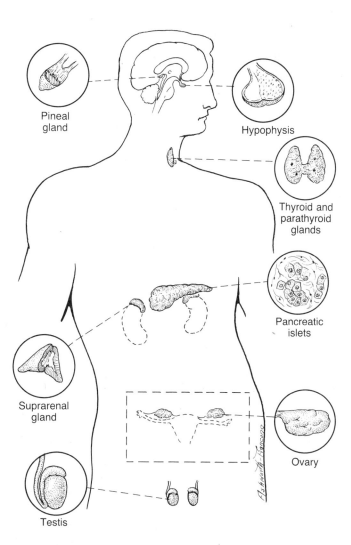

Figure 7–1 Location of eight glands of internal secretion.

Pineal gland

Hypophysis

Thyroid and parathyroid glands

Pancreatic islets

Suprarenal gland

Ovary

Testis

What Is a Hormone?

A *hormone* is a chemical substance (or stimulant) secreted by one part of the body (an endocrine gland) that controls or helps to control a function elsewhere in the body. The term "hormone" is derived from the Greek word *hormaein*, meaning to activate or set in motion.

Hormones pass (are secreted) directly into the blood through the capillaries running through each of the endocrine glands and are taken to other parts of the body through the blood stream.

Some hormones act *generally*, stimulating a specific activity over the whole body. For instance, insulin stimulates the absorption of glucose from the blood by the cells throughout the body. Other hormones directly affect only a *limited* area—these areas are called *target organs* for the hormone. For example, ADH (antidiuretic hormone) causes the renal tubules to increase their rate of water reabsorption. The direct effect of ADH on other tissues in the body is negligible.

An excess or deficiency in the secretion of a particular hormone may result in a specific disease state. For instance, diabetes mellitus is a condition in which insulin secretion is deficient.

THE PITUITARY GLAND

What Is the Pituitary Gland?

The *pituitary* (pi-too'i-tar"e) *gland* is a small, pea-sized organ located below the hypothalamus in the midbrain. Another name for the pituitary is the *hypophysis* (hi-pof'i-sis), from the Greek word meaning an undergrowth—so named because the gland seems to be growing on a stalk underneath the hypothalamus (Fig. 7–2). The pituitary, or hypophysis, is really two distinct and independently operating endocrine glands. The front half of the organ is called the *anterior lobe*, or also the *adenohypophysis*; the back half is called the *posterior lobe*, or the *neurohypophysis* ("neuro-" because it is more directly associated with the nervous tissue of the hypothalamus above).

What Does the Anterior Lobe of the Pituitary Gland Do?

The anterior lobe of the pituitary gland has been found to secrete at least *six hormones* of major importance. Five of these are commonly referred to by their abbreviated names: GH, ACTH, TSH, FSH, and LH. All these letters may seem a little overwhelming at first glance, but notice that each abbreviation ends with an H, and this always stands for hormone. In learning these hormones you should initially take the time to recall, out loud, the full name whenever you encounter the sequence of letters—this practice will help you to learn the full names in a short time.

The anterior lobe (adenohypophysis) has often been called the "master" endocrine gland, or the "leader of the endocrine orchestra," since four of its hormones act on other endocrine glands to control both their growth and rate of secretion. In other words, four hormones from the anterior pituitary have other endocrine glands as their "target organs." These include adrenocorticotropic hormone (ACTH), which acts on the adrenal cortex, and thyroid-stimulating hormone (TSH), which acts on the thyroid gland. Two hormones influence the ovary: follicle-stimulating hormone (FSH), which stimulates growth of the follicles of the ovaries, and luteinizing hormone (LH), which acts on one ovarian follicle each month (the one releasing the ovum) to stimulate its development into the corpus luteum.

ACTH   Adrenocorticotropic (ad-re"-no-kor"te-ko-trop'ik) *hormone* regulates the growth and activity of the cortex (outer portion) of the adrenal glands—the adrenal cortex— as indicated by the name. The suffix *-tropic* comes from the Greek word meaning to help to grow or act. The literal translation of "adrenocorticotropic hormone," then, is "the hormone that helps the adrenal cortex to grow and act." ACTH stimulates the adrenal cortex (itself an endocrine gland, considered below) to grow and secrete cortisol (hydrocortisone) and similar substances.

TSH   Thyroid-stimulating hormone controls the growth of the thyroid gland and the secretion of the thyroid hormones.

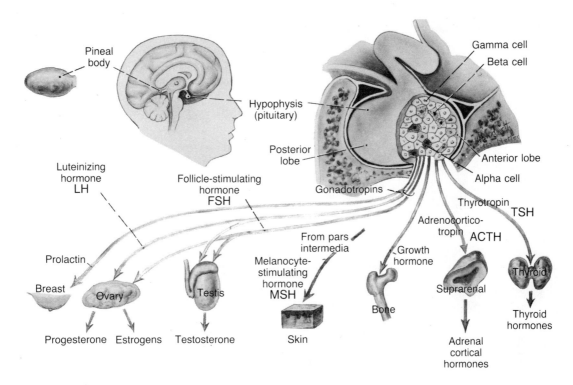

Figure 7-2   The adenohypophysis produces several hormones, some controlling the activity of other endocrine glands (thyroid, adrenal cortex, and gonads).

FSH and LH   *Follicle-stimulating hormone* and *luteinizing hormone* are called *gonadotropic* (gon"ad-do-trop'ik) hormones, since they control the development and level of activity of the ovaries (female gonads) in the female and the testes (male gonads) in the male. FSH in the female stimulates the growth of the graafian follicles to the point of maturity each month, until one ruptures and releases its ovum. FSH also stimulates the ovarian follicle cells to produce and secrete the female sex hormones, the estrogens and progesterone. In the male, FSH influences the development of spermatozoa.

Luteinizing hormone in the female also stimulates the growth process of the follicles. At the point of maturity, there is an additional sudden increase in LH secretion from the anterior pituitary, which causes *ovulation* (rupture of the follicle and release of the mature ovum). After ovulation, LH influences the ruptured follicle to develop into the *corpus luteum*. This latter process is called *luteinization* (loo"te-in"i-za'shun) and is the function that earned LH its name, luteinizing hormone. In the

male, LH stimulates the testes to produce the basic male sex hormone, *testosterone* (tes-tos'te-ron).

GH and Prolactin   The two hormones secreted by the anterior lobe of the pituitary gland that do not work directly on other endocrine glands are growth hormone (GH) and prolactin, or lactogenic hormone.

The mechanisms by which *growth hormone* (also referred to as *somatotropin*, abbreviated STH) accelerates growth are incompletely understood. Generally speaking, it alters the metabolism of cells, influencing them toward increased reproduction. One key discovery, however, is that GH promotes the movement of amino acids (protein building blocks) into the cells. This action seems to stimulate the cells to increase production of proteins—a major step in the reproductive and growth sequences. GH is also known to affect carbohydrate and fat metabolism, increasing the use of fat and decreasing the cellular uptake of glucose. Underproduction of growth hormone in adult life leads to

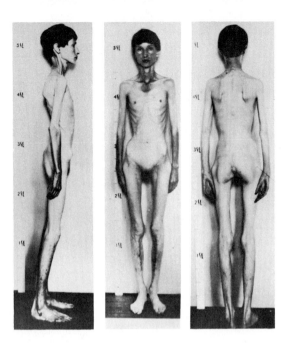

Figure 7–3 Simmonds' disease. (Courtesy of Escamilla and Lisser: California & West Med 48:343, 1938.)

Simmonds' disease (Fig. 7–3). Overproduction of growth hormone in adolescence leads to gigantism and, in adult life, to acromegaly (Fig. 7–4).

Prolactin promotes the growth of breast tissue during pregnancy, and operates in the maintenance of *lactation* (milk production) after the birth of the child. More specifically, the suckling reflex stimulates the secretion of prolactin, and prolactin, in turn, stimulates the production of more milk. Prolactin's other name, *lactogenic* hormone, means milk-producing hormone (*lact-* is Latin for milk; *-genic* means to make).

What Does the Posterior Lobe of the Pituitary Gland Do?

The posterior lobe of the pituitary gland does not really function alone as an endocrine gland but operates in close association with the hypothalamus. The two hormones they release — oxytocin (ok"se-to'sin) and antidiuretic hormone (ADH) — are actually produced and secreted by neurons in the hypothalamus. The posterior pituitary serves as a reservoir for these hormones until their eventual release. The hormones are released into the blood in response to nerve impulses from the hypothalamus.

Oxytocin This hormone stimulates the uterus to contract at the time of childbirth and stimulates the *release* of breast milk from the mammary glands into the ducts for suckling. Oxytocin (from the Greek *oxys*, swift, + *tokos*, childbirth) acts on the smooth muscle of the pregnant uterus to maintain labor and to decrease hemorrhage after delivery (by forcing stronger uterine contraction). Another function of oxytocin is to influence the glandular cells of the lactating breast to release the formed milk into the ducts. Suckling by the infant, in turn, stimulates additional secretion of oxytocin.

ADH *Antidiuretic hormone* stimulates cells in the kidney to draw (or reabsorb) water out of the forming urine and to replace it into the blood stream. The effect is to decrease the amount of water loss from the body into the urine. When the body has very low levels of water (dehydration), ADH stimulates the body to retain water by preventing further loss of water in urine formation. When there is an excess of body water, ADH secretion drops to almost nothing, and as a result urine (water) output greatly increases until a proper water balance in the body is reached. Then ADH secretion returns to a level that stimulates normal production of urine. The term "diuretic" comes from the Greek words *dia*, meaning intensive, and *uresis*, meaning urination. So "diuretic" refers to intensive urination and "antidiuretic" refers to nonintensive or low production of urine. *Antidiuretic hormone, then, is the hormone that decreases the rate of formation of urine in order to save water.*

Diabetes Insipidus Diabetes insipidus is a disease caused by an abnormal decrease in the production of ADH. The result is excessive output of urine — up to 20 liters a day. The term "diabetes" comes from the Greek word for siphon. It is intended to indicate excessive urination. The term "insipidus" is Latin and means "tasteless," which distinguishes diabetes insipidus from diabetes mellitus, in which the urine tastes sweet, since it contains glucose (a sugar). Diabetes mellitus is a disorder in which insulin production by the pancreas is impaired; it will be discussed later in the chapter. Although both types of diabetes have the common symptom of excessive urination, the underlying disorders are quite different.

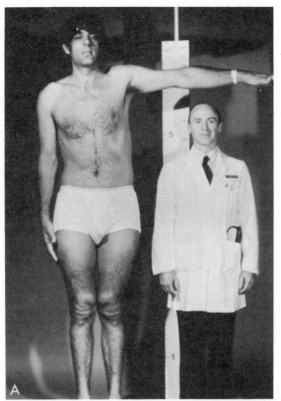

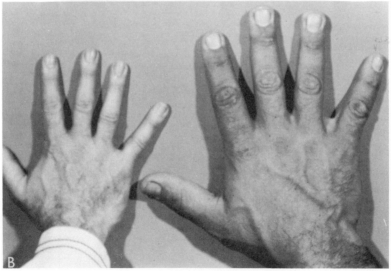

Figure 7–4 Gigantism with acromegaly in a male aged 28. *A*, Height approximately 7 feet, 6 inches. *B*, Hand of same individual as compared with normal-sized hand.

THE THYROID GLAND

What Does the Thyroid Gland Do?

The thyroid gland is located in the neck, in front of the trachea, with its major portion lying on either side of the trachea (windpipe) (Fig. 7–5). The thyroid gland produces and secretes two hormones, *thyroid hormone*, also called *thyroxin*, and *calcitonin*, also called *thyrocalcitonin.*

The growth and level of activity (secretion) of thyroid hormone is controlled by the anterior pituitary gland secretion of thyroid-stimulating hormone (TSH).

Thyroid hormone (thyroxin) stimulates all the cells of the body to be more active. It has been called the "metabolism-activating hormone." When secretion of thyroid hormone increases, the entire energy metabolism (and consequently all cellular activity) of the body speeds up. When thyroid hormone secretion decreases, all cellular (and therefore bodily) activity slows down. In abnormal thyroid conditions, excessive secretion of thyroid hormone can cause the patient to be nervous, jumpy, and *hyperactive. Exophthalmos* (ek"sof-thal'mos) (Fig. 7–6) is indicative of hyperthyroidism. If an abnormally low amount of thyroid hormone is secreted, the person tends to slow down considerably and to have little energy; in adults, this is referred to as *myxedema* (mik-se-de'mah) (Fig. 7–7).

One of the chemicals necessary for production of thyroid hormone is *iodine.* If iodine intake is too low, the thyroid gland enlarges in an attempt to prevent any further loss of iodine from the body. This is one cause of *goiter,* an enlargement of the thyroid gland that causes the front of the neck to have a puffy appearance. The term "goiter" is from the Latin word for throat.

Calcitonin (kal"si-to'-nin) is a hormone that is associated with the thyroid gland. There is some question, however, as to whether it is actually produced by thyroid gland cells, and its secretion does

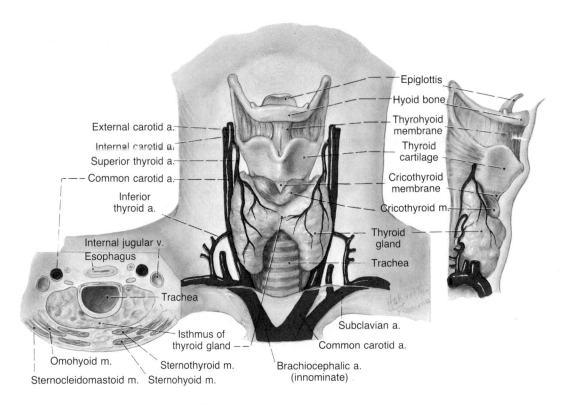

Figure 7–5 Thyroid gland: its blood supply and relations to trachea, in cross section, anterior, and right lateral views.

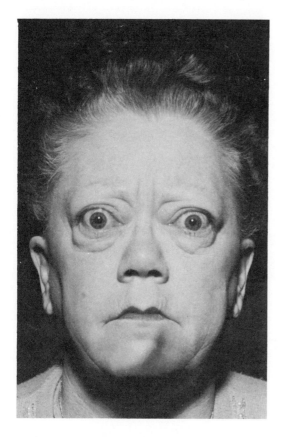

Figure 7-6 Exophthalmos. Note startled appearance and loss of eyebrows.

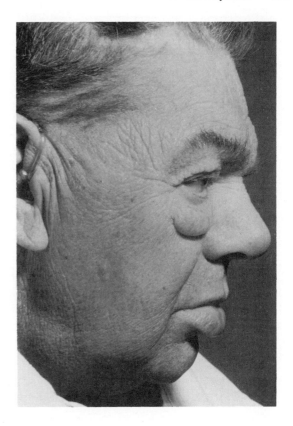

Figure 7-7 Myxedema. Note thick lips, baggy eyes, loss of hair, and dry skin.

not seem to be controlled by TSH. Calcitonin is secreted when the calcium level in the blood gets too high. Somehow, calcitonin works to decrease, and bring back toward normal, the concentration of calcium in the blood. It has an effect opposite to that of parathyroid hormone from the parathyroid gland.

THE PARATHYROID GLANDS

What Do the Parathyroid Glands Do?

There are four small parathyroid glands, and they are located on the back side of the thyroid gland (Fig. 7-8). They secrete only one hormone, which is called *parathyroid hormone*, or *parathormone* for short.

Parathyroid hormone is secreted when the calcium concentration in the blood becomes too low. It has the effect of increasing the blood calcium concentration by promoting the reabsorption of solid calcium deposits from the bones into the blood. Calcitonin has the opposite effect of promoting deposition.

Parathyroid hormone has also been shown to stimulate the uptake (absorption) of ingested calcium from the intestines into the blood. Absorption of calcium from the intestines is even more immediately dependent on the presence of vitamin D.

Parathyroid gland disorders can be very serious, since nerve and muscle cells are extremely sensitive to the concentration of calcium in the blood. With too much calcium in the blood—from excessive secretion of parathormone—brain and heart

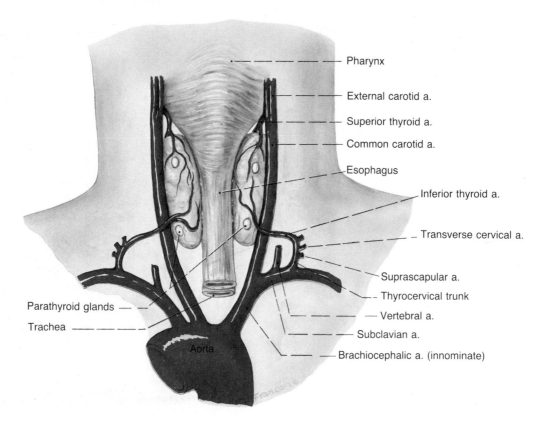

Pharynx

External carotid a.

Superior thyroid a.

Common carotid a.

Esophagus

Inferior thyroid a.

Transverse cervical a.

Suprascapular a.

Thyrocervical trunk

Vertebral a.

Subclavian a.

Brachiocephalic a. (innominate)

Parathyroid glands

Trachea

Aorta

Figure 7–8   Posterior view of the neck and thyroid gland, showing the approximate location of the parathyroid glands.

cell activity becomes *depressed*, and a person will become less responsive; and eventually the heart will stop. With too little calcium—from too little parathormone secretion—the nerve and muscle cells become *hypersensitive*, or overresponsive, resulting in severe jerkiness, muscle spasms, and cramps. This condition is known as *tetany* (tet'ah-ne). The term "tetany" derives from the Greek word meaning convulsive tension.

THE ADRENAL GLANDS

There are two *adrenal glands*, one above each kidney (Fig. 7–9). They have another name, *suprarenal* (literally, above + kidney) glands. Each adrenal gland has a cortex, or outer portion, and a medulla, or inner portion. The cortex and medulla of each adrenal gland are actually different in both embryonic origin and function. They are in reality two separate and distinct glands. Does this two-glands-in-one arrangement remind you of another endocrine gland?

What Does the Adrenal Cortex Do?

The *adrenal cortex* secretes three general types of substances: *mineralocorticoids*, represented principally by *aldosterone*; *glucocorticoids*, represented chiefly by *cortisol* (also called hydrocortisone); and *androgens*, represented by *testosterone*.

The *mineralocorticoids* (min"er-al-o-kor'ti-koids) help to control the amounts of several *mineral salts* in the bodily fluids. Aldosterone is the most active mineralocorticoid. It stimulates the kidney to retain (or reabsorb from the forming urine) sodium. It also has the opposite effect for potassium. A de-

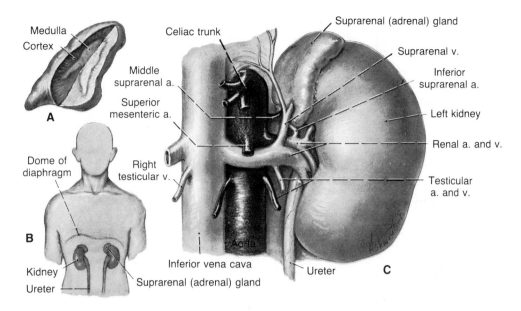

Figure 7–9 *A*, Suprarenal gland sectioned to show the medulla. *B*, Anatomic position of kidneys and suprarenal glands. *C*, Anterior aspect of left kidney, showing adrenal gland and vascular supply.

crease in normal aldosterone secretion has the reverse effect of increasing sodium loss and retaining potassium.

The *glucocorticoids* (gloo″ko-kor′ti-koids), chiefly the hormone *cortisol*, have an effect similar to that of thyroid hormone, that is, they stimulate the energy metabolism of the body. Normal amounts of the glucocorticoids are necessary for normal cellular metabolism. Equally important is the role of increased glucocorticoid secretion during periods of *stress*. During such periods, cortisol secretion leads to a breakdown of proteins into amino acids. These amino acids then circulate through the blood to the liver, where they undergo *gluconeogenesis* (gloo″ko-ne″o-jen′e-sis) — the process of making new glucose out of amino acids. This results in an immediate new supply of glucose to the blood for the quick energy needed to cope with stressful situations.

Surgery, hemorrhage, infections, severe burns, and intense emotions are examples of extreme stimuli that produce stress. Glucocorticoids are sometimes called the stress hormones. Persons with poorly functioning adrenal cortexes have a lower survival rate through periods of stress.

Androgens produce masculinization. The most important androgen is testosterone, which is secreted primarily by the testes. Adrenal androgens are of minor importance, except when an adrenal tumor develops, in which case excessive quantities of androgenic hormones are produced. This can cause a child or even an adult female to take on an adult, masculine (male) appearance, including growth of the clitoris to resemble a penis, growth of a beard, a change in the voice quality to bass, and increased muscular development.

What Does the Adrenal Medulla Do?

The adrenal medulla produces and secretes *epinephrine* (ep″i-nef′rin) (also known as adrenaline) and *norepinephrine* (also known as noradrenaline), with constant proportions of each for every species. The human adrenal medulla secretes ten times as much epinephrine as norepinephrine.

The adrenal medulla functions in conjunction with the sympathetic nervous system (part of the autonomic nervous system). The medullary hormones are released in response to sympathetic nervous system stimulation, which typically occurs in situations in which a person is prepared to fight or flee. Epinephrine operates to supercharge the body very quickly. It increases heart rate, blood pressure, and blood glucose levels. In times of stress and excitement the adrenal medulla will quickly infuse (literally squirt) large amounts of epinephrine into the blood.

THE PANCREAS

What Do the Pancreatic Islets Do?

The *pancreatic* (pan"kre-at'ik) *islets* are small clumps of specialized cells scattered throughout the pancreas (Fig. 7–10). The term "islet" (i'let) means little island. These islets were discovered by a German pathologist, Paul Langerhans, and are sometimes referred to as the *islets of Langerhans.* They operate independently of the exocrine portion of the pancreas, which secretes digestive juices via a duct into the duodenum during digestion.

The pancreatic islets contain two types of cells: beta cells, which produce and secrete *insulin,* and alpha cells, which produce and secrete *glucagon.*

Insulin regulates the cellular uptake of glucose from the blood, and as a consequence serves to regulate the concentration or amount of glucose present in the blood. Insulin is secreted most heavily after a meal, when glucose is being absorbed from the small intestine into the blood. This stimulates the cells to take up the glucose from the blood and ensures that an excessive buildup of glucose in the blood does not occur. Insulin secretion decreases when the concentration of glucose in the blood decreases (between meals). In *diabetes mellitus,* the beta cells of the pancreatic islets do not secrete enough insulin (or none at all), and as a result the blood glucose level rises dangerously; this leads to mental confusion, coma, and eventually death (Fig. 7–11). The kidneys attempt to rid the blood of the excess glucose by producing large amounts of urine.

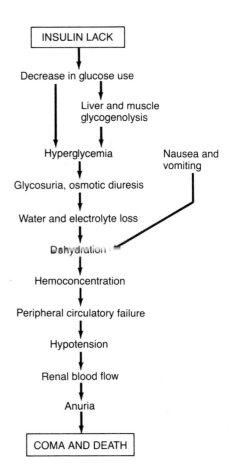

Figure 7–11 Progressive symptoms resulting from lack of insulin. (From Tepperman: *Metabolic and Endocrine Physiology.* Chicago, Year Book Medical Publishers, 1962.)

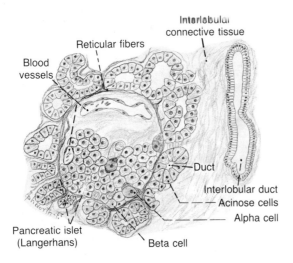

Figure 7–10 Microscopic section of pancreas showing a pancreatic islet (of Langerhans).

Prostaglandins

Prostaglandins are short-lived, hormonelike chemicals produced in the cells of many tissues. Because they exert their effects at or near the sites of synthesis they have also been characterized as "local hormones." They are like hormones in that they are chemical effectors. But they are unlike hormones in that they are produced by a wide range of cells in different types of tissues. The discovery of prostaglandins clearly extends our understanding of the chemical communication/action system of the body, complementary to the more obvious nervous system designed to transmit electrical impulses.

Although prostaglandins were first detected in 1930 as a component of secretions from the male prostate gland (whence the name prostaglandins), recent research has established them as powerful, short-range actors operating throughout the body. Derived from essential fatty acids, the precursor molecules are attached to the cell membranes. In at least some instances a local stimulus leads the cell to release these precursors. Extracellular enzymes convert them into the active prostaglandin form.

Among the local effects observed by scientists so far are lowering of blood pressure, decreasing gastric acid secretions, stimulation of intestinal smooth muscles, uterine stimulation, increasing salt and water clearance by the kidneys, regulating the secretion of certain hormones, modulating synaptic transmission by norepinephrine, and regulating the aggregation of platelets.

There are at least 16 known prostaglandins (PGs), often abbreviated PGE, PGF, PGA, and PGB, with numerical subscripts according to structure. The principal precursor for the synthesis of prostaglandins is arachidonic acid, a polyunsaturated fatty acid that is formed from linoleic acid. It has been suggested that some of the consequences of essential fatty acid deficiency may be due in part to the inability to synthesize prostaglandins.

Because prostaglandins are short acting it is not surprising that the same individual types of prostaglandins have been observed to produce very different effects in different tissues.

The discovery of the prostaglandins has improved our understanding of a variety of phenomena. For instance, some prostaglandins are known to be involved in the mechanisms that produce local pain and inflammation. And it was through this discovery that we first came to understand the pharmacologic action of aspirin: it inhibits the production of prostaglandins. Additional research has resulted in the development of a whole range of antiprostaglandin drugs; for instance, the nonsteroidal antiinflammatory drugs (NSAIDs; an example is ibuprofen), all act in one way or another to inhibit prostaglandin synthesis.

It is likely that interuterine devices (IUDs) inserted in the uterus for birth control work through stimulating the release of prostaglandins. Severe menstrual cramping and pain (primary dysmenorrhea) have also been linked to overproduction of prostaglandins. Prostaglandins normally rise sharply toward the end of the menstrual cycle. In women with primary dysmenorrhea, production of prostaglandins by the uterus is excessive. Their concentration in menstrual fluid is two to three times higher than normal. The concentration is highest when menstrual pain is most severe, on the first or second day of menstruation. In clinical trials, dysmenorrhea has been successfully treated in some cases with drugs that inhibit prostaglandin synthesis.

The term "diabetes" means excessive urine. The term "mellitus" comes from the Latin word meaning honeylike; this is appropriate because the glucose in the urine gives it a sweet taste. (Tasting the urine was the method used by the ancients to diagnose diabetes mellitus.) Glucose is not normally passed into the urine by the kidney. Diabetes insipidus, which results from deficient antidiuretic hormone (ADH) secretion by the posterior pituitary, also results in excessive urination, but the urine does not taste sweet—thus the appropriateness of the term "insipidus," which means tasteless.

Glucagon has an effect on the blood glucose concentration that is the opposite of insulin. Glucagon works to increase the amount of glucose in the blood. Secretion of glucagon is stimulated by a decrease from normal glucose levels. Glucagon accomplishes its task by acting on liver cells to promote the breakdown of *glycogen* and release of the resulting glucose. Recall that glycogen is a large storage molecule made up of many glucose molecules.

The major stimulant, then, for the release of either insulin or glucagon is a change in the circulating blood glucose concentration. Elevation of blood glucose results in insulin secretion; similarly, a fall in blood glucose stimulates secretion of glucagon.

THE PINEAL GLAND

What Does the Pineal Gland Do?

The *pineal* (pin'e-al) *gland* is located in the midbrain area. Its precise function is still somewhat of a mystery. One suggestion is that it influences the activity of the anterior pituitary gland. Most recently, investigators have suggested that the pineal gland may secrete a hormone called *melatonin* (mel"ah-to'nin), which somehow serves as a "biologic clock" for regulating the activities of the ovaries. At this time, however, these suggestions are merely interesting speculation.

THE GONADS (SEX GLANDS)

What Is the Endocrine Function of the Ovaries?

The ovaries are two medium-sized ovoid glands located in the pelvic portion of the female abdomen and attached to a supporting broad ligament. The outer layer of the ovary consists of a specialized germinal epithelium that produces *ova*. Two types of hormones are produced and secreted by the ovaries, the *estrogens* and *progesterone*. These are female sex hormones. The structure and function of these two endocrine glands will be discussed more fully in Chapter 14, The Reproductive System.

What Is the Endocrine Function of the Testes?

The testes are two medium-sized, ovoid glands suspended by the spermatic cord and surrounded and supported, below the pelvic region, by the *scrotum*. Two major types of specialized tissue are found in testicular substance. Tubules containing germinal epithelium function in the formation of spermatozoa. *Interstitial* (in"ter-stish'al) *cells* produce and secrete *testosterone*, the "masculinizing hormone." The structure and function of the testes will be discussed more fully in Chapter 13, The Urinary System.

CLINICAL CONSIDERATIONS

Anterior Lobe of Pituitary Gland

Since this is the source of several hormones that directly control other endocrine glands, abnormal increases or decreases in the production of these hormones will inevitably affect these target endocrine glands.

Overproduction of anterior pituitary hormones in adolescence leads to *gigantism* and, in adult life, *acromegaly* (see Fig. 7–4). In gigantism, the target endocrine glands as well as the whole body increase in size; metabolism is increased, and there are disturbances in glucose utilization. In acromegaly (ak"ro-meg'ah-lee), similar increases in organ sizes occur, with metabolic disturbances as well as noticeable growth and thickening of the skeletal framework. In both disorders, the oversecretion of growth hormone is thought to produce the most serious clinical symptoms.

Underproduction of anterior pituitary hormones, commonly known as *Simmonds' disease*, can occur at any age but is most frequent in adults. In children, it results in *dwarfism* or *Froehlich's syndrome* (obesity and lack of sexual development). In adults, the clinical syndrome is represented by insufficiency of the secondary target organs, particularly the adrenals, thyroid, and gonads. Patients gain weight, have metabolic disturbances, and are easily fatigued. It is remarkable that most patients survive many years, with the average duration of the disease 30 to 40 years.

Posterior Lobe of Pituitary Gland

Oversecretion of posterior pituitary hormones, principally antidiuretic hormone (ADH), is rare and is almost always associated with a cancer of the gland. It results in excessive retention of water and a condition of water intoxication.

Diabetes insipidus is a disease caused by an abnormal decrease in the production of ADH. The result is excessive output of urine — up to 20 liters a day.

Thyroid Gland

Hyperthyroidism, an excessive secretion of thyroxin, produces a marked increase in metabolic rate that is reflected by an increase in pulse rate, temperature, and blood pressure, accompanied by extreme nervousness, irritability, weight loss, and fatigability. *Exophthalmos* (see Fig. 7–6) is indicative of hyperthyroidism. Skeletal decalcification has been noted, which may be due to overproduction of the relatively recently discovered hormone *calcitonin*.

Hypothyroidism, insufficiency of thyroid hormone, produces *myxedema* — puffiness and edema of the face with a slowing of all metabolic activities and weight gain.

Parathyroid Glands

Oversecretion of parathormone causes an abnormal increase in the calcium concentration of the blood. Since nerve and muscle cells are very sensitive to calcium ion concentration, the brain and heart activity soon become *depressed*, and the patient becomes less responsive.

Undersecretion of parathormone results in an abnormal decrease in blood calcium. The nerve and muscle cells become *hypersensitive*, or overresponsive, resulting in severe jerkiness, muscle spasms, and cramps. This condition is known as tetany. The term "tetany" derives from the Greek word meaning convulsive tension.

Adrenal Cortex

A common type of oversecretion of adrenal cortical hormones is known as *Cushing's disease* and involves a complex of effects. Cushing's disease is characterized by development of a humped back, puffiness of the face, masculinizing effects, hypertension, and increased concentration of blood glucose (Fig. 7–12).

Hypersecretion of individual hormones produces more selective effects. *Aldosteronism*, involving overproduction of the sodium-retaining hormone aldosterone, results in water retention (edema), hypertension, excessive loss of potassium, and a tendency toward excessive concentrations of sodium. Oversecretion of cortisol, which is rare by itself, produces disturbances of protein, lipid, and glucose metabolism; in extreme cases a humped back develops. Adrenogenital syndrome results from oversecretion of the adrenal sex hormones (androgens), leading to intense masculinizing effects throughout the body.

Addison's disease, or insufficient production of the adrenal cortical hormones, has several consequences corresponding to the lack of each of the

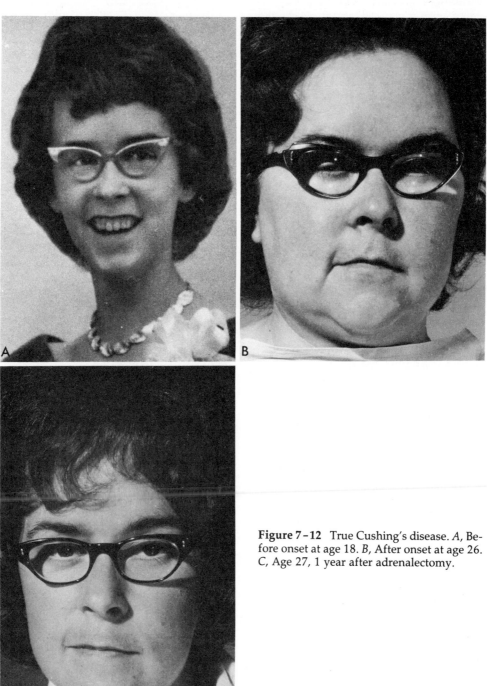

Figure 7-12 True Cushing's disease. *A*, Before onset at age 18. *B*, After onset at age 26. *C*, Age 27, 1 year after adrenalectomy.

specific hormones. Lack of aldosterone secretion allows large amounts of sodium ions (and water) to be lost into the urine. Loss of cortisol secretion makes it impossible for a person with Addison's disease to control blood glucose levels; mobilization of both proteins and fats is also reduced. Generally speaking, the most detrimental effect is the lack of responsiveness to the energy needs of the body. This leads to serious complications during periods of stress, such as diseases, surgery, or emotional crisis. Even a mild respiratory infection can sometimes cause death.

Adrenal Medulla

Hypersecretion of the adrenal medulla is rare and is almost always a result of cancer of the gland. The main consequence of oversecretion by the hormones (epinephrine and norepinephrine) is hypertension.

The adrenal medulla does not seem to be essential to life or normal functioning; as a consequence, no disorders of undersecretion have been described.

Pancreas

The primary disease of the endocrine portion of the pancreas is *diabetes mellitus.* When an insufficient amount of insulin is secreted, the blood glucose level rises markedly. As a result, the kidneys attempt to rid the blood of the excess glucose by producing large quantities of urine. Glucose in the urine is a major clinical sign of diabetes mellitus, since glucose does not normally pass into the urine.

Occasionally, the insulin-producing cells of the pancreatic islets have not been destroyed but are merely inactive, causing a mild form of diabetes. In such cases, the patient can be maintained on islet cell–stimulating drugs, which can be taken orally. In the more common cases of diabetes in which the cells are destroyed, injections of insulin are necessary. Insulin cannot be taken orally, since it is broken down in the digestive system before reaching the blood.

SUMMARY

A. The endocrine system, along with the nervous system, controls and coordinates the component parts of the body.
  1. The endocrine system is responsible for more general and longer lasting coordination than that effected by the nervous system.
  2. The endocrine system is made up of a collection of endocrine glands.
  3. The endocrine glands operate by secreting appropriate levels of hormones directly into the blood stream.
  4. Exocrine glands secrete special substances (usually enzymes) into ducts.
B. A hormone is a chemical substance (or stimulant) secreted by one part of the body (an endocrine gland) to control a function elsewhere in the body.
  1. Hormones enter the blood through the capillaries running through the endocrine gland.
  2. Hormones are carried throughout the body by the blood stream.
  3. Some hormones act generally on all (or most) cells in the body.
  4. Other hormones influence only a limited area or target organ.
C. The pituitary gland (or hypophysis) is a small pea-sized organ located below the hypothalamus.
  1. The pituitary is really two distinct glands operating independently.
    a. The front half, the anterior lobe, is also called the adenohypophysis.
    b. The back half, the posterior lobe, is also called the neurohypophysis.
    c. The neurohypophysis is more directly associated with the nervous tissue of the hypothalamus above.
  2. The anterior lobe of the pituitary secretes at least six major hormones.
    a. The anterior lobe is the "master" endocrine gland because four of its hormones have other endocrine glands as their target organs: ACTH, TSH, FSH, and LH.
    b. Adrenocorticotropic hormone (ACTH) regulates the growth and activity of the adrenal cortex.

c. Thyroid-stimulating hormone (TSH) controls the growth and activity of the thyroid gland.

d. Follicle-stimulating hormone (FSH) is a gonadotropic hormone.
   i. In females it stimulates growth of the follicles until one matures each month.
   ii. In females it also stimulates production and secretion of female sex hormones.
   iii. In males it stimulates development of spermatozoa.

e. Lutenizing hormone (LH) is a gonadotropic hormone.
   i. In females it stimulates follicle growth.
   ii. At follicle maturity, in a sudden increase, it stimulates ovulation.
   iii. After ovulation it influences the ruptured follicle to develop into the corpus luteum.
   iv. In the male, LH stimulates the testes to produce testosterone, the basic male sex hormone.

f. Growth hormone (GH), or somatotropin (STH), alters the metabolism of cells toward an increased reproduction.

g. Prolactin, or lactogenic hormone, promotes the growth of breast tissue during pregnancy.
   i. After birth, suckling stimulates secretion of prolactin.
   ii. This secretion of prolactin after birth stimulates production of more milk (lactation).

3. The posterior lobe of the pituitary secretes two hormones.
a. Oxytocin stimulates the uterus to contract at the time of childbirth.
   i. After birth, oxytocin stimulates the release of breast milk into the ducts.
   ii. Suckling by the infant stimulates additional secretion of oxytocin.
b. Antidiuretic hormone (ADH) stimulates cells in the kidney to reabsorb water out of forming urine.
   i. ADH decreases water loss from the body.
   ii. When there is excess water, ADH secretion drops to zero.
   iii. Diabetes insipidus is a disease caused by an abnormal decrease in production of ADH.

D. The thyroid gland, located in front of and on either side of the trachea (windpipe), produces and secretes two main hormones.
1. The growth and level of activity of the thyroid gland is controlled by thyroid-stimulating hormone secreted from the anterior pituitary.
2. Thyroid hormone, or thyroxin, stimulates all the cells of the body to be more active.
   a. Excess thyroid hormone (hyperthyroidism) causes hyperactivity and exophthalmos.
   b. Lack of thyroid hormone (hypothyroidism) results in myxedema, characterized by little energy and a slowing down.
   c. Goiter is a thyroid gland enlargement in response to low levels of thyroid hormone due to inadequate iodine levels.
3. Calcitonin decreases the level of calcium in the blood.
   a. It is secreted when calcium levels in the blood become too high.
   b. Its effect is opposite that of parathyroid hormone.

E. The four small parathyroid glands, located on the back side of the thyroid gland, secrete only one hormone.
1. Parathyroid hormone, or parathormone, is secreted when the calcium concentration in the blood is too low.
   a. Calcitonin has the opposite effect.
2. Parathyroid hormone also promotes absorption of ingested calcium.
3. Excessive parathormone, resulting in too much calcium in the blood, depresses nerve and muscle cell activity.
4. Too little parathormone, resulting in too little calcium in the blood, creates a state of hyperactivity, referred to traditionally as tetany.

F. Each of the two adrenal (or suprarenal) glands, one above each kidney, is in reality two separate and distinct glands.
1. The cortex (outer portion) and the medulla (inner portion) of each adrenal gland have different functions.
2. The adrenal cortex secretes three general types of substances.
   a. The mineralocorticoids help control the

amount of certain mineral salts in the bodily fluids.

    i. Aldosterone is the most important, stimulating the kidney to retain sodium.

    ii. Aldosterone has the opposite effect on the kidney for potassium.

  b. The glucocorticoids, chiefly cortisol, stimulate energy metabolism and thus function like thyroid hormone.

    i. Normal amounts are needed for normal energy metabolism.

    ii. During stress, cortisol leads to breakdown of proteins for gluconeogenesis in the liver.

  c. Androgens produce masculinization.

    i. Testosterone is the most important androgen and is secreted primarily in the testes.

    ii. Androgens from the adrenal cortex are of minor importance except when an adrenal tumor occurs, and hypersecretion may occur.

  3. The adrenal medulla produces and secretes epinephrine (adrenaline) and norepinephrine (noradrenaline).

    a. Ten times as much epinephrine is secreted as norepinephrine.

    b. The medullary hormones are released in response to "fight or flight" stimulation from the sympathetic nervous system.

      i. Epinephrine rapidly supercharges the body.

      ii. It increases heart rate, blood pressure, and blood glucose levels.

G. The pancreatic islets (of Langerhans), small clumps of specialized cells scattered throughout the pancreas, operate as an endocrine gland.

  1. The islets contain two types of cells.

    a. Beta cells produce and secrete insulin.

    b. Alpha cells produce and secrete glucagon.

  2. Insulin regulates the cellular uptake of glucose from the blood.

    a. As a consequence it regulates the level of glucose in the blood.

    b. Insulin is secreted most heavily after a meal.

      i. This prevents excessive glucose buildup.

      ii. Insulin secretion decreases when the glucose level in the blood decreases (as between meals).

    c. In diabetes mellitus, beta cells do not secrete enough insulin, and glucose levels rise dangerously.

      i. This can lead to mental confusion and coma.

      ii. The kidney attempts to rid the blood of excess glucose by producing large amounts of urine.

  3. Glucagon works to increase the amount of glucose in the blood — the opposite of what insulin does.

    a. Release of glucagon is stimulated by a decrease from normal glucose levels.

    b. Glucagon acts on liver cells to promote breakdown of glycogen to release the stored glucose molecules.

H. The pineal gland, located in the midbrain, produces and secretes melatonin.

  1. The pineal may affect the activity of the anterior pituitary and the rhythm of the ovaries.

  2. Melatonin release is linked to the "biologic clock."

I. The gonads in the male are the testes, suspended below the pelvis; in the female they are the ovaries, located in the abdomen.

  1. The outer layer of the ovaries is a specialized germinal epithelium that produces ova.

  2. The ovaries produce and secrete two female sex hormones: the estrogens and progesterone.

  3. Tubules in the testes, containing specialized germinal epithelium, produce spermatozoa.

  4. Interstitial cells in the testes produce and secrete testosterone, the masculinizing hormone.

J. There are a number of disorders of the endocrine system.

  1. Overproduction of anterior pituitary hormones leads to gigantism and, in adult life, to acromegaly.

  2. Underproduction of anterior pituitary hormones leads to Simmonds' disease or, in children, to dwarfism.

  3. Overproduction of posterior pituitary hormones is rare and usually indicates a cancer.

  4. Underproduction of posterior pituitary hormones results in diabetes insipidus.

  5. Cushing's disease is a common type of oversecretion of adrenal cortical hormones.

6. Addison's disease is due to an insufficiency of adrenal cortical hormones.
7. Hypersecretion by the adrenal medulla is rare and usually indicates a cancer.
8. Hyposecretion by the adrenal medulla has not been described.

K. Prostaglandins are short-lived, hormonelike chemicals produced in the cells of many tissues.
1. There are at least 16 known prostaglandins.
2. Nonsteroidal anti-inflammatory drugs (NSAIDs; such as ibuprofen) act by inhibiting synthesis of prostaglandins.

REVIEW QUESTIONS

1. Explain how the endocrine system and the nervous system are each specialized in the functions of control and coordination.
2. Distinguish between the products and modes of delivery of endocrine glands and exocrine glands.
3. Define hormone.
4. Some hormones act generally on all cells of the body, others act on limited target organs. Give two examples of each.
5. Explain why the anterior pituitary is sometimes referred to as the leader of the endocrine orchestra.

How do tropic hormones differ from other hormones?
6. Define negative feedback and explain how it regulates hormone levels in the blood.
7. Construct and label a diagram identifying the locations of each of the endocrine glands.
8. Explain the different actions of FSH and LH in males and in females.
9. Distinguish the action of prolactin from oxytocin in the process of providing milk for a newborn.
10. Outline the actions of calcitonin and parathormone in the regulation of calcium levels in the blood.
11. What are known as the stress hormones?
12. What are the fight or flight hormones?
13. What hormone is thought to be important in the regulation of the body's biologic clock?
14. What are the effects of glucagon, cortisol, epinephrine, and insulin on blood levels of glucose?
15. Name two hormones that are closely involved in the regulation of salt and fluid balance in the body. Explain their effects.
16. Distinguish between diabetes mellitus and diabetes insipidus.
17. A simple goiter is not caused by hypersecretion or hyposecretion of the thyroid. What causes it?
18. Identify the hormone and whether it is hypersecreted or hyposecreted in each of the following endocrine disorders: tetany, myxedema, exophthalmos, Simmonds' disease, Addison's disease, acromegaly, and Cushing's disease.

E I G H T

The Blood

The aim of this chapter is to enable the student to do the following:

- Describe the major constituents of whole blood.

- Distinguish the different types of blood cells and their primary functions.

- Identify the four main proteins found in plasma and describe their functions.

- Explain the blood groupings and their interactions.

- Describe the characteristics of the universal donor and universal recipient.

- Interpret the results of the following blood tests: hematocrit, blood count, and typing and crossmatching.

- List in sequence the basic steps of blood clotting.

- Explain the basis of transfusion reactions.

- Describe the characteristics of the main blood disorders.

BLOOD: WHAT IT DOES, WHAT IT CONTAINS

What Is the Function of the Blood?

The primary function of the blood is the internal transportation of cellular nutrients and wastes. Digested nutrients absorbed from the intestines and oxygen collected in the lungs are carried by the blood to all the cells in the body. The major waste product, carbon dioxide, is carried to the lungs for expulsion, whereas other wastes and excesses of cellular activity are carried to the kidneys for selective elimination.

Another function of the blood is accomplished principally by the white blood cells; they play a central role in the prevention of infection.

The blood also transports *hormones,* which are chemical messengers or stimulants secreted directly into the blood by special glandular cells. The function of hormones is discussed in more detail in Chapter 7, The Endocrine System.

Keeping balance of water. temperature regulation.

What Are the Major Constituents of the Blood?

The general appearance of blood might lead one to suppose that it is one simple substance. However, when blood is examined under a microscope or analyzed chemically, it is found to be composed of many distinct components (Figs. 8–1 and 8–2).

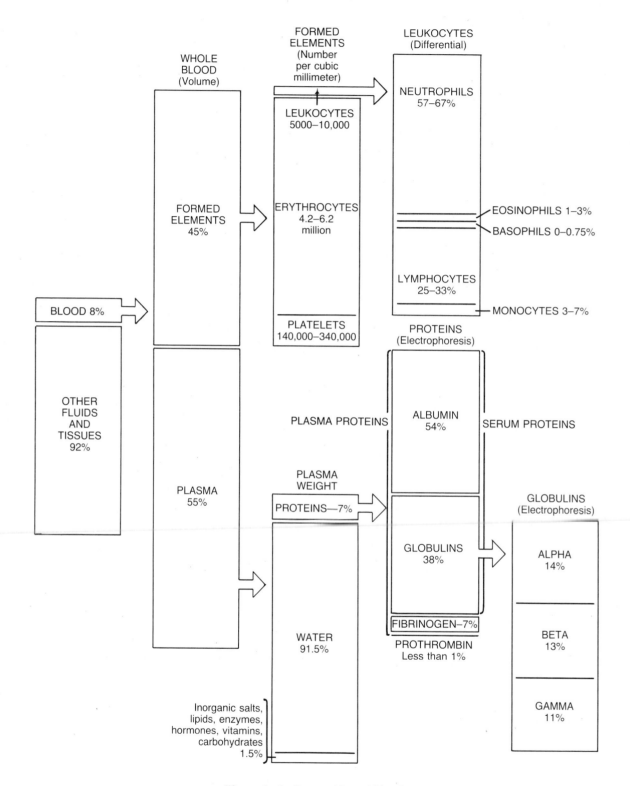

Figure 8-1 Composition of blood.

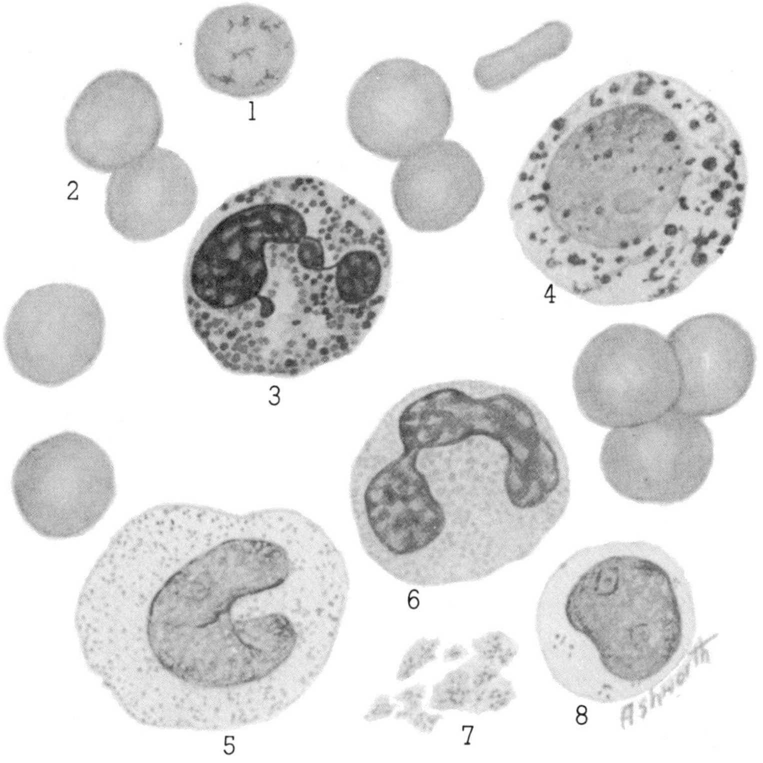

Figure 8–2 Blood cells:
1, reticulocyte;
2, erythrocyte;
3, eosinophil;
4, basophil;
5, monocyte;
6, neutrophil;
7, platelets;
8, lymphocyte.
Numbers correspond to those in Figure 8–4, illustrating the stages of blood cell formation.

One simple way to separate blood is by use of the centrifuge (sen'tri-fuj). A few minutes of low-speed spinning yields, in the lower portion, the *formed elements* (cells, etc.) and in the upper portion, the straw-colored *plasma* (plaz'mah). This centrifuge procedure is used for a standard type of blood test — to determine the percentage of formed elements in a person's blood. The term *hematocrit* (he-mat'o-krit) refers to the percentage of formed elements in the blood by volume (Fig. 8–3). Thus, if the percentage of formed elements in the centrifuge tube turns out to be 45, then the hematocrit is reported as 45. The word hematocrit is derived from the Greek words *haimat*, meaning blood, and *crino*, meaning to separate; literally, then, it means to separate the blood.

What Are the Formed Elements? What Functions Do They Perform?

The formed elements consist of the red blood cells, the white blood cells, and the platelets (Fig. 8–2). All the formed elements develop and mature from the same basic type of cell, known as a hemocytoblast (cell from which blood grows).

The *red blood cells*, or *erythrocytes* (e-rith'ro-sits), function to transport oxygen from the lungs to the cells throughout the body. The name erythrocyte is derived from the Greek words *erythros*, which means red, and *kytos*, which means hollow or cell. This oxygen-carrying task is accomplished through the action of a special protein, *hemoglobin* (he'mo-glo"bin), which is a major constituent of erythrocytes.

There are several types of *white blood cells*, or *leukocytes* (*leukos* means white and *kytos* means cell). The general function of leukocytes (loo'ko-sits) is to provide a defense against any virus, bacterium, or other foreign protein substance that enters into the blood stream or tissues. Two types of leukocytes, *neutrophils* (nu'tro-fils) and *monocytes*, operate by devouring any microorganisms or foreign protein. For example, the pus found around an infected wound is made up primarily of leukocytes that have died in combating the infection. Neutro-

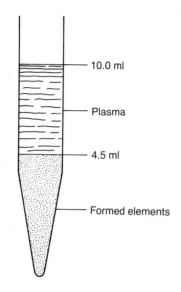

Figure 8-3   Demonstration of hematocrit.

phils comprise about 56 to 67 per cent of the white blood cells. Two other types of white blood cells are eosinophils and basophils.

Lymphocytes (lim'fo-sits) make up about 25 to 33 per cent of the leukocytes and operate to protect us from infection by a process known as immune response. A great deal of research is being done in an attempt to understand fully the immune response system. Very generally, one can say that when a virus, bacterium, or foreign protein, known generally as an antigen (an'ti-jen), enters the body, the immune system produces a special substance (antibody) that either destroys or alters the antigen to make it harmless. Understanding the immune response is of major concern in current cancer research. The term "antigen" derives from *anti,* body, + the Greek word *gennan,* meaning "to produce." In other words, an antigen is anything that will lead to the production of antibodies.

Platelets are the tiny cell-like parts that originate with the breakup or partial disintegration of the hemocytoblasts. As we will see below, *platelets* function in the mechanism of blood clotting (coagulation).

What Is Plasma? What Is Serum?

Blood *plasma* is a straw-colored liquid composed of a solution of water (91 per cent) and var-

ious chemical substances (9 per cent), primarily special blood proteins. Plasma is obtained by removing the formed elements from *whole* (complete) *blood,* usually by means of spinning whole blood in a centrifuge. Plasma can only be stored if an anticoagulant is added to prevent coagulation. (Coagulation, or clotting, is the process by which blood or plasma changes from a liquid state to that of a soft, jellylike solid.)

Blood *serum* is obtained from plasma by first causing or allowing the plasma to coagulate and then by removing the fibrous clotting material. This last step, which removes the clotted fibrous material from the solution, leaving serum, is commonly achieved by further use of a centrifuge. Serum is then identical to plasma except that the clotting factor has been removed. Serum can be stored almost indefinitely and there is, of course, no need to add an anticoagulant.

What Are the Functions of the Four Major Plasma Proteins?

The plasma proteins are dissolved proteins, not directly associated with formed elements. The plasma proteins are so called because they will always be found in blood plasma in solution, that is, after the formed elements are removed. Proteins dissolve in water in the same way that sugar dissolves. The four major plasma proteins are albumin, globulin, fibrinogen, and prothrombin.

Albumin (al-bu'min) is the most plentiful plasma protein (54 per cent). It is crucial in maintaining the proper osmotic balance between the blood and the interstitial (between cells) fluids. If albumin concentration decreases for any reason, the amount of water in the blood also decreases, making the blood thicker. In injury, such as a severe burn, albumin leaks from the damaged capillaries to the interstitial fluids. As a result, water cannot be kept in the blood compartment, and blood volume drops, leading to thickening of the blood. If the loss is severe, shock results. Treatment to counteract this disorder includes intravenous infusion of *serum albumin* (serum containing a high concentration of albumin).

Globulin (glob'u-lin) is important, because it contains antibodies involved in the body's immune (infection-fighting) mechanisms. When examined chemically, globulin can be separated into three groups: alpha, beta, and gamma. The *gamma globulin* is the most active antibody factor. Gamma globulin injections from previously affected persons have been used in the control and prevention of epidemics of some infectious diseases such as infectious hepatitis (liver inflammation).

Fibrinogen (fi-brin'o-jen) and *prothrombin* (prothrom'bin) are present in lesser amounts than those of albumin and globulin. These plasma proteins function in the coagulation process discussed as follows. Since these two proteins are used up in the coagulation process, would you expect to find them in serum? Albumin and globulin are both found in serum.

How Are Blood Cells Formed?

Development of blood cells within the bones begins during the fifth month of fetal life (Fig. 8–4).

Blood-forming elements initially appear in the centers of the bone marrow cavities; the blood-forming centers later expand to occupy the entire marrow space. This widely dispersed blood cell formation continues until puberty, when the marrow in the ends of all the long bones becomes less cellular and more fatty. In the adult, only the skull, vertebrae, ribs, sternum, pelvis, humerus, and femur retain active red marrow formation. In elderly individuals, areas of bone marrow once occupied by active cell production become fat laden. This helps to explain the difficulty elderly individuals experience in regenerating lost blood; it is because they have very little active red bone marrow remaining.

Two types of blood cells are not formed in the bone marrow. Lymphocytes and monocytes are formed by lymphatic tissue, chiefly in the lymph nodes and the spleen.

All blood cells originate from undifferentiated cells called hemocytoblasts (literally "blood-forming cells"). As these primitive cells mature, they un-

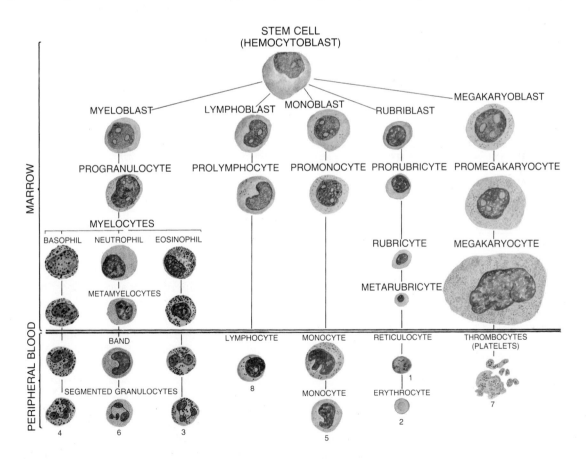

Figure 8–4 Stages in the formation of the peripheral blood cells. Numbered cells correspond to cell types in Figure 8–2.

dergo alterations in nuclear and cytoplasmic characteristics, producing the red blood cells, white blood cells, and platelets (Fig. 8–2).

What Factors Stimulate an Increase in the Rate of Blood Cell Formation?

Red blood cell production is stimulated by any factor that lowers the oxygen available to bone marrow or body tissue. Thus, high altitude, hemorrhage (blood loss), nutritional deficiencies, and respiratory disturbances may stimulate increased red blood cell formation. The life span of erythrocytes is approximately 80 to 120 days. When their usefulness is impaired with age, the red cells are destroyed by the spleen, liver, and bone marrow. Two to ten million red cells are destroyed each second, yet, because of replacement, the number of circulating cells remains remarkably constant.

Many diseases are characterized by a change in the number of circulating white cells (leukocytes). An increase in white cell count usually indicates an acute infection. More generally, anything that stimulates an immune response will increase the rate of white blood cell formation.

PROTECTION AGAINST BLOOD LOSS

What Are the Three Mechanisms in Stopping Blood Loss?

There are three separate mechanisms involved in checking the flow of blood from an injury: formation of the platelet block, contraction of the related blood vessels, and formation of a fibrin clot (Fig. 8–5).

First, when a vessel is cut or damaged, platelets rapidly accumulate at the site of blood loss. This collection of platelets forms a temporary plug that is capable of stopping blood loss in small arteries and veins.

Second, soon after the first step begins, there is a contraction of the blood vessels around the immediate area of the injury. This reduces the amount and

rate of blood flow around the wound. Later, a more generalized constriction of vessels occurs, resulting in an overall decrease in the flow of blood to the area.

Third, next begins the actual process of blood clotting, or coagulation. This takes place with the formation of the insoluble fibrin clot through a conversion of the normally soluble plasma protein fibrinogen into insoluble *fibrin.* This occurs at the point at which the platelets have built up earlier. Notice the Greek suffix *-gen,* meaning "to produce," in the word fibrino*gen;* this means "that which produces fibrin," which is precisely the outcome of the coagulation process — soluble fibrinogen turns into insoluble, fibrous, or fiberlike, fibrin.

The three essential steps in this third stage, the coagulation (or clotting) stage, are the following: (1) thromboplastin is formed by platelet-plasma interaction; (2) this stimulates conversion of prothrombin to thrombin; and, finally, (3) fibrinogen undergoes conversion to fibrin, which is dependent on the presence of thrombin (Fig. 8–6).

What Are Two Common Abnormalities of the Clotting Mechanism?

Two common abnormalities of the clotting mechanism are internal clotting, also called thrombosis (throm-bo'sis), and hemophilia (he"mo-fil'e-ah).

Thrombosis   The term thrombosis, derived from the Greek word *thrombos,* meaning clot, describes clotting inside a "normal" blood vessel. A clot, or thrombus, forming in the blood vessels of the leg or arm may cause some minor local damage. However, if an internal clot should block the blood supply to the heart or brain, it can be fatal. An *embolus* (Greek for plug) is an internal clot that has become dislodged from its place of origin and has lodged elsewhere in the body. The condition is spoken of as *embolism.*

Hemophilia   This is a hereditary bleeding disease that is characterized by delayed coagulation of the blood. It results from a diminished coagulation factor in the plasma. There are actually several types of hemophilia, classified according to which coagu-

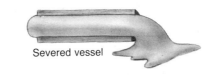
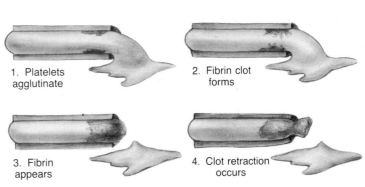

Figure 8-5 Formation of clot following injury.

Severed vessel

1. Platelets agglutinate

2. Fibrin clot forms

3. Fibrin appears

4. Clot retraction occurs

lation factor is deficient. Treatment consists of transfusions with fresh blood or administration of the deficient factor.

BLOOD TYPES AND TRANSFUSIONS

How Are Blood Groupings Related to Transfusions?

The transfusion of whole blood from one person to another can be a lifesaving procedure. However, the safe administration of whole blood from donor to recipient requires typing and crossmatching. These procedures are necessary, since a patient receiving blood of a type that reacts with his own will experience a serious, and sometimes fatal, reaction. The potential reaction is due to the presence of the *immune response system*, which attacks and alters foreign proteins that enter the blood. Whether one person's blood will be foreign to another person (or to his immune response system) depends on the types of proteins that make up the blood cells and other blood factors. If the proteins of the donor blood are foreign to the recipient's, then this will trigger an immune response, and already existing or newly produced antibodies will attack the transfused blood. Since the amount of blood transfused is usually large (one pint or more), a very serious or fatal condition can result from this reaction.

The systems of blood classification are based, therefore, on the presence of specific, known antigens (proteins foreign to some people in the population) in the red blood cells and on the presence of specific antibodies in the plasma or serum. The primary classification system identifies antigens A and B, antibodies anti-A and anti-B, and a factor known as Rh (see Table 8-1 and Fig. 8-7).

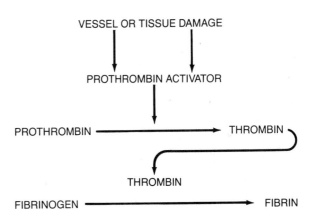

Figure 8-6 Phases of coagulation.

| | | TABLE 8–1   BLOOD GROUPING | | |
TYPE	PERCENTAGE OF POPULATION	RED CELL ANTIGENS	PLASMA ANTIBODIES
ABO			
A	41%	A	Anti-B
B	10%	B	Anti-A
AB	4%	A, B	
O	45%	*	Anti-A, anti-B
Rh (D)			
Positive	85%	Rh	
Negative	15%		†

* An individual with type O blood is sometimes called the "universal donor," since type O blood does not contain agglutinogens A and B.

† Anti-Rh does not occur naturally in blood, but will result if an Rh negative individual is given Rh positive blood.

How Are the Different Blood Types Related?

Blood groups are named for the protein antigens contained in the red blood cells. Blood type A contains A-type protein (also called A antigen), and type B blood contains B-type protein (also called B antigen). Type AB blood has both these protein antigens, and type O blood has neither.

The potential problem of a transfusion reaction arises because of the additional presence of antibodies to these antigens (A and B). If A antigen is contacted by antibody A (also called anti-A), a serious problem arises; the antagonism between these substances leads to a clumping or *agglutination* (ah-gloo"ti-na'shun) of the red blood cells—a very dangerous condition (Fig. 8–7).

The antibodies for A and B antigens are distributed on a sort of opposite or reciprocal basis. That is, type A blood contains type B antibody. And type B blood contains type A antibody. As a result, people with type A blood cannot receive type B blood, nor is the reverse possible.

Type AB blood, which contains both A and B antigen, does not contain either A or B antibodies. That is, it has no antibodies relevant to the ABO classification system for transfusions. As a consequence, any of the other blood types can be given to a person with type AB blood. An individual with type AB blood is referred to as the *universal recipient*.

Type O blood has *both* A and B antibodies, but contains neither A nor B antigen. A person with type O blood cannot receive type A, which contains A antigen, type B, which has B antigen, or type AB, which has both antigens but neither A nor B antibody. A person with type O blood can receive only type O blood. However, since it has no antigens, type O blood can be given to persons with any of the other types. An individual with type O blood is called the *universal donor*.

The antibodies contained in the blood that is actually transfused seem to have a negligible effect outside their host body. So what is important is the donor's antigens and the recipient's (host) antibodies.

What Is the Rh Factor?

The Rh factor, so named because it was first found in the blood of the Rhesus monkey, is a system consisting of 12 antigens. Of these, "D" is the most antigenic; the term Rh positive, as it is generally employed, refers to the presence of agglutinogen "D." The Rh negative individual does not naturally possess this D antigen, and consequently will form D antibodies (by means of the immune response system) when he receives blood cells containing D.

The anti-D antibody does not occur naturally in the blood (recall that A and B antibodies occur natu-

RECIPIENT'S BLOOD GROUP
(Plasma or serum tested)

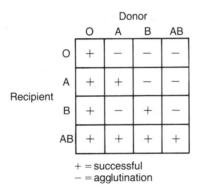

		AB	A	B	O
Donor's	AB				
Blood	A				
Group	B				
Red Cells Tested	O				

	Donor			
	O	A	B	AB
Recipient O	+	−	−	−
A	+	+	−	−
B	+	−	+	−
AB	+	+	+	+

+ = successful
− = agglutination

Figure 8–7 Crossmatching of blood types is necessary before blood from donor is administered to recipient. If the two types are not compatible, agglutination, a serious or fatal reaction, may occur.

rally). As a result, the initial transfusion of Rh positive blood into an Rh negative individual may merely sensitize the recipient and cause development of antibodies (somewhat like a vaccination), but without the occurrence of severe symptoms. However, once sensitized, the recipient will probably experience a severe reaction to subsequent infusions of Rh positive blood. Rh negative blood can always be given to an Rh positive person. Why?

Because Rh negative blood does not have the antigen (D).

The same reaction often occurs during pregnancy when the fetus of an Rh negative mother is Rh positive. Some positive red cells in the fetus leak across the placenta into the Rh negative blood of the mother, which produces antibodies in response to this invasion. The maternal antibodies then cross the placenta to the fetus and cause a reaction. When a woman is sensitized by this process during the first pregnancy, the first child is often normal and only in subsequent pregnancies does any severe reaction occur.

Many other antigenic factors have been discovered in the blood of various individuals, but their occurrence is relatively rare. Nonetheless, in any transfusion there remains a substantial danger of an immune reaction. Because of the sensitizing process of the immune response, people receiving transfusions again after several weeks, months, or years are in greater danger.

CLINICAL CONSIDERATIONS

What Can Blood Counts Tell Us?

A *blood count* is the number of either white or red blood cells per cubic millimeter of whole blood and is arrived at by counting under a microscope the number of cells in a sample of blood in a given area.

As noted earlier, many diseases are characterized by an increase in the white (cell) blood count. Normally, the total white cell count ranges from 5000 to 10,000 per cubic millimeter; however, it may be as high as 500,000 per cubic millimeter in leukemia.

Leukemia   Derived from the Greek words meaning white blood, this disease is characterized by a rapid and abnormal growth of white blood cells (leukocytes) in the peripheral blood. It is generally thought of as a blood cancer (malignant disease). The word "benign" is derived from the Latin word meaning "to be kind" and is opposed to the word "malignant," which is derived from the Latin word meaning "to be malicious (unkind)."

Infectious Mononucleosis (mon"o-nu"kle-o'sis)   This is a benign disease associated with an increase in mononuclear leukocytes (the type of leukocytes with a *single* nucleus—*mono* means one). It usually occurs in children and young adults and is believed to be caused by a virus. The patient with infectious mononucleosis evidences a slightly elevated temperature, enlarged lymph nodes, fatigue, and a sore throat.

Anemias   Normal red blood cell count is approximately 5,400,000 per cubic millimeter in males and 4,900,000 per cubic millimeter in females. In other words, there are about 500 to 1000 red cells for every white cell in the blood. A reduction in the total number of red cells or in the amount of hemoglobin in the body results in anemia. *Anemia* (from the Latin words meaning "lack of blood") is defined as a decrease in the capacity of the blood to transport oxygen to the tissues. Two common types are pernicious anemia and iron deficiency anemia. In *pernicious* (per-nish'us) *anemia,* there is a decrease in the total number of erythrocytes, and those that are produced are large, oddly shaped, and fragile. *Iron deficiency anemia* usually follows a loss of blood or occurs during other periods when the demand for iron is unusually great. Without iron, hemoglobin formation is retarded.

Sickle cell anemia is a condition in which the red blood cells are abnormally shaped and do not function properly. It is genetically based, affecting a primarily black population. Its prevalence has recently been explained by the fact that persons carrying one gene for sickle cell are more resistant (and thus better adapted) to malaria, a virus that is common in areas of predominantly black population. Persons with only one gene for sickle cell who are resistant to malaria do not develop sickle cells. However, persons with two sickle cell genes will probably die young because they will develop sickle cell anemia.

SUMMARY

A. The primary function of the blood is internal transportation of nutrients and wastes.
  1. Digestive nutrients and oxygen are carried to all cells.
  2. Carbon dioxide is carried to the lungs for expulsion.
  3. Other wastes are carried to the kidneys for selective elimination.
B. The white blood cells function to prevent infection.
C. Whole blood is easily separated into plasma and formed elements.
  1. The percentage of formed elements is termed the hematocrit.
  2. The formed elements all develop and mature from the same basic type of cell: the hemocytoblast.

D. The formed elements consist of the red blood cells, the white blood cells, and the platelets.
   1. The red blood cells, or erythrocytes, transport oxygen through the action of a special protein, hemoglobin.
   2. The white blood cells, or leukocytes, provide defense against any virus, bacterium, or other foreign substance.
      a. Neutrophils and monocytes devour any microorganism or foreign protein.
      b. Eosinophils and basophils are less prominent white blood cells.
      c. Lymphocytes carry out the immune response, producing antibodies specifically to attach foreign substances, which are also known as antigens.
   3. Platelets function in the mechanism of blood clotting (coagulation).
E. Blood plasma is 91 per cent water and about 9 per cent special blood proteins.
   1. Plasma is obtained by removing the formed elements from whole blood.
   2. Blood serum is obtained by removing the fibrous clotting material from plasma.
   3. Albumin, the most plentiful protein, maintains proper osmotic balance.
   4. Globulin contains antibodies involved in the body's immune response mechanism.
   5. Fibrinogen and prothrombin function in the coagulation process.
F. All blood cells originate from undifferentiated cells called hemocytoblasts.
   1. As hemocytoblasts mature, they differentiate into red blood cells, white blood cells, and platelets.
   2. Most blood formation occurs in the red bone marrow.
   3. Lymphocytes and monocytes are formed by lymphatic tissue, chiefly in the lymph nodes and spleen.
G. The blood cell formation and maturation process is stimulated by any factor or situation that uses or requires more blood cells.
   1. Red blood cell production is stimulated by anything that lowers the amount of oxygen to the tissues.
   2. Anything that stimulates an immune response will increase the rate of white blood cell formation.
H. There are three separate mechanisms involved in checking the flow of blood from a wound.

   1. Platelets form a temporary plug at the site of blood loss or vessel damage.
   2. Vessels local to the injury site contract, decreasing the flow of blood to the area.
   3. Blood clotting, or coagulation, forms an insoluble fibrin clot by converting soluble fibrinogen into insoluble fibrin. The three steps in this process are as follows:
      a. Platelet-plasma interaction forms thromboplastin.
      b. Prothrombin is converted to thrombin.
      c. Fibrinogen is converted to fibrin.
I. Two common abnormalities of the clotting mechanism are thrombosis and hemophilia.
   1. Thrombosis is internal clotting inside a normal blood vessel.
   2. An embolus is an internal clot that has become dislodged and lodged somewhere else in the body.
   3. Hemophilia is characterized by delayed clotting.
J. The safe transfusion of whole blood requires typing and crossmatching.
   1. The potential reaction is an immune response attacking the transfused blood as foreign.
   2. The blood classification system is based on the presence of specific protein antigens and antibodies, which are known to cross-react.
   3. A person with type AB blood is referred to the universal recipient.
   4. A person with type O blood is referred to as the universal donor.
   5. Because of the sensitizing process, people receiving multiple transfusions over weeks or years are at increased danger of a serious reaction.
K. A blood count is the number of white or red blood cells per cubic millimeter of whole blood.
   1. Normal white blood cell count ranges from 5000 to 10,000.
      a. In leukemia white blood count may go as high as 500,000.
      b. Leukemia involves a rapid, uncontrolled growth of white blood cells.
      c. Infectious mononucleosis is a virus-caused disease associated with an increase in mononuclear leukocytes.
   2. Normal red blood cell count is 5,400,000 in males and 4,900,000 in females (500 to 1000 red cells for each white cell).
      a. In pernicious anemia the number of red

blood cells is decreased, and those present are abnormal.

   b. Iron deficiency anemia follows blood loss or unusual demand for iron. Hemoglobin requires iron.

   c. Sickle cell anemia is a genetic disorder of the hemoglobin molecule.

      i. Persons with one sickle cell gene are protected from malaria.

      ii. Persons with two sickle cell genes develop sickle cell anemia.

REVIEW QUESTIONS

1. Briefly describe the functions of red blood cells, white blood cells, and the platelets.

2. Define hematocrit.

3. Distinguish among whole blood, plasma, and serum.

4. Name the four major plasma proteins and explain their functions.

5. What is the life span of a red blood cell? How is the production of red blood cells regulated?

6. What does an increase in the number of circulating white cells usually indicate?

7. Distinguish three mechanisms that function to stop blood loss.

8. Describe the steps involved in the process of blood coagulation.

9. Define thrombosis. What is an embolism?

10. What is hemophilia?

11. What is the basis of blood groups? What happens when blood groups are mixed?

12. Explain the danger of an Rh negative mother giving birth to an Rh positive baby.

13. What is the normal range for number of white blood cells? For red blood cells?

14. Characterize leukemia.

15. Distinguish and characterize three types of anemias.

N I N E
The Circulatory System, The Lymphatic System, and Accessory Organs

---

O B J E C T I V E S

The aim of this chapter is to enable the student to do the following:

- Describe the overall circulation of fluids in the body, distinguishing the blood and lymphatic systems.

- Construct and label diagrams showing the gross anatomy of the heart.

- Trace the route of the blood through the heart.

- Enumerate the steps of the cardiac cycle.

- Explain the origin of the heart beat.

- Explain cardiac output and list the factors that affect it.

- Distinguish the pulmonary, systemic, and portal circuits.

- Describe what information can be gained from an electrocardiogram (ECG).

- Compare the structure and function of arteries, veins, and capillaries.

- List the major factors affecting and/or determining blood pressure.

- Identify the major arteries and veins and the region of the body served by each.

- Explain the functions of the lymphatic system and describe its functional relation to the cardiovascular system.

- Describe the functions of the lymph nodes, tonsils, thymus, and spleen.

THE CIRCULATORY SYSTEM

What Is the Function of the Circulatory System?

The circulatory system is the transportation system of the body. It provides a link — either direct or indirect — between each individual cell and the major homeostatic organs. By way of the circulatory system each cell in the body has fairly rapid communicative access to the lungs for oxygen (or for elimination of carbon dioxide), to the digestive tract for nutrients, and to the kidneys for elimination of cellular wastes.

The circulatory system itself should be considered as primarily a homeostatic organ system. The successful operation of each of the other homeostatic organ systems (respiratory, digestive, urinary) is inseparable from the effective operation of the circulatory system.

The circulatory system also performs two other "helping" functions. First, it helps the endocrine system by transporting the substances secreted by the endocrine glands. These substances help to regulate bodily processes; for example, one substance regulates growth, whereas others stimulate sexual development at puberty. These endocrine substances (hormones) are all delivered to their site of action by the circulatory system. The second, additional "helping" function performed by the circulatory system is in the bodily process that protects against infection. The circulatory system transports antibodies and specialized bacteria-fighting white blood cells to the area of possible infection.

What Structures Make Up the Circulatory System?

Strictly speaking the expression "circulatory system" should refer to both the *blood circulating system* and the *lymph circulating system*. In actual practice the expression "circulatory system" usually refers to the blood circulating system alone; this is particularly true in medicine, since the traditional concern and most immediate medical problems are with the blood system. The lymph circulating system is usually referred to separately as the *lymphatic* (lim-fat'ik) *system*.

The blood circulatory system is made up of the blood, the heart, and the blood vessels and capillaries. The lymphatic system is made up of lymph (the plasmalike tissue fluid), the lymph nodes, and

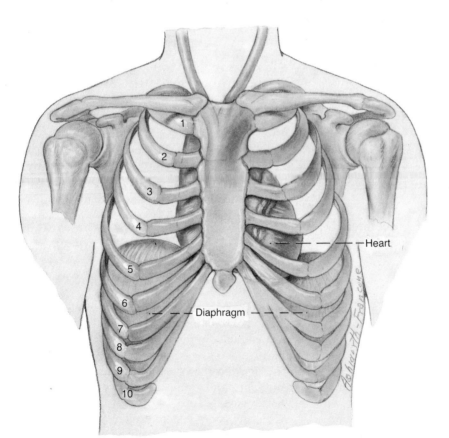

Figure 9–1 Relationship of the heart and diaphragm to the rib cage.

the lymph vessels. The lymphatic system has no pump corresponding to the heart in the blood system.

In the first part of this chapter we will consider the blood circulating system, which we shall refer to as the circulatory system unless otherwise specified. In the latter part of the chapter the lymphatic system will be considered.

THE HEART

What Is the Heart?

The heart is the pump of the circulatory system. It is a four-chambered muscular organ lying in the thoracic cavity between the two lungs (Fig. 9–1). The structures of the heart include the *pericardium* (*peri* means "around," and *cardium* means "heart"), the wall surrounding the heart; the *valves* associated with the chambers; and the *cardiac arteries* and *veins* that supply blood to the heart tissue.

The pericardium is a saclike structure surrounding and supporting the heart. It consists of two layers, an external fibrous layer called the *parietal* (pah-ri'e-tal) *pericardium,* and an inner serous (from Latin, meaning water) layer, which adheres to the heart and becomes its outer layer, called the

visceral (vis'er-al) *pericardium* (also called the epicardium (*epi* = upon, *cardium* = heart). Serous fluid found between these two layers lubricates the two membranes with every beat of the heart as their surfaces glide over each other (Fig. 9–2).

The wall of the heart consists of three distinct layers — the epicardium (external layer), the myocardium (middle layer), and the endocardium (inner layer). The *epicardium* (visceral pericardium) is a serous layer containing some connective tissue and stored fats. The *myocardium* (from Greek, *mys* = muscle; *cardium* = heart) is the muscular layer of the heart and consists of interlacing bundles of cardiac muscle fibers. This layer is responsible for the ability of the heart to contract. The *endocardium* (*endo* = internal, *cardium* = heart) lines the cavities of the heart, covers the valves, and is continuous with the lining membrane of the large blood vessels; that is, it is one continuous internal lining of the heart and major vessels.

What Are the Four Chambers of the Heart?

The heart is divided into right and left halves by a lengthwise *septum* (Latin for wall or partition) or wall of tissue. Each half is subdivided into two chambers. The upper chambers on each side are called the *atria* (a'tre-ah), singular *atrium* (Latin for

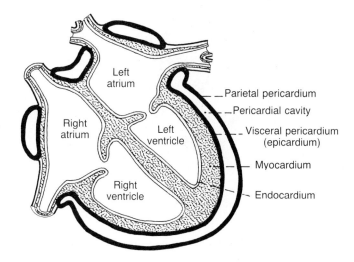

Figure 9–2 Heart wall and pericardium. (Note the thickened left ventricular wall.)

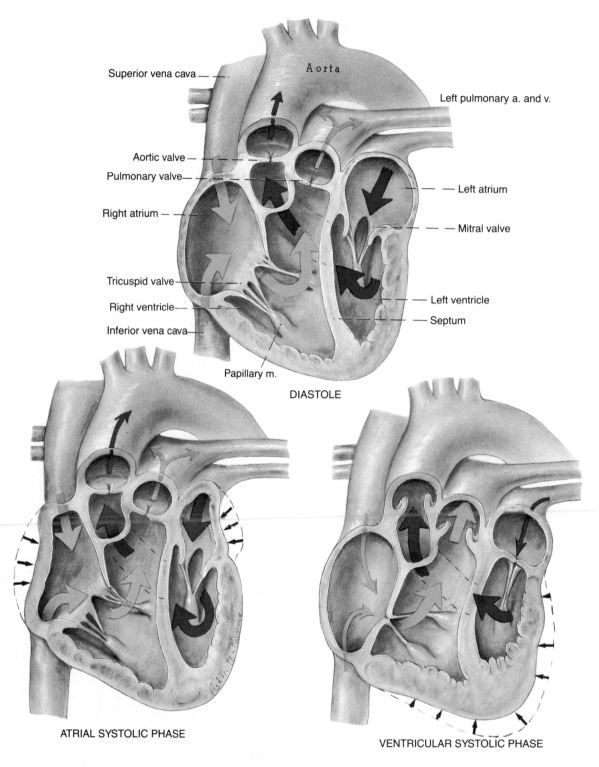

Figure 9-3 Phases of the cardiac cycle. The size of the arrows indicates the volume of blood flow.

entrance hall), and the larger, lower chambers are called the *ventricles* (from the Latin for belly or cavity). Figure 9–3 shows the four chambers and the phases of the cardiac cycle.

The atria serve as receiving chambers for blood from the various parts of the body and pump blood into the ventricles. Since the distance the atria pump their blood is short (into the adjoining ventricles), they are less muscular. The *right atrium* is a thin-walled chamber that receives blood from all parts of the body except the lungs. Three large veins empty into the right atrium: the *superior vena cava,* bringing venous blood from the lower portion of the body; the *inferior vena cava,* bringing venous blood from the lower portion of the body; and the *coronary sinus,* draining blood from the heart itself. The right atrium pumps the deoxygenated (bluish) venous blood into the right ventricle.

The *right ventricle* is a thick-walled, muscular chamber that pumps the blood, received from the right atrium, out of the heart through the *pulmonary* (from Latin for lung) *artery* into the lungs. This chamber must be very powerful to push the blood through the thousands of capillaries in the lungs and back to the left atrial chamber of the heart.

The *left atrium* receives the now oxygenated (bright red) blood from the lungs through the four *pulmonary veins.* From this receiving chamber the blood is then pumped into the left ventricle.

The *left ventricle* is the most muscular chamber. Its walls are three times as thick as those of the right ventricle. This powerful pumping chamber forces the oxygenated blood out through the *aorta* to all parts (upper and lower portions) of the body except the lungs. The blood returns to the heart at the left atrium.

What Are the Valves? What Is Their Function?

The four heart valves are membranous structures designed to prevent *backflow* (in the wrong direction) of blood during the heart's pumping cycle. There are two types of valves: the atrioventricular valves and the semilunar valves.

The *atrioventricular* (a"tre-o-ven-trik'u-lar) *valves* are thin, leaflike structures between the atria and ventricles. They prevent backflow from the ventricles to the atria during the period when the ventricles are pumping (contracting). Between the right atrium and the right ventricle is the *tricuspid* (*tri* = three, *cuspid* = cusps) *valve,* so called because it consists of three irregularly shaped flaps (or cusps) formed mainly of fibrous tissue. The opening between the left atrium and the left ventricle is

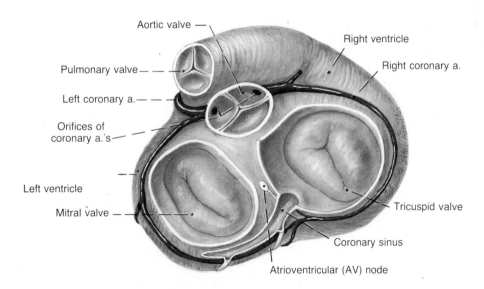

Aortic valve —
Pulmonary valve— —
Left coronary a.— —
Orifices of coronary a.'s—
Left ventricle
Mitral valve — —
Right ventricle
Right coronary a.
Tricuspid valve
Coronary sinus
Atrioventricular (AV) node

Figure 9–4 A view of the heart from above, showing the valves, coronary arteries, and sinus.

guarded by the *mitral* or *bicuspid valve,* so named because it consists of two flaps. The bicuspid valve is stronger and thicker, since the left ventricle is a more powerful pump (Fig. 9–4).

Blood is propelled through the tricuspid and bicuspid valves when the atria contract. When the ventricles contract, the valves close, resisting any pressure of the blood that might force them open into the atria.

The *semilunar (semi* means half, *lunar* means moon) *valves* are pocketlike structures attached at the points at which the pulmonary artery and aorta leave the ventricles. The *pulmonary valve* guards the opening between the right ventricle and the pulmonary artery (which leads to the lung). The *aortic valve* guards the opening between the left ventricle and the aorta. Figure 9–5 is a radiograph showing implanted artificial valves.

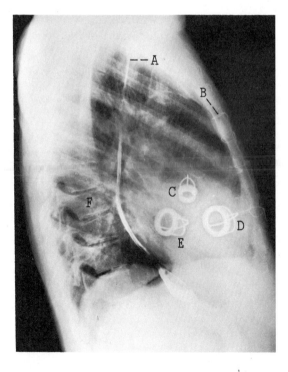

Figure 9–5 Three artificial valves implanted in a patient's heart by Dr. A. Starr of the University of Oregon Medical School. *A,* esophagus; *B,* wire sutures in sternum; *C,* aortic valve; *D,* tricuspid valve; *E,* mitral valve; and *F,* vertebral column.

What Causes the Valves to Open and Close?

When electrical impulses spread through the ventricular muscle of the lower heart, the two ventricles contract at the same time. This contraction of the ventricle is referred to as *ventricular systole* (sis'to-le); the term "systole" is from the Greek word meaning a contracting. This results in a rise in the ventricular pressure—the pressure inside the ventricular chambers. When ventricular pressure exceeds atrial pressure, the atrioventricular valves (tricuspid and bicuspid) are forced shut.

When the ventricular pressure builds up to exceed the pressure in the pulmonary artery and the aorta, the semilunar (pulmonary and aortic) valves open.

The period of ventricular contraction is followed by relaxation of the ventricular muscle and an abrupt fall in the ventricular blood pressure. When ventricular pressure falls below pulmonary (artery) and aortic pressure, the pulmonary and aortic valves are forced shut, preventing backflow. Further relaxation of the ventricles follows, resulting in a drop of ventricular pressure below that of atrial pressure. At this point the atrioventricular valves open, and the ventricles begin filling again as the atria contracts.

In short, the heart valves open and close as the pressure of the blood on either side of the valves changes. And this pressure difference is primarily due to the action of the powerful ventricles.

What Produces the Heart Sounds?

The characteristic heart sounds are caused by the sudden deceleration of the blood when the heart valves close. The first sound occurs when the tricuspid and bicuspid valves close. It has a characteristic dull quality and low pitch and has been described classically by the syllable "lubb." The second heart sound is produced when the pulmonary and aortic valves close. It is described by the syllable "dupp" and is of a snapping quality. The first heart sound is followed after a short pause by the second. A pause about two times longer comes between the second sound and the beginning of the next cycle. The opening of the valves is silent.

What Are the Elements of the Heart's Electrical Stimulating System?

Specialized sections of the myocardium initiate the sequence of events in the cardiac cycle and control the cycle's regularity. The *sinoatrial* (si"no-a'tre-al) *node* (SA node) is located in the wall of the right atrium. Its regular rate of electrical (electrochemical) discharge sets the rhythm of contraction for the entire heart, and for this reason it is known as the *pacemaker.*

The atrioventricular node (AV node), located in the lower right wall (septum) between the atria, conducts the electrochemical impulses set up by the SA node to the *bundle of His,* named after its discoverer, Wilhelm His, Jr. The bundle of His conducts the electrochemical impulses from the AV node to the ventricles and activates depolarization—an electrochemical process that causes the cardiac muscle fibers to contract (Figs. 9–6 and 9–7).

What is the Cardiac Rate and Rhythm?

The normal heart *rate* is 60 to 100 beats per minute at regular rhythmic intervals. *Tachycardia* (tak"e-kar'de-ah) is a condition characterized by a rhythmic beat at a rate of over 100 per minute; the term tachycardia is from the Greek, *tachys,* meaning quick, and *cardia* = heart. This occurs because the sinoatrial (SA) node is stimulated to set the pace at an increased rate. It can follow exercise or emotional disturbances, or it can result from disease. When the sinoatrial node has a rate of less than 60 beats per minute, *bradycardia (brady* = slow, *cardia* = heart) is present. This rate may be normal in some individuals, particularly in well-conditioned athletes.

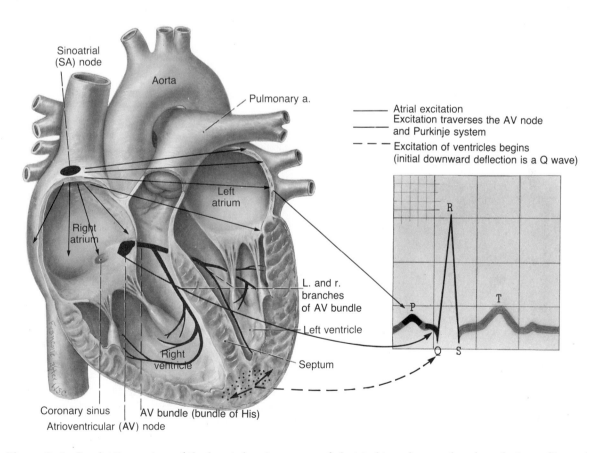

Figure 9–6 Conducting system of the heart showing source of electrical impulses produced on electrocardiogram.

ELECTROCARDIOGRAM

The wave of excitation spreading through the heart wall is accompanied by electrical changes.
The record of these changes is an ELECTROCARDIOGRAM (ECG)

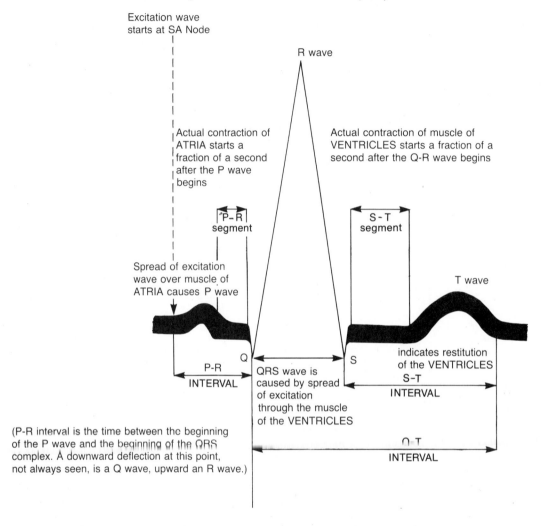

Excitation wave
starts at SA Node

R wave

Actual contraction of
ATRIA starts a
fraction of a second
after the P wave
begins

Actual contraction of muscle of
VENTRICLES starts a fraction of a
second after the Q-R wave begins

P-R
segment

S-T
segment

Spread of excitation
wave over muscle of
ATRIA causes P wave

T wave

Q

P-R
INTERVAL

S

QRS wave is
caused by spread
of excitation
through the muscle
of the VENTRICLES

indicates restitution
of the VENTRICLES
S-T
INTERVAL

(P-R interval is the time between the beginning
of the P wave and the beginning of the QRS
complex. A downward deflection at this point,
not always seen, is a Q wave, upward an R wave.)

Q-T
INTERVAL

Figure 9–7 Electrocardiogram.

What Factors Determine Cardiac Output?

Cardiac output is the volume of blood pumped by the heart over a given interval, usually calculated for a minute; that is, the number of beats per minute times the average volume, or the sum total of the volumes of all the beats in a minute. Under normal resting conditions, cardiac output approximates *4 to 5 liters per minute* — an amazing fact considering the total blood volume of an average man is only 5 to 6 liters. The average volume of blood ejected by each beat of the heart is 60 to 70 millimeters; this is referred to as the *stroke volume*.

The cardiac output over a specific period depends on several factors, including the volume of the venous blood returning to the heart, the number of beats per minute, and the force of each contraction.

Venous Return Cardiac output increases with an increase in venous return. Venous return is influenced by the following factors: contraction of skeletal muscles squeezing the associated veins and forcing the blood to move and an increase in arterial or capillary blood pressure. With decreased blood, as in hemorrhage, venous return is lowered, and consequently cardiac output tends to decrease.

Heart Rate Frequency of heart beat influences cardiac output. However, even with a constant heart rate, an increased venous return will increase cardiac output. In order to accomplish this the heart must work harder, pumping a greater volume with each stroke.

Force of Contraction The force or power of each cardiac contraction depends, interestingly, on the initial length of the cardiac muscle fibers. *Starling's Law of the Heart* states that "the energy of contraction is proportional to the initial length of the cardiac muscle fiber." As venous return increases, it tends to expand the heart. This increases the strength of contraction, producing an increased output without any change in rate.

The heart could handle increased venous return by speeding up, but it seems to prefer to be stretched and contract harder instead. During exercise and periods of excitement, both mechanisms operate; that is, there are more beats and stronger and bigger (more voluminous) contractions.

THE BLOOD VESSELS

What Are the Three Kinds of Blood Vessels?

There are three kinds of blood vessels: the arteries, the capillaries, and the veins.

Arteries The arteries (from the Greek word for pipe) carry oxygenated blood away from the heart. They are thicker than the other vessels and are composed of three layers of tissue, the most functional of which is made up of smooth muscle fibers and elastic connective tissue. The inner layer is made up of *epithelial* tissue, which is continuous through all the vessels and the heart (endocardium). The largest artery in the body is the *aorta,* which leaves from the powerful left ventricle of the heart. Slightly smaller arteries branch off the aorta, and still smaller arteries branch off these. The smallest arteries are called *arterioles,* and they pass the blood into the tiny capillaries (Figs. 9–8 and 9–9).

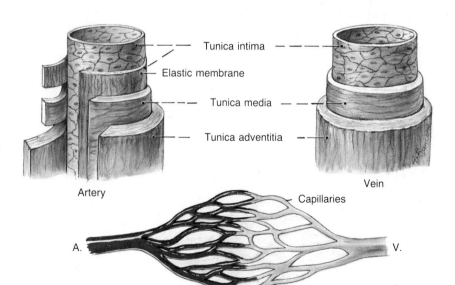

Figure 9–8 Component parts of arteries and veins.

Tunica intima

Elastic membrane

Tunica media

Tunica adventitia

Artery

Vein

Capillaries

A.

V.

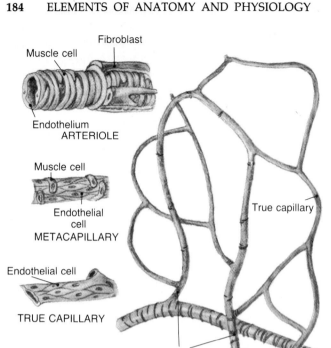

Figure 9-9 Diagrammatic representation of a portion of a capillary bed typical of many tissues. Blood flows into the bed through an arteriole and out through a venule. Connecting the arteriole and venule is a metacapillary, from which blood flows into true capillaries. Precapillary sphincters regulate the flow of blood from the metacapillary into the true capillaries.

Capillaries   There are literally thousands of miles of tiny capillaries supplying the tissues of the body; if all of them were laid end to end, they would form a tube 62,000 miles long. The term "capillary" is derived from the Latin word for hair, indicating their thinness; however, capillaries are actually several times thinner than a human hair and can be seen only through a microscope. The wall of a capillary is only one layer of *epithelial cells* thick, and most capillaries are just large enough in diameter to allow cells of blood to pass through in single file. The exchange of waste products for oxygen and nutrients is constantly occurring between the blood and the tissue spaces through the thin walls of the capillaries. The capillaries are, in this sense, the secret of the success that the circulatory system has in linking the individual cells to the major homeostatic organs (lungs, digestive system, kidneys). At the ends of the capillary beds, the deoxygenated blood flows into the smallest veins, the *venules* (ven'uls).

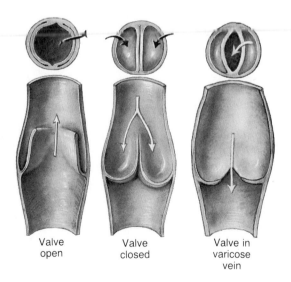

| Valve open | Valve closed | Valve in varicose vein |

Figure 9-10 Veins contain bicuspid valves that open in the direction of blood flow but prevent regurgitation of flow when pockets become filled and distended.

Veins The venules empty blood into veins, and these in turn drain into still larger veins. The veins (Latin for vines), like the arteries, are composed of three layers, but they are thin walled and less muscular than the arteries. The veins also contain small *valves* along their length to prevent *backflow* of blood during periods when the blood pressure changes (Fig. 9 – 10). If the valves break down, *varicose* (var'i-kos) *veins* result; "varicose" is Latin for dilated vein.

CIRCULATION

What Are the Three Main Circuits of the Circulatory System?

The term "circulation" comes from the Latin word *circulatio*, referring to movements in a circle or through a circular course. The overall circulatory

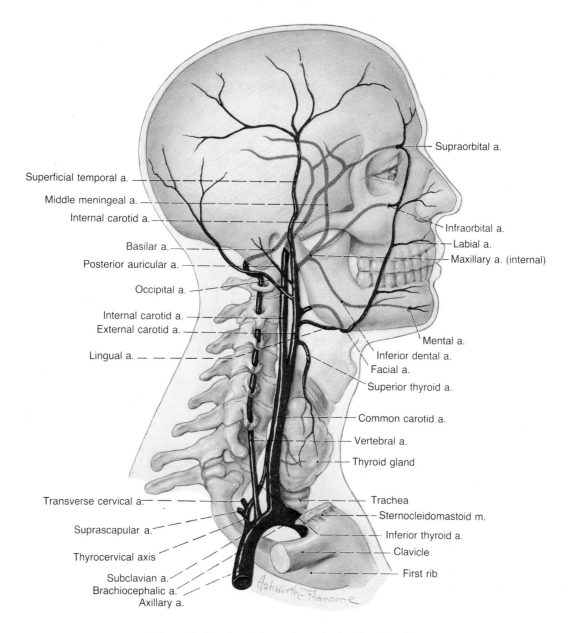

Figure 9–11 Arterial supply to the head and neck.

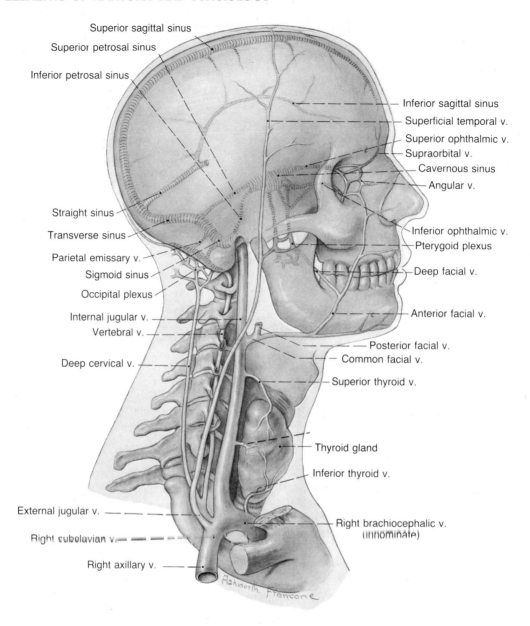

Superior sagittal sinus
Superior petrosal sinus
Inferior petrosal sinus
Inferior sagittal sinus
Superficial temporal v.
Superior ophthalmic v.
Supraorbital v.
Cavernous sinus
Angular v.
Straight sinus
Transverse sinus
Parietal emissary v.
Sigmoid sinus
Occipital plexus
Internal jugular v.
Vertebral v.
Deep cervical v.
Inferior ophthalmic v.
Pterygoid plexus
Deep facial v.
Anterior facial v.
Posterior facial v.
Common facial v.
Superior thyroid v.
Thyroid gland
Inferior thyroid v.
External jugular v.
Right subclavian v.
Right axillary v.
Right brachiocephalic v. (innominate)

Figure 9–12 Venous drainage of the head and neck.

system can be studied in terms of three smaller, interrelated flow circuits: the pulmonary system, the systemic system, and the portal system (Figs. 9–11 to 9–22).

Pulmonary Flow The pulmonary system carries blood from the heart to the lungs and back to the heart again; more specifically, the blood travels

from the right ventricle through the *pulmonary artery* to the lungs. Upon entering the lungs the pulmonary arteries quickly branch down to capillaries, which surround the air sacs (alveoli), exchanging oxygen and carbon dioxide. Gradually, the capillaries reunite, taking on the characteristics of veins. The veins join to form the *pulmonary veins*, which carry oxygenated blood from the lungs to the left

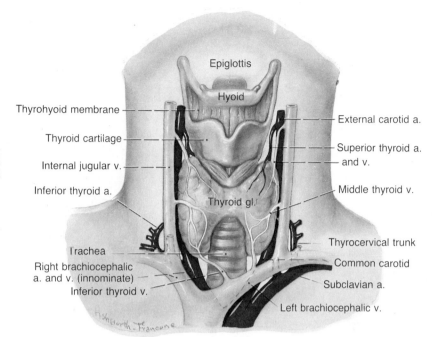

Figure 9–13 Arterial supply and venous drainage of the thyroid gland.

atrium. Figure 9–23 shows the relationship between the systemic and pulmonary circuits.

Systemic Flow The systemic (sis-tem'ik) circulation is the main flow circuit, as its name implies. It carries the oxygenated blood from the heart to all areas of the body except the lungs, and then back again to the heart. All systemic arteries spring from the *aorta*. The veins of the systemic circulation flow into either the inferior vena cava or the superior vena cava, which in turn empties into the right atrium.

Portal Flow The portal (Latin for gate) system is really part of the systemic circulation but is distinguished by the fact that blood from the spleen, stomach, pancreas, and intestines first passes through and branches out into the liver before going on to the heart. The liver then receives blood from two major vessels, the *hepatic* (Greek for liver) *artery* (20 per cent) and the *portal vein* (80 per cent). The hepatic (he-pat'ik) artery supplies the liver with the necessary oxygenated blood. The blood from the intestinal tract, which is rich in newly absorbed nutrient substances, passes into the liver through the portal veins. The liver cells are very active in taking up nutrients from the portal blood after a meal. The blood leaving the liver flows through the hepatic vein, which empties into the inferior vena cava.

BLOOD PRESSURE

What Is Blood Pressure?

Blood pressure is the pressure exerted by the blood against the walls of the vessels as it is forced through the circulatory system. The term applies properly to arterial, capillary, and venous pressure.

Most commonly the expression "blood pressure" refers to the pressure existing in the large arteries — usually the *brachial* (bra'ke-al) *artery*, just above the elbow, where external measurement is relatively easy. The blood pressure is highest in the brachial artery at the time of contraction of the ventricles — ventricular systole (recall systole means contraction). This level is known as *systolic* (sis-tol'ik) *pressure*. Pressure during ventricular *diastole* (Greek for dilation or relaxation) is called *diastolic* (di"ah-stol'ik) *pressure*. Blood pressure is usu-

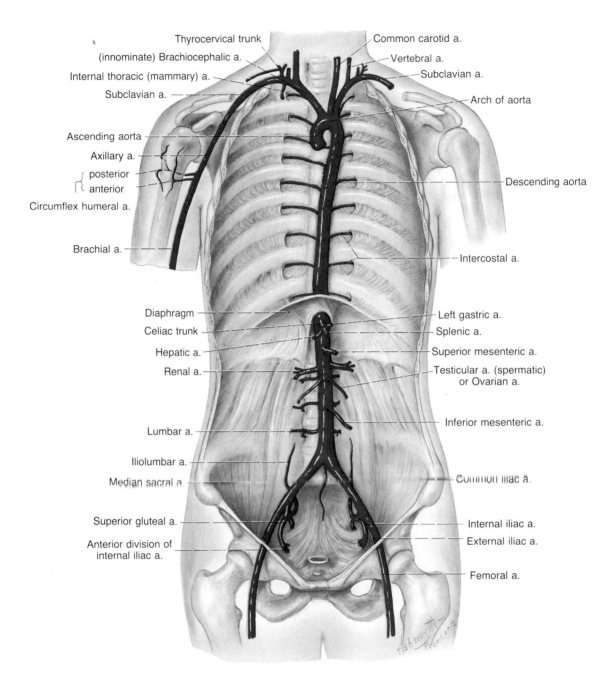

Figure 9–14 The aorta and its major branches.

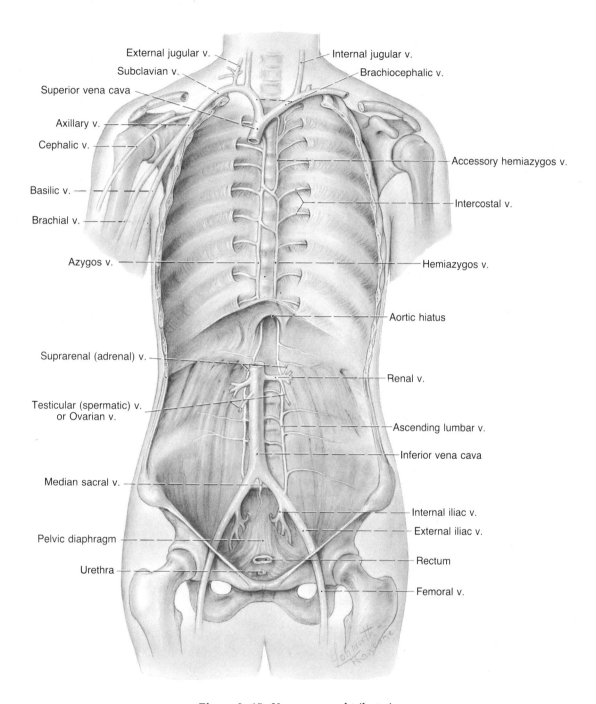

Figure 9-15 Vena cava and tributaries.

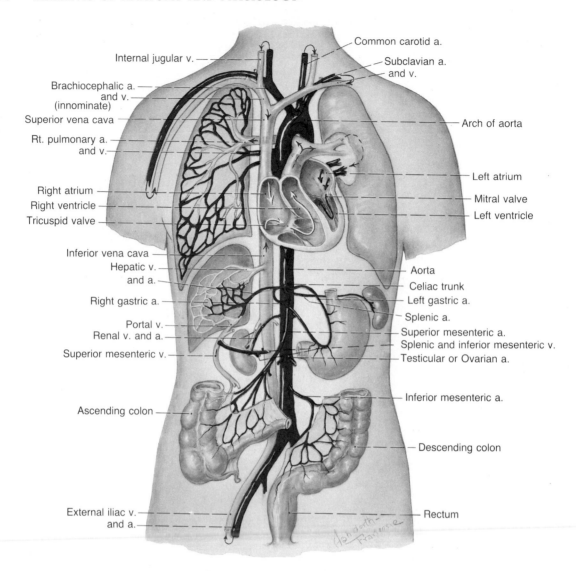

Figure 9–16 Arterial supply and venous drainage of organs.

ally expressed as a fraction: for example, 120/80, in which 120 represents systolic pressure and in which 80 represents diastolic pressure. The units are in terms of millimeters of mercury, abbreviated as mm Hg.

The blood pressure decreases as the blood passes from the aorta into the arteries to the arterioles and capillaries and venules and veins, until finally, at the left atrium when it enters the heart, the blood pressure is close to zero (Fig. 9–24).

What Is a Normal Blood Pressure?

Blood pressure is subject to fluctuations. In general, the healthy individual has a systolic pressure of 100 to 120 mm Hg and a diastolic pressure of 60 to 80 mm Hg. Variations in systolic blood pressure are expected in normal persons. Exercise may cause a rise in systolic pressure.

A blood pressure difference of 10 to 15 mm Hg

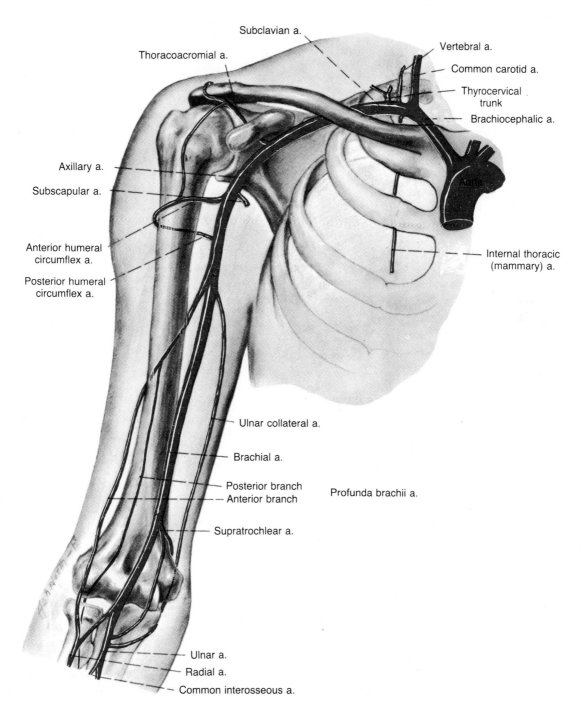

Figure 9-17 Arteries of the right shoulder and upper arm.

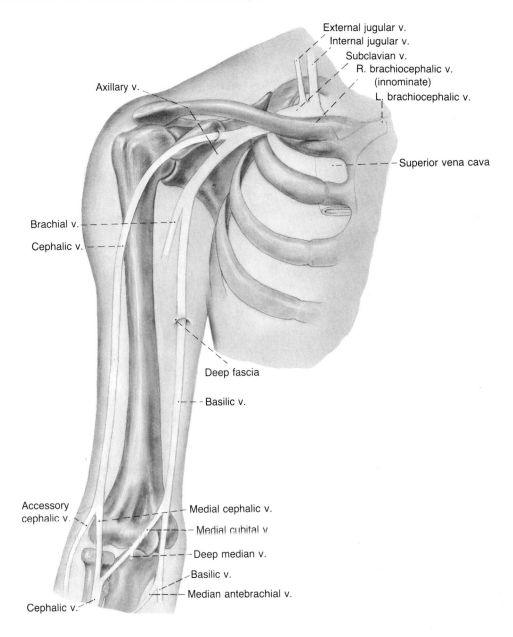

Figure 9-18 Veins of the right shoulder and upper arm. The basilic vein pierces the deep fascia in the region of the middle of the arm.

often exists between the two arms of an individual. The higher pressure is usually found in the right arm. A pressure difference greater than 10 to 15 mm Hg should arouse suspicion, since it might be the result of a congenital (from the Latin word meaning born with) narrowing of the aorta between the beginnings of the right and left subclavian arteries. This narrowing condition is known as a *coarctation* (ko"ark-ta'shun), from the Latin word meaning to press together.

The upper limits of normal blood pressure are usually defined as 140 mm Hg systolic and 90 mm Hg diastolic. Pressures above this level (hypertension) shorten life expectancy.

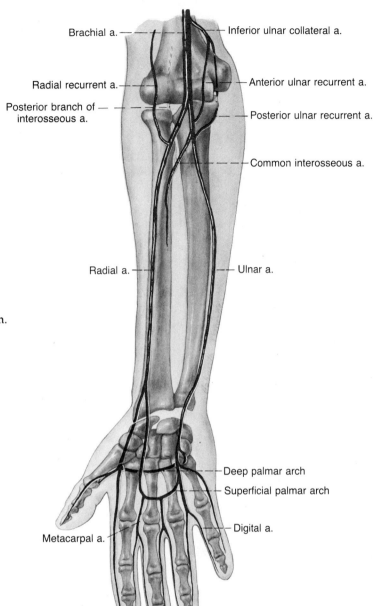

Brachial a.

Inferior ulnar collateral a.

Radial recurrent a.

Anterior ulnar recurrent a.

Posterior branch of interosseous a.

Posterior ulnar recurrent a.

Common interosseous a.

Radial a.

Ulnar a.

Deep palmar arch

Superficial palmar arch

Digital a.

Metacarpal a.

Figure 9-19 Arteries of the right lower arm.

What Are the Factors That Influence Blood Pressure?

The blood pressure is influenced by a number of factors. Normal regulation is the responsibility of the nervous system and, somewhat independently, the heart.

The nervous system can bring about rapid changes in blood pressure and blood flow by stimulating the muscular contraction of the blood vessels, particularly the arterioles. When the vessels constrict they become smaller in diameter, and this causes the blood pressure to increase. The *vasomotor* (*vaso* means vessel, *motor* indicates an activating center) *center* in the medulla of the brain is the area

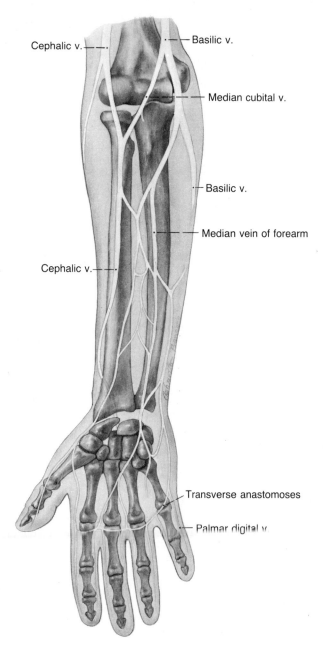

Figure 9-20 Venous drainage of the right forearm and hand.

that activates vessel constriction. It is also capable of influencing heart rate and strength of contraction. However, the heart itself can affect blood pressure by increasing its rate and strength of contraction, and this seems to occur independently of the vasomotor center activity.

The vasomotor center receives sensory signals from a number of sources that influence its regulatory action on the blood pressure. The *baroreceptors* (pressure sensitive receptors) located in the large arteries monitor blood pressure for the vasomotor center. The baroreceptors are sensitive to the stretching of the artery walls caused by changes in blood pressure inside the arteries. Other receptors, *chemoreceptors,* are sensitive to the concentrations of various substances in the blood, such as oxygen, carbon dioxide, and pH (acid content). If carbon dioxide concentration becomes too high, this will cause the vasomotor center to increase cardiac output and blood pressure, which serves, along with an increased respiration, to accelerate carbon dioxide release in the lungs.

CLINICAL CONSIDERATIONS OF THE BLOOD CIRCULATORY SYSTEM

What Is Shock?

Shock is an impairment (disorder) of the circulation resulting from stress or injury; the damage reduces the output of blood from the heart to a level below that needed for normal cellular function. Another way to characterize the condition is as a loss of effective circulating volume in the heart and vessels, leading to a sort of circulatory panic. The symptoms of shock are apprehension, cold skin, reduced blood pressure, shallow respiratory activity, sweating, and rapid pulse.

What Conditions May Lead to Shock?

A reduction of blood volume frequently produces shock. A loss of over 40 per cent of the blood volume causes collapse of the arteries. This condition frequently does not respond to blood transfusions and is sometimes referred to as "irreversible shock." Sudden losses of small quantities of blood can produce consequences more serious than slow losses of larger volumes. Massive injury to the heart (as in heart attack) leading to an inadequate cardiac output is an important cause of shock.

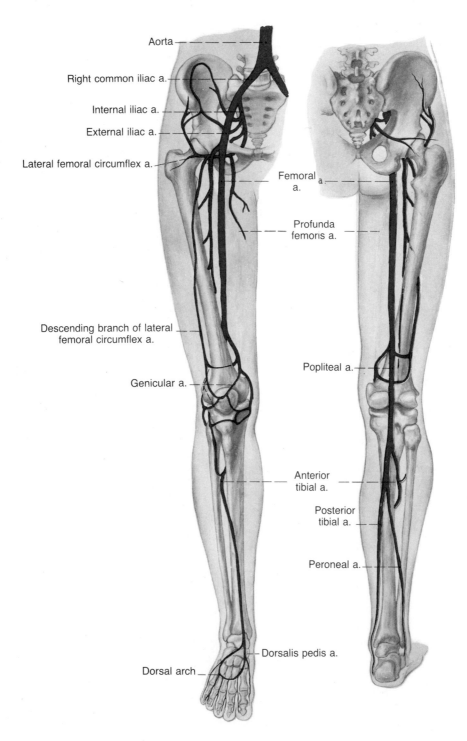

Aorta

Right common iliac a.

Internal iliac a.

External iliac a.

Lateral femoral circumflex a.

Femoral a.

Profunda femoris a.

Descending branch of lateral femoral circumflex a.

Genicular a.

Popliteal a.

Anterior tibial a.

Posterior tibial a.

Peroneal a.

Dorsalis pedis a.

Dorsal arch

Figure 9–21 Arteries of the right pelvis and leg.

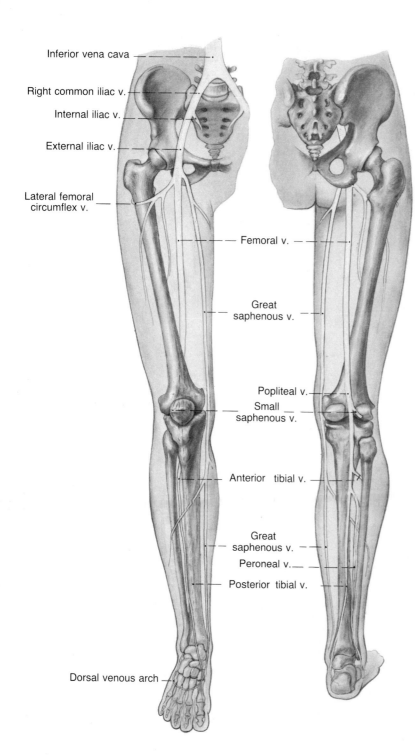

Inferior vena cava

Right common iliac v.

Internal iliac v.

External iliac v.

Lateral femoral
circumflex v.

Femoral v.

Great
saphenous v.

Popliteal v.

Small
saphenous v.

Anterior tibial v.

Great
saphenous v.

Peroneal v.

Posterior tibial v.

Dorsal venous arch

Figure 9–22 Veins of the right pelvis and leg.

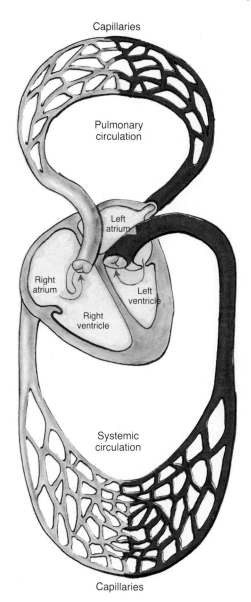

Capillaries

Pulmonary
circulation

Left
atrium

Right
atrium

Left
ventricle

Right
ventricle

Systemic
circulation

Capillaries

Figure 9-23 Schematic drawing showing relationship between systemic and pulmonary circulatory circuits. Observe that in this drawing of the pulmonary circuit the veins are colored red and the arteries gray to denote the higher level of oxygenation of the blood in the pulmonary veins.

the capillary walls, actual plasma loss, and, popularly, the pooling of blood in the peripheral capillary beds.

What Is Arteriosclerosis?

Arteriosclerosis (ar-te″re-o-skle-ro′sis) is a condition characterized by a depositing of material, called plaque (plak), on the walls of the arteries, especially at the junctions. The disease frequently leads to a progressive blockage of blood vessels. Occasionally, part of the deposit will break off and rapidly block a vessel (Fig. 9 – 25). This can produce an acute coronary or a cerebral seizure, if the blocked vessel is in the heart or brain, respectively.

Excessive fat in the diet can be an important factor leading to arteriosclerosis, although the disease also seems to run in families. This disease is the number one medical problem in the United States.

Why Take the Pulse?

The pulsation felt when the fingertips are placed over an artery close to the body surface is generally referred to as simply the *pulse.* Pulse rate corresponds to heart rate, one pulse for every ventricular systole (Fig. 9 – 26).

The pulse is described according to several characteristics: *rate,* fast or slow; *size,* large or small; *type of wave,* abrupt or prolonged; and *rhythm,* regular or irregular. An increase in pulse rate is normal during and after exercise and after eating. It is decreased during sleep. In most diseases associated with fever the pulse rate is increased, usually at an average of five beats for every degree Fahrenheit. An increased pulse rate is usually present in severe anemias, and pulse rate become markedly increased after severe hemorrhage.

What Are Two Forms of Heart Disease?

If the myocardium receives an inadequate oxygen supply, it cannot function properly. A primary sign of this inadequate supply is a peculiar, severe type of chest pain called *angina pectoris.* Angina pectoris is relieved by rest or the administration of

In the absence of hemorrhage or actual damage to the heart, the reason for loss of effective circulating volume — typical of shock — is not clearly understood. Three widely held views that attempt to explain this blood loss are increased permeability of

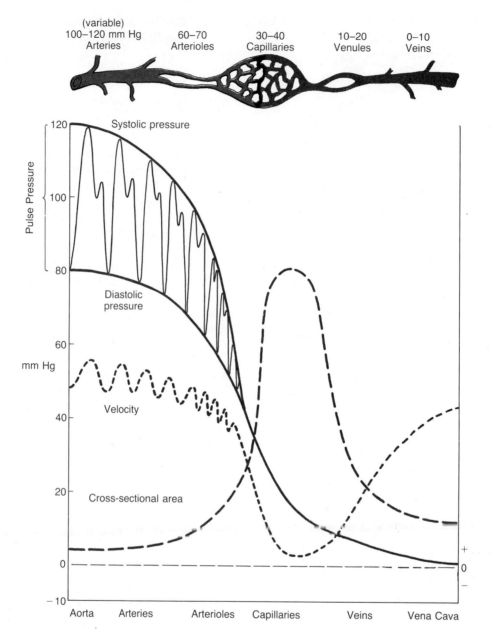

Figure 9–24 Blood pressure, blood velocity, and cross-sectional area of the vascular tree in various segments of the circulatory system. (Modified from Zoethout and Tuttle: *Textbook of Physiology*, 12th ed. St. Louis, C. V. Mosby Co., 1955.)

nitrites. Attacks of angina pectoris are usually precipitated by exertion or emotional tension. The pain, frequently described as a feeling of tightness, pressure, aching, or heaviness below the sternum, may radiate to the left shoulder and arm and neck. The pain is of short duration, usually lasting 3 to 5 minutes.

The pain of *myocardial infarction* (from the Latin for disorder) causes more prolonged chest pain than angina pectoris. In this case, there is actual blockage

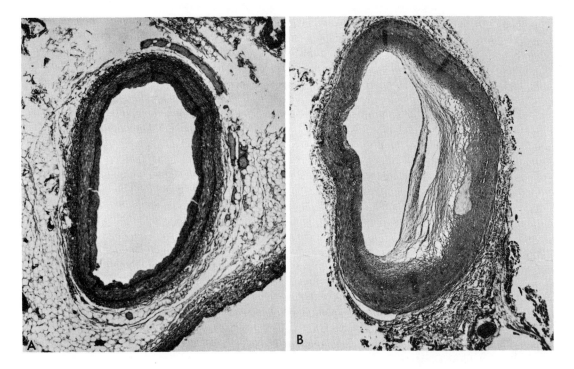

Figure 9-25 These photomicrographs show *(A)* a normal artery seen in cross section and *(B)* a diseased artery in which the channel is partially occluded by atherosclerosis. (By permission of David M. Spain, M.D.; previously published in Scientific American, August 1966.)

of some part of the arterial supply to the myocardium, resulting in death of a portion of the heart muscle.

THE LYMPHATIC SYSTEM

What Is the Lymphatic System?

The lymphatic system is made up of a network of vessels, beginning with *lymphatic capillaries,* which lead into larger and larger lymphatic vessels. This network of vessels drains and filters tissue fluid, which is then returned to the blood stream. Tissue fluid in the lymphatic vessels is called *lymph.* The term "lymph" is from the Latin word *lympha,* meaning clear spring water. The larger lymphatic vessels have valves that permit lymph to flow in only one direction. All lymph vessels are directed toward the thoracic cavity. They converge into either the *right lymphatic duct* or the *thoracic (left lymphatic) duct.* Both ducts empty into large veins in the upper chest area (Fig. 9-27).

What Are Lymph Nodes?

Lymph nodes are small, oval bodies found at intervals in the course of the lymphatic vessels (Fig 9-28).

Lymph passes through several groups of nodes before entering the blood. Within the nodes, the lymph is filtered and receives lymphocytes, globulin, and antibodies, which are manufactured by the specialized tissue of the lymph node. Lymph nodes serve as efficient filters for red blood cells and bacteria but are ineffective barriers against viruses. Lymph enters the nodes through several channels and leaves through one or two channels.

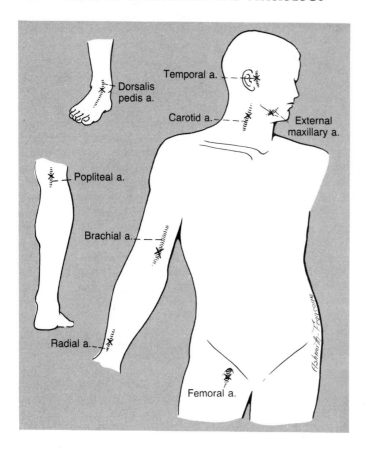

Dorsalis pedis a.

Temporal a.

Carotid a.

External maxillary a.

Popliteal a.

Brachial a.

Radial a.

Femoral a.

Figure 9–26 The pulse is readily distinguished at any of the indicated pressure points.

Where Are the Lymph Nodes Located?

Lymph nodes usually appear in groups. The *superficial nodes* are located near the body surface in the neck, armpit, and groin. The *deep nodes* are located in the internal groin area and adjacent to the lumbar vertebrae, at the root of the lungs, attached to the tissue surrounding the small intestines, and in association with the liver (Fig. 9–29).

What Are the Specific Functions of the Lymphatic System?

The most important function of the lymphatic vessel system is that it returns to the blood stream vital substances—chiefly proteins—that have leaked out of the blood capillaries.

Lymph vessels also provide drainage channels into lymph nodes. The lymph nodes themselves have several specific functions. They filter and isolate products resulting from bacterial and nonbacterial inflammation, and prevent these products from entering the general circulation. This process often produces tenderness and swelling in nodes in an infected area. The special tissue of the lymph nodes also produces lymphocytes, globulin, and antibodies and releases them into the blood, where they function in producing immunity to disease.

The intestinal lymph vessels have an additional special function. Lymph is generally a clear (plasmalike) liquid, but lymph from the intestines becomes milky after a meal. The milky appearance results from the presence of minute fat globules collected from the digestive tract. The lymphatic system distributes these fat globules to the tissues where they are stored, occasionally in excessive amounts.

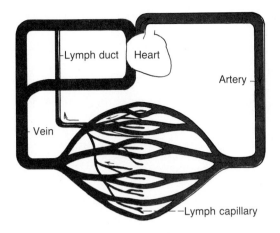

Figure 9-27 Diagrammatic representation of lymphatic system showing its relationship to the circulatory system.

THREE ACCESSORY ORGANS (IMMUNE RESPONSE)

What Are the Tonsils?

Several groups of *tonsils,* forming a ring of lymphatic tissue, guard the entrance to the digestive and respiratory tracts from bacterial invasion (Figs. 9–30 and 9–31).

Chronic infection of the tonsils is not so common as was once suspected. The term "chronic tonsillitis" is frequently misused to indicate any type of sore throat occurring when the tonsils are still present. With tonsillitis, enlargement and tenderness of the anterior lymph nodes in the neck are common. The tonsils may be enlarged and red or covered with pus. If both tonsils and adenoids are infected, the lymph nodes in the posterior triangle of the neck enlarge.

Fewer tonsillectomies (*-ectomy* means removal) and adenoidectomies are being performed today than were done 30 years ago. This is because recent knowledge indicates that removal of tonsils and adenoids may not significantly lower the incidence of upper respiratory infection unless the tonsils themselves have been infected. Tonsils form a protective barrier for the mouth, throat, larynx, trachea, and lungs. They may also be important in the development of immune bodies; however, true recurrent infection of the tonsils is still an indication for their removal by operation.

What Is the Thymus?

The *thymus* is a flat, pinkish-gray, two-lobed organ lying high in the chest under the sternum and in front of the aorta (Fig. 9–32).

This gland is one of the central controls of the

Figure 9-28 Diagrammatic drawing of a lymph node in the area of an infected ulcer.

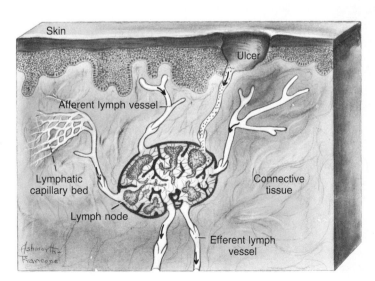

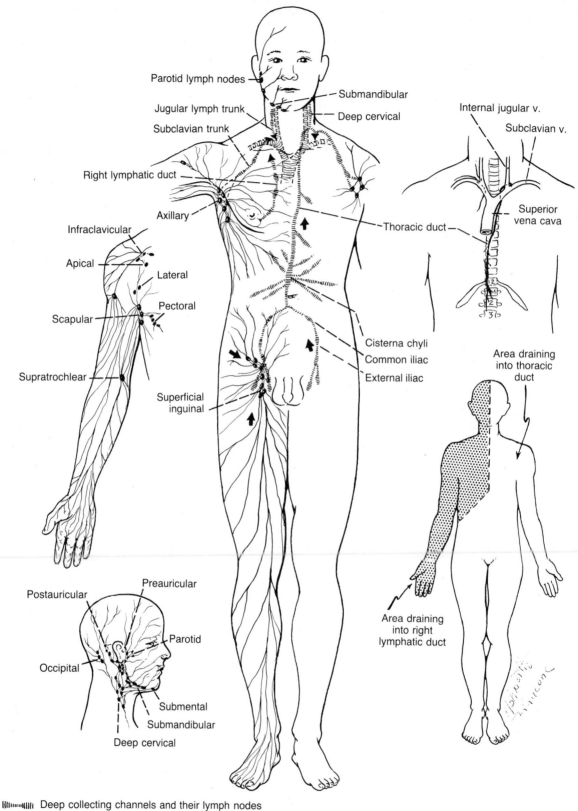

Parotid lymph nodes

Jugular lymph trunk

Subclavian trunk

Right lymphatic duct

Axillary

Infraclavicular

Apical

Scapular

Supratrochlear

Superficial inguinal

Submandibular

Deep cervical

Internal jugular v.

Subclavian v.

Superior vena cava

Thoracic duct

Cisterna chyli

Common iliac

External iliac

Lateral

Pectoral

Area draining into thoracic duct

Area draining into right lymphatic duct

Preauricular

Postauricular

Parotid

Occipital

Submental

Submandibular

Deep cervical

‖⌇⇥⇥‖‖ Deep collecting channels and their lymph nodes

◗━━━ Superficial collecting channels and their lymph nodes

Figure 9–29 The lymphatic system and drainage.

202

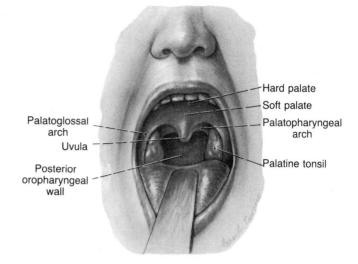

Figure 9–30 Relationship of tongue, uvula, and palatine tonsils.

Hard palate
Soft palate
Palatoglossal arch
Palatopharyngeal arch
Uvula
Palatine tonsil
Posterior oropharyngeal wall

body's immunity system. The term "immunity" derives from the Latin word meaning exempt or free from. If someone is immune to a disease, it means that they have the necessary protective devices to fight the disease easily. Recent evidence indicates that the thymus performs two functions. First, early in life it releases a substance that prepares the lymphatic tissue throughout the body for immune response. Second, the thymus processes lymphocytes, which help to populate the other lymphatic tissues of the body.

It was reported in 1961 that removal of the thymus from an animal just after birth resulted in great impairment of its immunologic responses to antigens in later life, and also impaired its ability to reject skin grafts.

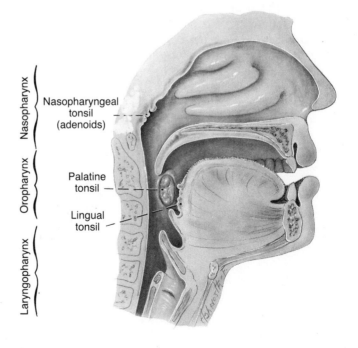

Figure 9–31 The nasopharyngeal tonsil extends from the roof of the nasal pharynx to the free edge of the soft palate; the palatine tonsils are attached to the side walls of the back of the mouth between the anterior and posterior pillars; the lingual tonsils are located on the dorsum of the tongue from the vallate papillae of the tongue to the epiglottis.

Nasopharynx
Oropharynx
Laryngopharynx

Nasopharyngeal tonsil (adenoids)
Palatine tonsil
Lingual tonsil

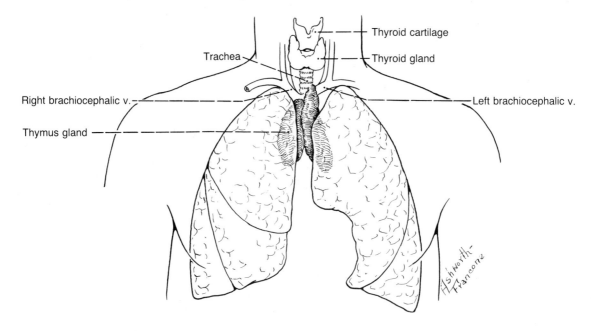

Figure 9-32 Location of thymus gland and relationship to lungs.

What Is the Spleen?

The spleen is a soft, vascular (having many blood vessels), oval body 5 inches long and 3 inches wide, weighing approximately 7 ounces. It lies in the left upper abdomen beneath the diaphragm and behind the lower ribs (Fig. 9-33).

The spleen has five major functions:

1.   Blood Destruction. Old red blood cells, having reached their normal life span of approximately 120 days, are destroyed and digested by special cells located in the spleen.
2.   Blood Production. The spleen exerts an effect on production and release of blood cells from bone marrow.
3.   Immunologic Function. The spleen is a source of production of antibodies and contains a large mass of lymphatic tissue.

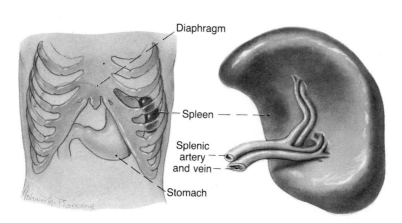

Figure 9-33 The spleen and its relationship to the stomach and rib cage.

4. Blood Storage. The spleen serves as a reservoir for blood. It undergoes rhythmic variations in size in response to physiologic demands such as exercise and hemorrhage and thus influences the volume of circulating blood.

5. Blood Filtration. The spleen serves as one of the body's defense mechanisms by filtering microorganisms from the blood.

SUMMARY

A. The circulatory system is the internal transportation system of the body.
   1. The circulatory system links the other major homeostatic systems: respiratory, digestive, and urinary.
   2. The endocrine system depends on circulation for delivery of hormones.
   3. Infection-fighting processes are also highly dependent on the circulatory system.

B. Strictly speaking, the circulatory system is made up of the blood circulatory system and the lymph circulatory system.

C. The heart is the four-chambered muscular pump of the circulatory system, lying in the thoracic cavity between the lungs.
   1. The pericardium is a saclike structure surrounding and supporting the heart.
   2. The wall of the heart consists of three distinct layers: the epicardium, myocardium, and endocardium.
      a. The epicardium is a serous layer of connective tissue and stored fats.
      b. The myocardium is the muscular layer.
      c. The endocardium is continuous with the inner lining of the cavities and major vessels.

D. The heart is divided into right and left halves by a lengthwise septum, or wall of tissue.
   1. The upper chambers on each side are called the atria.
      a. The left atrium receives blood from the lungs through the pulmonary veins.
      b. The right atrium receives blood from the rest of the body through the superior and inferior vena cava.

2. The more muscular lower chambers on each side are called the ventricles.
   a. The right ventricle pumps blood received from the right atrium through the pulmonary artery to the lungs.
   b. The left ventricle is the most muscular, pumping the oxygenated blood received from the left atrium through the aorta to all parts of the body except the lungs.

E. The four heart valves are membranous structures designed to prevent backflow of the blood.
   1. The atrioventricular valves prevent ventricular to atrial backflow.
   2. The semilunar valves prevent backflow from the pulmonary artery and the aorta.
   3. Heart valves open and close as the pressure of the blood on either side of the valves changes.

F. The characteristic heart sounds are caused by the sudden deceleration of the blood when the heart valves close.
   1. The first dull, low-pitched "lubb" sound occurs when the atrioventricular valves close.
   2. The second, snappy "dupp" sound occurs with closure of the semilunar valves.

G. The heart's electrical stimulating system initiates the sequence of the cardiac cycle and controls its regularity.
   1. The sinoatrial node (SA node), or pacemaker, discharges regularly, setting the rhythm of the heart.
   2. The atrioventricular node (AV node) conducts electrochemical impulses from the SA node to the bundle of His.
   3. The bundle of His conducts the electrochemical impulses from the AV node to the ventricles, activating contraction.

H. Normal cardiac heart rate is 60 to 100 beats per minute.
   1. Tachycardia occurs with a rate over 100 per minute.
   2. Bradycardia is a rate less than 60 per minute.

I. Cardiac output is the volume of blood pumped by the heart in one minute: beats per minute times average volume per beat.
   1. Normal resting cardiac output is 4 to 5 liters/minute.
   2. Cardiac output is affected by volume of

venous blood returning, number of beats per minute, and the force of each contraction.

3. Starling's Law of the Heart states that the "energy of contraction is proportional to the initial length of the cardiac muscle fiber."

J. The electrocardiogram (ECG) is a record of the electrical impulses traversing the heart, initiating the heart's contraction.

K. The three main kinds of blood vessels are the arteries, veins, and capillaries.

1. The arteries carry oxygenated blood away from the heart.
   a. One exception: the pulmonary artery carries deoxygenated blood from the heart to the lungs.
   b. Arteries are thicker than other vessels.
   c. The three layers are made up of smooth muscle, elastic connective tissue, and an inner lining of epithelial tissue.
   d. The largest artery is the aorta, and the smallest arteries are called arterioles.

2. The exchange of wastes for nutrients and oxygen occurs across the walls of the capillaries.
   a. The thin walls are single-layer epithelial tissue.
   b. Capillaries are just large enough in diameter to allow a single file line of blood cells.

3. The veins receive the blood from the capillaries and in turn drain into still larger veins.
   a. The veins have three layers but are thin walled and less muscular.
   b. The largest vein is called the vena cava, and the smallest veins are called venules.
   c. The veins have small valves to prevent backflow.
   d. Varicose veins occur when the valves break down.

L. The overall blood circulatory system consists of three smaller, interrelated flow circuits.

1. The pulmonary flow carries blood from the heart to the lungs and back to the heart again.

2. The systemic flow carries oxygenated blood to all areas except the lungs, and then back again to the heart.

3. The portal flow is distinguished because blood from the spleen, stomach, pancreas, and intestines first passes through and branches out into the liver before going to the heart.

M. Blood pressure is the internal pressure exerted by the blood against the walls of the vessels.

1. Systolic pressure is the blood pressure in the arteries during cardiac systole (norm = 120).

2. Diastolic pressure is the blood pressure in the arteries during cardiac diastole (norm = 80).

3. Normal systolic/diastolic is 120/80.

4. A number of factors affect blood pressure.
   a. Vessel contraction raises the pressure inside.
   b. The heart influences pressure by increasing rate or strength of contraction.
   c. Baroreceptors and chemoreceptors signal the vasomotor portion of the brain that stimulates vessel contraction.

N. Shock is a disorder of the circulatory system characterized by a loss of effective circulating volume.

1. The symptoms of shock include apprehension, cold skin, reduced blood pressure, shallow respiratory activity, sweating, and rapid pulse.

2. Shock may be caused by large losses of blood or by sudden, smaller losses of blood.

3. Shock is also common following massive injury to the heart, as in a heart attack.

4. Shock also occurs in other circumstances, probably as a result of pooling of blood in the peripheral capillaries.

O. Arteriosclerosis involves the deposition of fatty plaque on artery walls and at junctions.

1. The disease leads to a progressive blockage of vessels, leading eventually to acute blockage.

2. Arteriosclerosis (the major medical problem in the United States) is caused by excessive fat in the diet.

3. Angina pectoris is a peculiar type of chest pain due to inadequate oxygen supply to the myocardium.

4. Myocardial infarction involves actual death of a portion of heart muscle.

P. Pulse rate corresponds to heart rate and can be felt with the finger tips as a regular pulsation over an artery close to the body surface.

1. Pulse is characterized by rate, size, type of wave, and rhythm.
2. Pulse rate increases with exercise and after eating.
3. Pulse rate increases in most diseases associated with fever and in injuries involving blood loss.

Q. The lymphatic circulatory system is a network of lymphatic capillaries and larger lymphatic vessels.
   1. This network of vessels drains and filters the lymph, a plasmalike tissue fluid.
   2. All lymph vessels flow toward the thoracic cavity, converging on either the right or left lymphatic ducts.
   3. Both ducts empty into large blood veins in the upper chest.

R. Lymph nodes are small oval bodies that filter the lymph.
   1. They are found at intervals along the lymph vessels.
   2. Lymph passes through several groups of nodes, where it also receives lymphocytes, globulin, and antibodies.
   3. The intestinal lymphatic system also functions to distribute fat globules to the tissues for storage.

S. Groups of tonsils, composed of lymphatic tissue, guard the entrance to the digestive and respiratory tracts from bacterial infection.

T. The thymus is one of the central controls of the body's immune system, stimulating lymphatic tissue and manufacturing lymphocytes (see Chapter 10).

U. The spleen has five major functions: blood destruction, blood production, immunologic function, blood storage, and blood filtration.

REVIEW QUESTIONS

1. Name three other organ systems that rely on the transportation function of the circulatory system to be effective and to reach the individual cells.

2. What are the two main subsystems of the circulatory system? What is the fluid circulated by each?

3. Describe the position of the heart in the thoracic cavity.

4. What is the relation between the visceral pericardium and the epicardium?

5. Construct a diagram of the heart, indicating the layers of the heart wall and the pericardium. Label the four heart chambers and the major vessels that enter and leave them and also show the location of the AV and SA nodes and the semilunar valves.

6. What is the function of the fluid that fills the pericardial sac?

7. What causes the heart valves to open and close?

8. What causes the "lubb" and the "dupp" heart sounds?

9. What is the ECG?

10. Distinguish the pulmonary and systemic circulations. What is the specific function of each?

11. Describe the path taken by a drop of blood entering the right atrium and eventually leaving the left ventricle.

12. What is the pacemaker? The bundle of His?

13. Define tachycardia and bradycardia.

14. Define cardiac output and stroke volume. About how long does it take for the heart to pump an amount of blood equal to the total volume of blood in the body?

15. Name three factors that influence cardiac output over a specific period of time.

16. With increased venous return does the heart prefer to increase its rate or pump greater volume with each stroke?

17. What is the function of the small valves located inside and along the length of the veins? What happens when they break down?

18. Why do the arteries need to be more muscular and elastic than the veins?

19. Describe the structure of the capillary wall and explain how this is functionally important.

20. What are the two exceptions to the rule that arteries carry oxygen-rich blood and veins carry oxygen-poor (carbon dioxide rich) blood?

21. Draw a diagram tracing the portal flow. What is the function of the portal system?

22. Define blood pressure and explain the difference between systolic and diastolic pressure.

23. What is pulse? What does it indicate?

24. What are the two ways in which the heart can

influence blood pressure? What other mechanisms function to alter blood pressure?

25. What is the number one medical problem in the United States?

26. What is angina pectoris? What is myocardial infarction?

27. Name the most general function of the lymphatic vessels and the lymph nodes. What is added to the lymph as it passes through the nodes?

28. Identify three locations of superficial lymph nodes.

29. What additional function is served by the intestinal lymph vessels?

30. What is the function of the tonsils? Where are they located? Why is the frequency of tonsillectomies being questioned?

31. What is the early function of the thymus and its later function? Where is the thymus located?

32. Draw a diagram of the upper body, indicating the approximate size and location of the spleen.

33. Name and briefly characterize the five major functions of the spleen.

T E N

The Immune System

The aim of this chapter is to enable the student to do the following:

- Describe the primary functions of the immune system.

- Identify three classes of phagocytes.

- List the two main types of lymphocytes and their subclasses.

- Explain the origin, processing, and distribution of lymphocytes.

- Define and distinguish humoral immunity and cell-mediated immunity.

- Define antibody and antigen.

- Describe the complement system.

- Explain the need for diversity in the immune system.

- Explain the need for rapid growth in the immune system.

- Define and characterize the following: allergens, urticaria, hay fever, asthma, and anaphylaxis.

- Explain how vaccination prevents disease.

- Define and characterize autoimmunity and transplantation.

- Define and characterize acquired immunodeficiency syndrome (AIDS).

FUNCTIONS AND STRUCTURES OF THE IMMUNE SYSTEM

What Are the Functions of the Immune System?

The primary function of the immune system is to defend the body from attacks by microorganisms. When unfriendly organisms, referred to as pathogens, gain access to the circulatory system or penetrate the body's deeper tissues, it is the task of the immune system to deactivate and remove the invaders. The body's capacity to resist almost all types of organisms or toxins that damage the tissues and organs is called immunity.

The immune system also maintains the integrity, or self-identity, of the body by removing damaged cells and by clearing debris, or foreign materials, from the body's internal environment. Normal body cells are frequently diseased or become damaged from mechanical traumas or exposure to toxic substances. Abnormal cells or their debris may interfere with the harmonious internal workings of the body and must be removed. Damaged cells that are not removed may eventually become cancerous.

What Are the Structures of the Immune System?

The immune system is composed primarily of individual cells and associated circulating protein molecules. In this way the immune system is similar to the circulatory system. The cells of the immune system, however, are warriors serving in the body's protective forces. Some of these immune system cells attack invaders directly, while others produce *antibodies,* the second main component of the immune system. Highly supportive of antibody activity is a group of circulating enzymes referred to as *the complement complex.*

The immune system is organized into three major subsystems: *the phagocytes, lymphocytes,* and *circulating antibodies plus complement.* These subsystems can all operate independently, but they are much more effective when they interact and aid one another to defect and remove invaders and damaged material.

What Are Antigens? What Are Antibodies?

By definition an *antigen* is any substance that can trigger a defensive response by the immune system. Antigens are typically foreign protein molecules. Most often antigens are present in the surface membranes of invading microorganisms. Another class of antigens is the *toxins,* or poisons, produced and released by some invading organisms.

Antibodies are relatively large protein molecules, frequently referred to as *immunoglobulins,* sometimes abbreviated "Ig." They are not cells; they do not grow or reproduce. Antibodies are produced and secreted into the lymph and blood by the B lymphocytes. Usually about 20 per cent of all the circulating plasma proteins are antibodies.

Since antibodies are not themselves living but are created by the living lymphocytes, one might think of them as small robot weapons launched into the lymph and blood by the B lymphocytes and individually designed to identify and attack a specific type of foreign invader. One area of each antibody molecule is specialized to bind to one specific type of antigen. The "fit" between a particular antibody and its specific antigen is very precise, like a lock and key (Fig. 10–1).

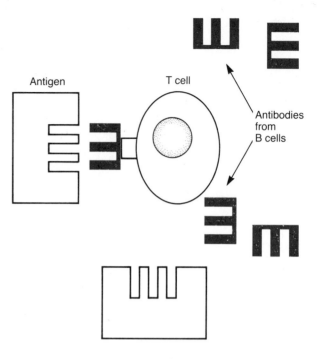

Figure 10–1 The "fit." Specific antibodies fit specific antigens like lock and key. Antibody receptors on T cells have the same key structure as circulating antibodies released by B cells.

What Are Phagocytes?

Phagocytes are the foot soldiers of the immune system. They are cells that ingest (phagocytize) and digest infectious and toxic agents as well as debris and damaged cells. There are several specialized types of phagocytes: *neutrophils, monocytes,* and *macrophages.*

Neutrophils and monocytes are white blood cells and originate in the bone marrow, becoming specialized for phagocytosis as they mature. Neutrophils are mature cells that can directly attack and destroy harmful bacteria and viruses by ingesting and digesting them.

Monocytes are immature until they enter the tissues and begin to grow and mature to much larger sizes to become tissue macrophages. As mature macrophages they are extremely capable of combating disease agents.

As neutrophils and monocytes move from the circulatory system into the tissues, the circulatory system stimulates the bone marrow to increase the production of neutrophils and monocytes.

A neutrophil can ingest 5 to 20 bacteria before the neutrophil becomes inactivated. Macrophages are capable of phagocytizing as many as 100 bacteria. Macrophages can even ingest whole red blood cells or malarial parasites.

Neutrophils and macrophages both have an abundance of lysosomes with enzymes especially geared for digesting bacteria and other foreign materials. Unfortunately, some bacteria have protein coats that are resistant to lysosomal digestion. Often, these bacteria, like the one that causes tuberculosis, are responsible for chronic diseases.

Neutrophils normally make up about 62 per cent of circulating white blood cells, and monocytes make up about 5 per cent. Macrophages reside almost exclusively in the tissues and lymph nodes.

How Do the Phagocytes Move Around?

When an unfriendly microorganism (pathogen) invades the body or when there is damage to normal body tissue, a number of special substances are released that attract the phagocytes to the area of the problem. This phenomenon is known as *chemotaxis.*

Macrophages residing in the local tissue migrate to the area. Circulating neutrophils and monocytes squeeze through the pores of blood vessels and move to the exact site of infection or tissue injury. This process is referred to as *diapedesis* (*dia* means through, *pedesis* means leaping). Using ameboid motion, they can all move through the tissues at a rate of several times their diameter each minute.

Although some macrophages are present in all body tissues, a sizable population of macrophages remains stationary in the tissue networks of the *lymph nodes.* Here, the macrophages are able to capture foreign particles as they circulate with the lymph through the nodes. Macrophages residing in the spleen and bone marrow help remove foreign particles and debris circulating in the blood.

How Do Macrophages and Neutrophils Respond to Inflammation?

The *inflammatory response* is triggered whenever tissue injury occurs, whether it is caused by bacteria, trauma, chemicals, heat, or any other phenomena. Over the next few hours after injury, the inflammed tissues are invaded by neutrophils and monocytes as well as local macrophages. They begin their scavenging functions, devouring infectious and toxic agents and cellular debris.

The macrophages already present in the area are the first line of defense. The mature neutrophils and immature monocytes present in the blood and bone marrow invade the inflamed area over a period of hours and days. Production of neutrophils and monocytes in the bone marrow increases dramatically, allowing the overall response to be sustained for many days, weeks, or even months.

All neutrophils and most macrophages eventually die after having ingested large numbers of bacteria and tissue debris. The accumulation of dead tissue, dead neutrophils, and dead macrophages forms a mixture commonly referred to as pus (or purulent matter).

What Are the Lymphocytes?

There are two types of lymphocytes, which are designated as *T lymphocytes* and *B lymphocytes,* or for short, T cells and B cells.

T cells produce special antigen-sensitive protein substances that reside in the T cell membranes. There are about 100,000 of these antigen-receptor sites located in the surface membrane of each T cell. When a T cell attaches to an invading organism, the specific antigen receptor in the membrane is the site of attachment. (The antigen is typically a protein molecule in the surface structure of the invading organism.)

B cells produce and secrete special antigen-sensitive protein molecules called antibodies, which circulate in the body fluids. These free-circulating antibodies attach to a specific antigen in an invading agent in a manner that parallels T cell attachment. The antigen-sensitive receptor sites on T cells are the same as those that are found on the antibody molecules produced by the B cells.

T cells are said to produce cell-mediated immunity, since the antigen-sensitive binding site remains with the T cell. B cells are said to produce *humoral immunity,* the system of circulating antibodies. In both cases the antigen-sensitive receptor sites are the same; in one case they are located in the T cell membrane, and in the other they are mounted on circulating antibody molecules.

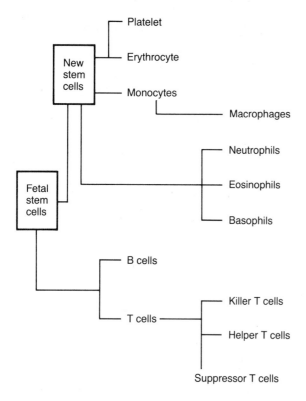

Figure 10–2 Origins. Stem cells are the original source of B cells and T cells and the continuing source of all other white and red blood cells.

which they migrate from the bone marrow shortly before the time of birth. While residing in the thymus, the primitive stem cells develop into T cells. T cells receive their designation "T" from this important association with the thymus.

Those fetal stem cells destined to become B cells also migrate from the bone marrow a few months before and after birth. The original research uncovering this fact occurred in chickens, in whom the primitive cells migrate to a structure called the bursa of Fabricius. The designation "B" arose from this association with the bursa.

Unfortunately, there is no bursa of Fabricius in humans. It is thought in humans that the primitive stem cells—soon to be B cells—migrate to structures associated perhaps with the liver. But because their function is the same, it has been decided to call them B cells in all species.

In summary, the lymphocytes do not originate in the lymphoid tissue but instead are transported to

ORIGIN AND FUNCTION OF LYMPHOCYTES

What Is the Origin of Lymphocytes?

Curiously, lymphocytes do not arise from lymphoid tissue, like the tonsils and lymph nodes, where they often reside. Instead, lymphocytes originate in the bone marrow.

Both T cells and B cells evolve from the same type of source cell as for all types of blood cells—known as fetal stem cells (Fig. 10–2). Lymphocytes then are in this sense white blood cells. However, the fetal stem cells by themselves are incapable of forming active lymphocytes. Additional processing is required.

The fetal stem cells that become T cells receive this additional processing in the thymus gland to

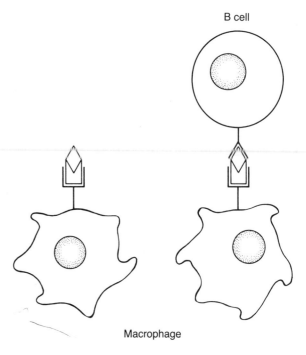

Figure 10–3 Cooperation among cells of the immune system. In one form of cooperation, macrophages pass antigens to T cells, improving the response time of lymphocytes to invaders. Interleukin-1 further stimulates the lymphocytes.

this tissue by way of the preprocessing areas of the thymus and probably, in mammals, the fetal liver.

How Are T Cells Activated?

T cells become activated, or sensitized, to a particular antigen when it binds to the corresponding antigen-sensitive receptor in the surface membrane of the T cell. The T cells often receive the antigen from a macrophage when both T cell and macrophage are located in a lymph node. The macrophage appears to ingest and digest the invading organism and then hand several of the antigens to the T cells (Fig. 10–3).

The sensitized T cells then multiply rapidly and are released from their residence in the lymphoid tissue to circulate in the lymph and blood. These mobilized T cells distribute themselves throughout the body, passing through capillaries into the tissue spaces, back into the lymph and blood once again, and circulating again and again, sometimes for

months or even years. This T cell system produces what is referred to as *cell-mediated immunity* (Fig. 10–4).

How Do T Cells Function To Produce Cell-mediated Immunity?

Recent research has revealed that there are three distinct types of T cells: (1) *killer T cells,* (2) *helper T cells,* and (3) *suppressor T cells.* The functions of each of these are quite distinct.

The killer T cell is the direct attack cell. It is capable of killing microorganisms and is frequently called the killer cell. The antigen-sensitive receptor sites on the surface of these T cells bind tightly to those organisms that contain their specific antigens. The process is parallel to the way in which the independent antibodies secreted from B cells bind to their antigens.

The killer T cells attack the invading cell by injecting cytotoxic substances into the attacked cell.

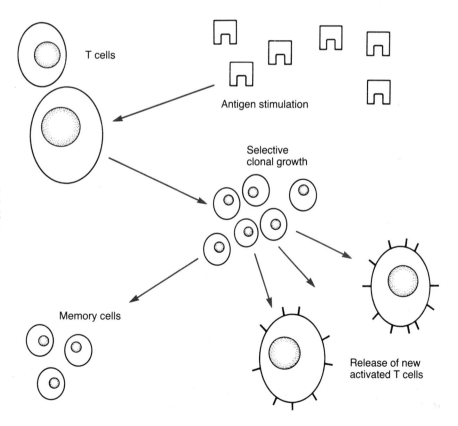

Figure 10-4 Cell-mediated immunity. Selected T cells grow and circulate following stimulation by a specific antigen.

"Cytotoxic" means poisonous to cells. Each of these killer cells can attack many different organisms instead of merely one, often without the killer cells themselves being harmed. The killer cells can attack the body's own cells that have been invaded by viruses. The killer cell detects the viruses that have become entrapped in the cell's membranes.

The killer T cells are also one of the most important operatives in maintaining the body's cellular integrity. They destroy precancerous as well as cancerous cells, cells and tissues transplanted from another person, or any other types of cells that are or become "foreign" to the person's own body.

What Are Helper and Suppressor T Cells?

The helper T cells are by far the most numerous of the T cells. As the name implies, they "help" other portions of the immune system function. For instance, they increase activation of B cells, killer T cells, and suppressor T cells and in addition enhance the effectiveness of macrophages.

The suppressor T cells, sometimes called regulator T cells, suppress the functions of other T cells, keeping them from undertaking excessive immune reactions. It is also probable that the suppressor T cells are important in preventing immune system attack on a person's own body tissues. This is called immune tolerance. Breakdown in immune tolerance may be a precipitating factor leading to autoimmune diseases.

How Are B Cells Activated?

One result of the original B cell processing around the time of birth is the creation of a wide diversity of B cells. Prior to stimulation by an antigen there is a roughly equal distribution of types among the billions of B cells.

A few immature B cells are activated when the specific antigen binds to the specific antigen-sensitive receptor sites in the B cell membrane. The first step here is almost identical to that which occurs in T cell activation. This specific, activated subpopulation, or *clone* of B lymphocytes, then begins to divide rapidly and repeatedly. As they divide and multiply, these B lymphocytes mature, developing into what are referred to as *plasma cells.*

Within 4 days each original activated B cell has multiplied to about 500 plasma cells. Each of these plasma cells produces and secretes antibodies into the lymph and blood at an extremely rapid rate— about 2000 molecules per second for each plasma cell. This process continues for several days or weeks until the death of the plasma cells.

The only real difference from T cell activation is that instead of whole activated T cells being released, hundreds of thousands of individual antibodies are released into the lymph. These antibodies released from B cells form the essence of humoral immunity (Fig. 10–5).

IMMUNE RESPONSE

How Do Antibodies Function?

Antibodies accomplish their defensive task by binding to specific antigens to form antigen-antibody complexes. Attachment by the antibody serves in several ways to make antigens and cells with surface antigens harmless. For example, antibodies that attach to the surfaces of invading cells frequently serve as a sort of glue, causing the invading cells to clump together. Other antibodies neutralize the effects of many toxic antigens.

The antibody molecules themselves often attack and alter the invader directly. Launched by the B lymphocytes, antibodies are like small robot weapons. However, this is only a minor initial attack compared with what comes next. When an antibody attaches to an antigen, the antibody changes shape and triggers the complement proteins.

What is Complement?

Complement is a group of about 11 different proteins normally present in the blood. They serve as a sort of second phase in the attack on invading microorganisms.

Complement is an extremely important part of humoral immunity. Complement is activated by and works in conjunction with the antibodies. Once an antibody has attached to the invader, the antibody signals and attracts the first complement pro-

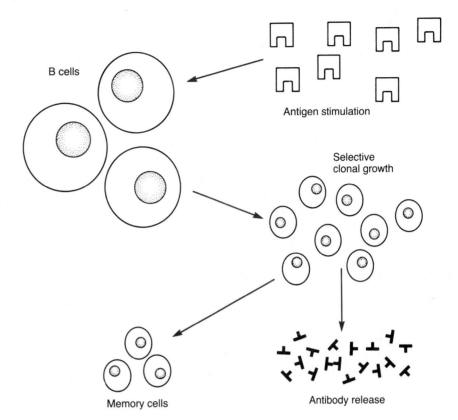

Figure 10-5 Humoral immunity. Selected B cells grow and release antibodies following stimulation by a specific antigen. Complement is also part of humoral immunity.

tein. This signal attracts the second complement protein and so forth until all 11 have linked up to form a doughnut-shaped structure on the surface membrane of the invader.

This doughnut-shaped structure then drills a hole in the invader's cell membrane. Fluid pours through the hole into the microorganism, swelling it, eventually to the point of bursting.

Humoral immunity should be thought of as the combination of circulating antibodies produced and secreted by the B cells and the 11-protein complement system.

IMMUNE STRATEGY

What Is the Role of Diversity and Rapid Growth in Immune Strategy?

To understand the overall function of the immune system, one needs to understand the nature of the enemy and its attack strategy. The primary enemy is an incredible diversity of bacteria and viruses. Their universal attack strategy is to reproduce faster than the victim can produce an effective defense.

The immune system is a brilliant strategic response by larger animals to the problem of combating the wide diversity of rapidly reproducing microorganisms. To prevent the possibility of some microorganism's being able to evade the immune system, there must be an equally wide range of defensive cells in the immune system.

When the T cells and B cells are processed, they divide in such a way as to produce a population of cells with incredible variety. Although it is estimated there are perhaps a trillion lymphocytes in the body, there may be a million distinct types of T cells and an equal number of B cell types.

The difference among T cells is in the antigen-sensitive receptor sites on the surface membrane. With some overlap, each T cell has a different range of receptors than the other T cells. Similarly, B cells differ in the range of antibodies that each produces.

Each type of T cell, by virtue of its surface receptors, is a specialist in attacking a large but limited selection of antigens. Each type of B cell is a specialist in producing and secreting its own large but limited selection of the many millions of possible antibodies.

This diversity of the T and B cells enables the body to develop immunity to an equally extensive range of organisms that might attack. However, this tremendous diversity means that for any specific invader, the number of lymphocytes originally available to respond to it must be quite small. Therefore, the diversity of the system creates a disadvantage in the other dimension of the problem—growth rates of the invading antigens.

Bacteria reproduce by dividing, doubling their numbers about every 20 minutes. Viruses reproduce inside cells, multiplying their numbers by a factor of thousands with each reproductive cycle. Whenever the body is invaded (infected) by one of these microorganisms, there is a race over which can reproduce faster, the invaders or the specific lymphocytes needed to defend and destroy the invaders.

The rapid growth of the invading microorganism population is met by the immune system with several strategies. First, because the immune system is made up of individual cells—phagocytes and lymphocytes—there is the potential for rapid reproduction.

The existing phagocytes and circulating antibodies are the first line of internal defense (Fig. 10–6).

The second internal line of defense arises as each invading organism activates the corresponding subgroup of lymphocytes; a reproductive race begins. Reproduction of the specific lymphocytic cells as well as more phagocytes is greatly accelerated to meet the challenge of the reproducing microorganisms. An additional strategy is the rapid production of antibodies specific to the organism's antigens by the already expanding population of B cells.

By using a special system that remembers previous attacks, the immune system is able to gain a tremendous advantage over the common microorganisms in its environment.

How Does the Immune System "Remember"?

When the lymphocytes are activated and rapidly reproducing, both the T lymphocyte clones and the B lymphocyte clones form a subpopulation of *memory cells*. These are identical to the plasma cells but are inactive. These T and B memory cells are formed in moderate numbers. They migrate throughout the body to be stored in the lymph nodes, where they wait for future invasions by the same organisms (antigen).

This means that among the trillion or so lymphocytes waiting for future activation, the number of T and B cells specific for that microorganism that recently activated the system is greatly increased. These memory cells remain dormant until activated once again by a new quantity of the same antigen.

Why Is the Second Response Better?

The first time the immune system encounters a specific invader or antigen the response is relatively slow, weak, and short lived. The memory system

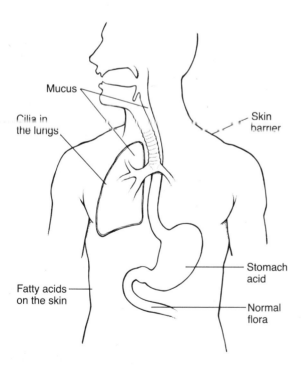

Mucus

Cilia in the lungs

Skin barrier

Fatty acids on the skin

Stomach acid

Normal flora

Figure 10–6 The first lines of defense. Protection from infection is provided by the external body surfaces, mucus, and the environment of the gastrointestinal tract.

What Is an Allergy?

Allergic reactions can be thought of as side effects of creating immunity. An allergy is a hypersensitivity to certain chemicals or biologic preparations. There are two main types: those that can occur in any person and those that can occur only in persons with a specific allergic tendency.

The common type of allergy that can occur in any person is also known as delayed-reaction allergy. No reaction occurs on first exposure. But after a few days to 2 weeks the subject becomes sensitive. Thereafter, the specific antigen, referred to as an allergen, evokes a reaction in minutes to hours. The severity depends on the quantity of allergen and route of entry. Common examples of this type of allergic reaction are skin eruptions following repeated exposures to some cosmetics and household chemicals. Skin eruptions caused by exposure to poison ivy is another example.

Delayed reaction allergy is caused by activated T cells and not by antibodies. Repeated exposure causes the formation of activated T cells.

Some persons have an "allergic tendency," which is passed from parent to child, and are characterized by having large quantities of a subclass of antibodies in their immune system — sensitizing antibodies. They constitute a nonordinary response of the immune system. When an allergen enters the body a reaction occurs with these sensitizing antibodies, and a subsequent allergic reaction takes place. These antibody-allergen complexes attach to specialized connective tissue cells called mast cells. The mast cells soon rupture, releasing histamine and other powerful substances. A variety of different types of abnormal tissue responses can occur at this point, depending on the type of tissue in which the allergen-antibody reaction occurs.

Urticaria, or "hives," is common when the reaction occurs in the skin. Histamine release causes a red flare and swelling. Antihistamine drugs prior to exposure can prevent the hives.

In hay fever, the allergen-antibody reaction occurs in the nose. Histamine release causes the nasal linings to become swollen and secretory. Antihistamine drugs can prevent this swelling. However, other released substances still produce irritation and the typical sneezing syndrome.

Asthma occurs when the allergen-antibody reaction occurs in the bronchioles of the lungs. Here, the most important substance released from the ruptured mast cells is referred to as "the slow-reacting substance of anaphylaxis." This substance causes constriction of the smooth muscles of the bronchioles. The result is that the person has trouble breathing until this substance has been removed. Antihistamine drugs have little effect in asthma because histamine is not the major factor causing the problem.

The most severe allergic reaction occurs when the allergen is injected directly into the circulation, producing a widespread reaction. This widespread reaction is called anaphylaxis and is triggered by the release of histamine inside the circulatory system. Release of "the slow-reacting substance of anaphylaxis" also produces severe asthmalike symptoms. This severe reaction can result in death from circulatory shock within a few minutes unless treated with norepinephrine (noradrenalin) to oppose the effects of the histamine.

gives the body a great advantage by enabling it to respond much more rapidly and vigorously the second time the microorganism is encountered.

The second response, based on the waiting army of preformed memory cells, begins more rapidly, is far more potent, and forms antibodies for many months rather than for weeks. The more frequently a microorganism is encountered, the quicker the immune system responds to it (Fig. 10–7).

The immune system never actually destroys or removes all the invaders. In healthy persons the mouth and the respiratory tract almost always contain various pneumococcal and streptococcal bacteria. The gastrointestinal tract regularly houses numerous colonic bacilli. And one can almost always find bacteria in the eyes, urethra, and the vagina. Even though it has gained the upper hand, the immune system must continue to produce the specific successful lymphocytes for months and years. The result is a balance between attackers and defenders.

This dynamic balance, with the few surviving, residual microorganisms, also serves to provide the body with another type of memory by continuing the activation of at least a few plasma cells over the long run, which keeps the immune system prepared for any second, or third, or subsequent invasion.

How Do the Subsystems Interact?

The phagocytes, lymphocytes, and antibodies all interact to stimulate or to regulate each other.

Macrophages residing in the lymph nodes, the first cells to encounter and ingest an invader, pass on digested portions of the invader to the lymphocytes residing in the lymph nodes. This cooperation improves the response time of the lymphocytes to these antigens (see Fig. 10–3).

At the time of digesting an invader, macrophages also secrete *interleukin-1,* an activating substance that promotes the growth and reproduction of the specific activated lymphocytes.

Most antigens activate both T lymphocytes and B lymphocytes at the same time. Some of the T cells that are formed, called helper cells, in turn secrete specific substances, called *lymphokines,* that further activate the B lymphocytes. Without the help of these helper T cells the quantity of antibodies

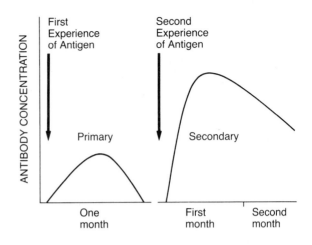

Figure 10–7 Primary and secondary antibody response. The antibody response on second contact with the antigen is more rapid and intense and lasts longer.

formed by the B cells is usually minor. One of the important lymphokines secreted by T helper cells is *interleukin-2.* T helper cells secrete another lymphokine that stimulates the macrophage system.

Substances released by the actions of the humoral immunity subsystem—antibodies and complement—also act to stimulate the phagocytosis and activation of lymphocytes.

CLINICAL CONSIDERATIONS

What Is an Autoimmune Disorder?

Autoimmunity occurs when the immune system attacks the body's own tissues. Diseases known to involve autoimmunity include the following:

1. *Rheumatic fever,* in which the body becomes immunized against tissues in the joints and heart, especially the heart valves, following exposure to a specific type of streptococcal toxin.
2. *Myasthenia gravis,* in which immunity develops against acetylcholine receptors at the junction between nerves and muscles, causing paralysis.
3. *Lupus erythematosus,* in which the person be-

comes immunized against many different body tissues at the same time in a disease that causes extensive damage and often rapid death.

Unfortunately, as people grow older they often lose some of their immune tolerance. This frequently occurs after some tissue destruction that releases considerable quantities of damaged protein molecules. These may then combine with other proteins from viruses and bacteria to form new antigens that can trigger an immune response. The resulting activated T cells and antibodies from B cells attack the body's own tissues.

What Is Vaccination?

Immunity against specific diseases has been artificially stimulated for many years in a process known as vaccination. Three main approaches are used: killed bacteria, altered toxins, or attenuated, live viruses.

In the first technique antigens are introduced by injecting dead organisms, which are no longer capable of causing disease. This type of vaccination is used to protect against typhoid fever, whooping cough, diphtheria, and many other types of bacterial disease.

Immunity against toxins can be achieved by introducing chemically altered toxin — deactivating its harmful effects — while leaving the antigens causing immunity intact. This procedure is used in vaccinating against tetanus and botulism.

Finally, immunity to viruses is often achieved by infecting a person with live viruses that have been "attenuated," or processed, to reduce their ability to cause disease while still carrying the specific antigens. This procedure is used to protect against poliomyelitis, yellow fever, measles, smallpox, and many other viral diseases.

What Is the Response to Transplantation?

Transplantation of tissues or organs from one person to another almost always produces an immune response in the recipient. The recipient's immune system reacts to some of the donor's proteins as foreign and rejects the tissue. This rejection involves formation of antibodies and eventual ingestion of the tissue by phagocytes. By suppressing the immune system with a drug like *cyclosporine*, successful kidney transplantation has become very common.

What Is AIDS?

Acquired immune deficiency syndrome (AIDS) is a sexually transmitted disease caused by a virus, referred to as human immunodeficiency virus (HIV). AIDS is also commonly transmitted among intravenous drug users through needle sharing. Because the virus attacks and disables some parts of the immune system, the body becomes vulnerable to invasion by a host of other microorganisms.

Persons with AIDS lack cell-mediated immunity. Examination of their blood reveals a depletion of T cells. AIDS patients are unable to protect themselves from certain forms of cancer and many viral, protozoal, and fungal diseases. This means that the actual overt symptoms can be quite varied, depending to a large extent on the secondary invaders.

The death rate for those who contract AIDS is quite high, close to 100 per cent, and will remain so until an effective therapy is discovered. It is estimated that several million people in the United States will have been exposed to the virus by 1991.

Treatment using antiviral drugs is promising. However, most antiviral drugs have serious short-term side effects. The long-term side effects of antiviral drugs are even less well understood.

Because of the unique characteristics of HIV, public health officials are suggesting that it may be a decade or more before a vaccine can be developed or a truly effective drug cure is found.

The best defense in the interim will be a strong public education effort aimed at prevention by reducing transmission through sexual contact and intravenous drug use practices.

SUMMARY

A. The immune system functions to defend the body and to maintain its self-identity.

1. It defends against invasion by harmful microorganisms.
2. It maintains bodily integrity by removing damaged cells, debris, and foreign material.

B. The immune system is made up of individual cells and circulating antibodies.
   1. The cells of the immune system can be divided into the phagocytes and the lymphocytes.
   2. The circulating antibodies are large protein molecules and are supported by the complement complex.
   3. These components are most effective when they work together to accomplish their tasks.

C. Antigens are substances that trigger an immune response.
   1. Antigens are usually foreign proteins.
   2. Antigens are often parts of the surface membrane of invading microorganisms.
   3. Toxins are also often antigenic.

D. Antibodies are large protein molecules that bind to antigens.
   1. They make up 20 per cent of the circulating proteins.
   2. Antibodies are antigen specific and work as a lock and key.

E. Phagocytes are cells that ingest and digest foreign organisms and materials as well as debris and damaged cells.
   1. Neutrophils and monocytes are white blood cells that specialize in phagocytosis.
      a. Neutrophils make up about 62 per cent of white blood cells.
      b. Monocytes make up about 5 per cent of white blood cells.
   2. Neutrophils are mature and directly attack and ingest foreign organisms and materials.
      a. They can ingest and digest 5 to 20 bacteria before dying.
      b. They use lysosomes to digest organisms and other materials.
   3. Monocytes are immature and circulate until attracted to enter the tissues.
      a. Once in the tissues they grow and mature to become macrophages.
      b. Maturing of monocytes to become macrophages stimulates production of monocyte in the bone marrow.
   4. Macrophages can ingest and digest as many as 100 bacteria before dying.

   a. They digest materials using powerful lysosomes.
   b. They do not normally circulate but rather reside in the tissues or lymph nodes.

F. By a process known as chemotaxis, phagocytes are attracted to the site of tissue damage by substances released from the area.
   1. Local macrophages migrate to the site.
   2. Neutrophils and monocytes squeeze through pores in blood vessels to arrive at the exact site.
   3. Phagocytes travel using ameboid movements.
   4. There is a special concentration of macrophages in the lymph nodes, spleen, and bone marrow.

G. The inflammatory response is triggered by tissue damage.
   1. Local macrophages are the first line of defense during the first hours.
   2. Existing neutrophils and monocytes arrive over the course of hours and days.
   3. Newly produced neutrophils and monocytes continue to arrive for days, weeks, or even months.
   4. Pus is an accumulation of dead phagocytes and tissue debris.

H. There are two main kinds of lymphocytes, which are referred to as T cells and B cells.
   1. T cells produce cell-mediated immunity.
      a. There are 100,000 different antigen-sensitive receptor sites on T cell surface membranes.
      b. T cells attach to antigens at the corresponding receptor sites.
      c. Other T cells perform supportive functions.
   2. B cells produce and secrete antibodies, the main component providing humoral immunity.
   3. The protein segments that bind to the antigens are the same for both T cells and the antibodies produced by B cells.

I. Lymphocytes originate as stem cells in the bone marrow.
   1. Around the time of birth they migrate to special processing areas.
      a. T cells are processed in the thymus gland.
      b. B cells are processed in chickens in the bursa of Fabricius.

c. In humans, B cells are probably processed in the fetal liver.

2. After processing, the newly formed lymphocytes migrate throughout the body, with special concentrations in lymphoid tissues.

J. T cells are activated, or sensitized, when an antigen binds to one of its antigen-sensitive surface receptors.

1. Antigens are often passed on to lymphocytes by macrophages residing in the same lymph node.

2. Once sensitized, the T cells multiply rapidly and are released into the blood and lymph.

3. Mobilized T cells move throughout the tissue spaces, back into the circulatory system, and so on for months or years.

K. Recent research reveals distinctions among killer T cells, helper T cells, and suppressor T cells.

1. Killer T cells directly attack invaders.

a. They bind to the invader and inject cytotoxic substances into it.

b. Each killer T cell may attack and kill numerous invaders and last for months.

c. Killer T cells devour cells that have been invaded and taken over by viruses.

d. They remove damaged precancerous as well as cancerous cells.

2. Helper T cells stimulate, or help, other portions of the immune system.

a. Helper T cells enhance the actions of the phagocytes.

b. They increase the activation of B cells, killer T cells, and suppressor T cells.

3. Suppressor T cells function to regulate, or suppress, the action of the other parts of the immune system.

a. They prevent excessive immune responses.

b. They are important in maintaining the immune system's tolerance of the body's own tissues.

L. B cells are activated when an antigen binds to a specific antigen-sensitive receptor site in the surface membrane of the B cell.

1. The activated B cells reproduce rapidly and mature into 500 plasma cells in about 4 days.

2. Each plasma cell produces and secretes about 2000 antibodies per second for days or weeks.

M. Antibodies attach to antigens, forming antigen-antibody complexes.

1. Antigen-antibody complexes clump together, incapacitating the invader.

2. Antibodies neutralize toxins.

3. Antibody attachment often causes damage to the surface of the invader.

N. Complement consists of a group of 11 proteins circulating in the blood.

1. They attach in sequence to antigen-antibody complexes.

2. The completed doughnut-shaped structure drills a hole in the surface membrane of the invading microorganism.

3. Fluid pours in through the hole until the invader bursts.

O. The immune system is confronted with a wide diversity of rapidly reproducing microorganisms.

1. T and B cells are processed to produce an incredible diversity of cells.

a. Each T cell is able to respond to some large but very limited range of antigens.

b. Each B cell produces and secretes a large but very limited range of antibodies.

2. Once activated the immune system accelerates reproduction of phagocytes.

3. The T and B lymphocytes are activated by the new antigens to begin rapid reproduction.

P. Activated T and B lymphocyte clones form subpopulations of identical but temporarily inactive memory cells.

1. Memory cells migrate throughout the body.

2. They are stored in the lymph nodes.

3. Memory cells serve to increase the numbers of lymphocytes of that type ready for activation.

a. The first immune response to a particular antigen is slow, weak, and short lived.

b. Memory cells make the second (and subsequent) immune responses quicker, more potent, and sustained.

4. Continuing plasma and memory cells form a dynamic balance with the few surviving residual microorganisms.

Q. The phagocytes, lymphocytes, antibodies, and complement systems all interact to stimulate and regulate one another.

1. Macrophages pass antigens from digested invaders to the lymphocytes.
2. Macrophages secrete interleukin-1, which promotes lymphocyte activity.
3. Helper T cells secrete interleukin-2, which greatly enhances antibody production by B cells.
4. Helper T cells also secrete a substance that stimulates the macrophages.
5. Substances released by activity of the humoral immunity serve to stimulate the lymphocytes and phagocytes.

R. An allergy is a hypersensitivity to chemicals or biologic preparations.
1. Delayed reaction allergies can occur in anyone.
   a. Repeated exposure to the allergen creates sensitivity in days to 2 weeks.
   b. Exposure provokes allergic reaction.
   c. Reaction is caused by T cell sensitization.
2. Some persons have an "allergic tendency."
   a. They have a large quantity of a special class of antibodies—the sensitizing type.
   b. Allergens attach to these antibodies.
   c. Allergen-antibody complexes attach to mast cells.
   d. Mast cells release histamine and other powerful substances into surrounding tissues.
3. Urticaria, or hives, occurs when the reaction is in the skin.
   a. Histamine release causes a red flare and swelling.
   b. Antihistamine drugs can prevent it.
4. Hay fever occurs when the reaction occurs in the nose.
   a. Antihistamines are helpful.
   b. Other substances cause irritation and sneezing.
5. Asthma occurs when the reaction takes place in the lungs.
   a. Antihistamine does not usually help.
   b. The slow-reacting substance of anaphylaxis causes smooth muscle spasm in the bronchioles.
6. Anaphylaxis occurs when the allergen-antibody reaction occurs in the circulatory system.
   a. Histamine release can cause shock and death in minutes.
   b. Norepinephrine (noradrenalin) can oppose the effect of the histamine.
   c. The slow-reacting substance of anaphylaxis causes asthmalike symptoms.

S. Autoimmunity occurs when the immune system attacks the body's own tissues.
1. In rheumatic fever the immune system attacks the joints and heart valves.
2. In myasthenia gravis, receptors at the nerve-muscle junction are attacked.
3. In lupus erythematosus many body tissues are attacked by the immune system.
4. Immune tolerance tends to decrease in general as people age.

T. Vaccination is an artificial means of stimulating immunity to a specific organism.
1. One approach is to use killed bacteria, as in vaccination against typhoid, whooping cough, and diphtheria.
2. Another approach uses altered toxins, as in vaccination against tetanus and botulism.
3. Another approach is to use live "attenuated" viruses, as in vaccination against polio, measles, and small pox.

U. Transplantation of tissue from one person to another almost always stimulates an immune response.
1. The recipient's immune system is said to reject the donor's tissue.
2. Drugs that suppress the activity of the immune system allow tissue and organ transplantation to be more successful.

V. Acquired immunodeficiency syndrome (AIDS) is a sexually transmitted viral disease.
1. The disease is caused by the human immune virus (HIV).
2. The virus attacks the immune system.
3. Persons with AIDS lack cell-mediated immunity.
4. Treatment with antiviral drugs does seem to help in some cases.

REVIEW QUESTIONS

1. What is the primary function of the immune system?

2. Describe the important secondary functions of the immune system.

3. What may happen to damaged cells that are not removed?

4. Explain why the immune system might be accurately characterized as a system of individual cells and circulating molecules. What other body system is most similar?

5. Define antigen.

6. Define antibody.

7. What is phagocytosis?

8. Where do neutrophils and monocytes come from?

9. Monocytes and macrophages are really the same cells. Describe the life history that relates them.

10. Which is the most powerful phagocyte? Which is the most numerous in the circulatory system?

11. Since phagocytes use lysosomes to digest ingested materials, some proteins are not as easily digested. How does this lead to problems?

12. How does inflammation serve to mobilize the phagocytes?

13. What is the composition of pus?

14. Compare and contrast T and B lymphocytes.

15. Describe the special processing involved in the maturation of lymphocytes.

16. How are T cells activated? Briefly characterize the functions of killer, helper, and suppressor T cells.

17. How are B cells activated? Once activated, what is the output of antibody molecules per hour by each cell?

18. Describe the actions of an antibody and some of its effects.

19. Once an antigen-antibody complex is formed, the complement sequence is activated. Describe what happens.

20. How is the ability to respond to diverse invaders built into the structure of the immune system? Are there any disadvantages to this strategy?

21. Explain how the immune system uses its memory system to gain a growth advantage on frequently encountered microorganisms.

22. Identify at least one way in which each subsystem (phagocytes, lymphocytes, and antibodies/complement) serves to enhance the activity of the others.

23. What are the functions of interleukin-1 and interleukin-2?

24. Characterize and distinguish the two main types of allergic reaction.

25. What is an allergen? What is a mast cell?

26. Why is it that antihistamine drugs do not have much benefit in asthma?

27. What is anaphylaxis? How can it be treated?

28. Define autoimmunity. Name and characterize three autoimmune disorders.

29. Describe the three different techniques used to prepare antigens for vaccinations for bacteria, viruses, and toxins.

30. Explain why tissue transplanted from one person to another is almost always rejected by the immune system of the recipient.

31. What is acquired immunodeficiency syndrome (AIDS)? How does it attack the immune system?

E L E V E N

The Respiratory System

The aim of this chapter is to enable the student to do the following:

- Explain the functions of the respiratory system and describe its relation to other homeostatic systems.

- Construct and label a diagram identifying the structures forming the upper respiratory tract.

- Explain how the respiratory muscles cause volume changes that lead to air flow into and out of the lungs (breathing).

- Define and compare the following respiratory volumes: tidal volume, vital

- capacity, and functional residual capacity.

- Describe the process of gas exchange in the lungs and tissues.

- Explain the respiratory processes that normally prevent severe acidosis and alkalosis.

- Identify the factors important in controlling respiration.

- Define the different types of abnormal breathing.

- Describe the characteristics of several respiratory disorders.

FUNCTION OF THE RESPIRATORY SYSTEM

What Does the Respiratory System Do?

The maintenance of life depends on a continuous supply of oxygen to, and removal of carbon dioxide from, the cells of the body. The transportation of these gases between the cells and the respiratory system (specifically the lungs) is accomplished by the circulatory system. The respiratory system functions in the exchange of gases between the blood circulating through the lungs and the external environment. It serves to bring in oxygen and eliminate excess carbon dioxide.

An additional related function of the respiratory system is to regulate the acid-base balance in the blood. This happens because carbon dioxide, when dissolved in blood, is an acid. Thus, when there is too much carbon dioxide in the blood, the blood becomes too acidic. And when there is too little carbon dioxide in the blood, the blood becomes too basic (or alkaline). Variations on the rate and depth of respiration serve to control the amount of carbon dioxide in the blood within a rather narrow range of concentrations.

STRUCTURES OF THE RESPIRATORY SYSTEM

The specific function of the respiratory tract is to bring air close enough to the blood to allow oxygen to get into the blood and carbon dioxide to get out. The *upper respiratory tract*, made up of the nose, pharynx, larynx, trachea, and bronchi, forms an open passage between the lungs and the exterior. The *lungs* are the essential organs of respiration. With their extensive network of capillaries, the lungs provide an adequate surface for a high volume of exchange of gases between the body and the external environment. The *muscular diaphragm* and *intercostal muscles* of the chest produce the mechanical force needed to fill and empty the lungs in the process called *breathing*.

What Is the Thoracic Cavity? The Pleural Cavity? The Mediastinum?

The *thoracic cavity*, or chest, is separated from the abdominal cavity by the diaphragm, a large sheet of muscle. The *mediastinum* (me"de-as-ti'num) is the middle compartment of the chest and is located between the two pleural cavities, which contain the lungs. The heart and its associated structures are located in the mediastinum.

Each *pleural cavity* contains one of the lungs. The wall of the pleural cavities is lined by membrane called the *pleura*. Each lung is covered by a second layer of *pleura*. These two pleural membranes (pleura) are moist and slippery, and between the two layers is found a special lubricating *serous fluid* (Fig. 11–1).

This double pleural membrane arrangement allows respiration with minimal friction. In the condition known as *pleurisy*, the pleura become irritated and inflamed, and breathing becomes painful.

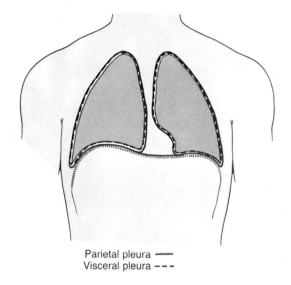

Parietal pleura ——
Visceral pleura - - -

Figure 11–1 Lungs and associated visceral and parietal pleurae.

What Is the Nose?

The term *nose* includes both the external nose —that part of the upper respiratory tract that protrudes from the face—and the *nasal cavity*. Only a small part of the nasal cavity is in the external nose; most of it lies over the roof of the mouth. The nasal cavity is composed of two wedge-shaped cavities separated by a *septum* (from the Latin word meaning partition or wall) (Figs 11–2 and 11–3).

The nasal cavity is lined with a thick mucous membrane containing a rich supply of tiny capillaries. This mucous membrane serves to warm and moisten the air on its way to the lungs. If the air is not warmed, the tissue lining the lower respiratory tract will function poorly. Absence of moisture for even a few minutes can destroy the delicate *cilia* (hairlike) in the lining of the respiratory tract.

The mucous membrane also captures bacteria and dust particles. Air currents passing over the moist mucosa in curved pathways deposit fine particles, powder, and smoke against the walls. These fine particles are subsequently moved to the pharynx by the wavelike action of the cilia. These cilia wave back and forth about 12 times per second, helping to move mucus toward the throat to be swallowed.

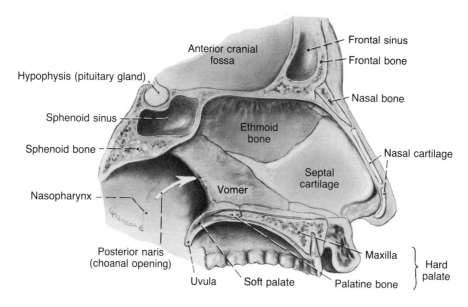

Figure 11-2 Sagittal section through the nose showing components of nasal septum.

The uppermost portion of the nasal cavity is lined with special nerve tissue containing *olfactory* (ol-fak'to-re) *cells,* which function in the sensation of smell. The location of the olfactory cells at the beginning of the upper respiratory tract is important in that it allows the brain to be alerted to the presence of poisonous substances in the air *before* they are inhaled.

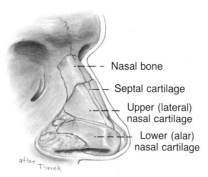

Figure 11-3 The lower portion of the external nose has a cartilaginous rather than a skeletal framework, consisting of a septal cartilage, two lateral cartilages, and a series of smaller cartilages.

What Are the Paranasal Sinuses? What Is Their Function?

The *paranasal sinuses* are air-containing spaces lined with mucous membrane that are connected at various points to the nasal cavity. These *paired* sinuses include the *maxillary, frontal, ethmoid,* and *sphenoid* sinuses (Fig. 11-4).

The primary function of the paranasal sinuses is to manufacture mucus for the air-cleansing activity of the nasal cavity. They serve secondarily to lighten the bones of the skull and to act as sound chambers for the production of sound.

What Is the Pharynx? What Is Its Function?

The *pharynx* (far'inks), or throat, serves as a passage for two systems — the digestive system and the respiratory system. Air can enter the pharynx either from the two nasal cavities or from the mouth. At the lower end, air proceeds to the larynx, while food is swallowed into the esophagus.

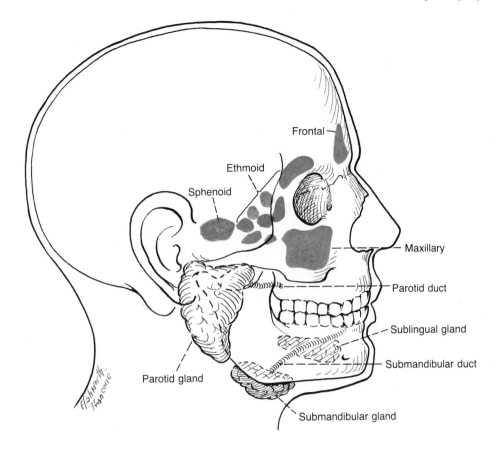

Figure 11–4 Lateral view of head showing sinuses and salivary glands.

The right and left *eustachian* (auditory) *tubes* open into the pharynx, connecting the middle ear with the upper respiratory tract. The tonsils and adenoids are located along the walls of the pharynx.

What Is the Larynx? What Is Its Function?

The *larynx*, or "voice box," connects the pharynx with the trachea. The larynx is broad at the top and shaped like a triangular box (Fig. 11–5). It is made up of nine pieces of cartilage and united by muscles and ligaments. The *thyroid cartilage*, or Adam's apple, is the largest cartilage in the larynx. In the male, the thyroid cartilage increases in size at

puberty. The leaf-shaped *epiglottis* (from *epi*, meaning on, and *glottis*, meaning mouth of the windpipe) is attached to the top border of the thyroid cartilage. It has a hinged, doorlike action at the entrance to the larynx. During swallowing, it acts as a lid to prevent food from entering the larynx.

The chief function of the larynx is the production of sounds. Two short, fibrous bands called *vocal cords* stretch across the interior of the larynx chamber (Fig. 11–6). The pitch (high or low) of the sound produced is determined by the shape and tightness of these cords. Long, loose cords produce low-pitched tones, while short, tense cords give higher tones. The voice is modified by the nose, mouth, and throat (pharynx) as well as by the sinuses, which act as sounding boards and vibrational (echo) chambers.

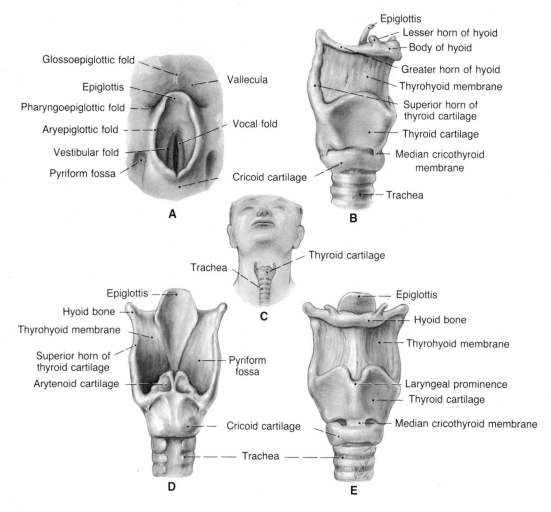

Figure 11–5   The larynx as viewed from above (A), from the side (B), in relation to the head and neck (C), from behind (D), and from the front (E).

What Is the Trachea? What Is Its Function?

The *trachea*, or "windpipe," is a cylindrical tube about 4 to 5 inches in length, consisting of circular rings of cartilage separated by fibrous and muscular tissue. The trachea functions as a simple passageway for air to reach the lungs. When it becomes blocked from swelling or from *aspiration* (breathing in) of some material, blocking the passage of air, a *tracheotomy* is necessary (Fig. 11–7).

What Are the Bronchi? What Is Their Function?

The two primary bronchi or *bronchial tubes* split from the trachea, each leading to one of the lungs. The right bronchus differs from the left in that it is shorter and wider and takes a more vertical course. Because of this vertical characteristic, foreign bodies entering the trachea usually enter the right bronchus (Fig. 11–8).

Moving down from the trachea through the

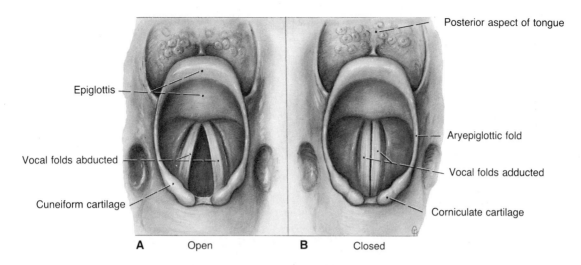

Epiglottis

Posterior aspect of tongue

Aryepiglottic fold

Vocal folds abducted

Vocal folds adducted

Cuneiform cartilage

Corniculate cartilage

A   Open   **B**   Closed

Figure 11-6 Superior view of vocal cords.

primary bronchial tubes and into the secondary bronchial tubes, the walls of the passage are composed of less cartilage and more smooth muscle.

What Are the Lungs? How Do They Work?

The lungs are two cone-shaped organs extending from the diaphragm to about 1½ inches above

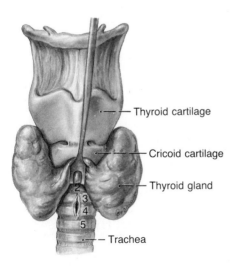

Thyroid cartilage

Cricoid cartilage

Thyroid gland

Trachea

Figure 11-7 Incision for a tracheotomy

the clavicle (Fig. 11-9). The large primary bronchi and the pulmonary arteries from the heart enter a slit in each lung called the *hilum.* This entry point at the root of each lung is the only real connection the lungs have to the body itself.

The right lung has three lobes, and the left lung has two lobes. The adult lung is a spongy mass and is frequently blue-gray in color because of inhaled dust and soot lodged in the respiratory lymphatics. In contrast, the lung of a baby is pink, since no foreign substances have yet entered. At birth the lungs are filled with fluid. When the first breath is taken the lungs begin to become spongy and eventually fill with air to a degree similar to that of an adult.

What Is An Alveolus?

The thousands of air passages resulting from the repeated branching of the primary bronchi into each lung form a structure resembling an upside-down tree. The smallest bronchial tubes (bronchioles) subdivide into very tiny twiglike tubes called *alveolar* (al-ve'o-lar) *ducts.* Each alveolar duct blossoms out into several *alveolar sacs,* resembling clusters of grapes. Each cluster is made up of numerous *alveoli,* each resembling a single grape in a cluster. The term "alveolus," which is the singular of

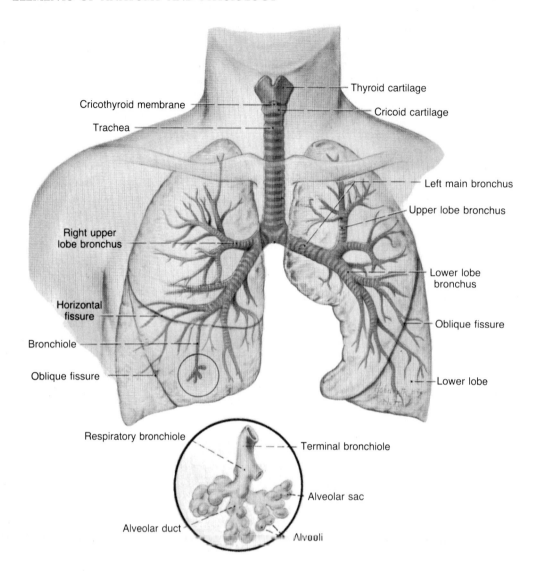

Figure 11–8   Distribution of bronchi within the lungs. Enlarged inset shows detail of alveolar ducts opening into clusters of alveoli, each cluster an alveolar sac.

alveoli, is from the Latin word meaning a small chamber or cavity.

A rich network of capillaries surrounds each alveolus, and it is at this point in the respiratory tract that the exchange of gases between the blood and inhaled air takes place (Figs. 11–10 and 11–11).

The interior surface of the lung is by far the most extensive body surface in contact with the environment; its area is many times greater than the skin. In the normal adult this internal lung surface area, when laid out, would cover a regular-sized tennis court.

BREATHING

The process of breathing involves two phases: inspiration and expiration. *Inspiration* requires coordinated muscular contractions that increase chest

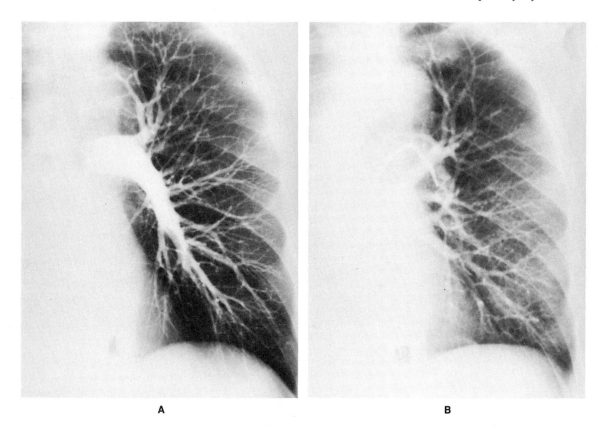

A   **B**

Figure 11–9 *A*, Angiograph of pulmonary arterial system. *B*, Angiograph of pulmonary venous system.

volume, drawing air into the lungs. *Expiration* is ordinarily entirely passive; the chest volume decreases and air is pushed out of the lungs.

What Are the Mechanisms of Breathing?

There are actually two different mechanisms for breathing; one is called *costal breathing* and the other *diaphragmatic* (di"ah-frag-mat'ik) *breathing*. Costal breathing is shallow and can be identified by the typical upward and outward movement of the chest. It is seen in runners at the conclusion of a race. Costal breathing involves primarily the use of the intercostal (between the ribs) muscles of the chest.

Diaphragmatic breathing, on the other hand, involves the use of the diaphragm rather than the intercostal muscles. Diaphragmatic breathing is deep and is identified by movement of the abdomi-

nal wall, caused by the contraction and descent of the diaphragm. This type of breathing is usually seen during sleep.

What Is Tidal Volume? Vital Capacity?

The normal resting chest volume in a man of average size is about 3 liters (there are 947 ml in a quart). Normal inspiration increases this volume by approximately 500 ml. Because this normal breathing volume of 500 ml comes and goes regularly like the tides of the sea, it is referred to as the *tidal volume* (TV). Forced maximum inspiration raises the overall chest capacity to 6 liters. Forced maximum expiration lowers the chest volume to approximately 1 liter. The largest amount of air that we can breathe in and out in one inspiration and expiration, about 5 liters, is known as the *vital capacity* (vc). This is about 10 times the tidal volume (Fig. 11–12).

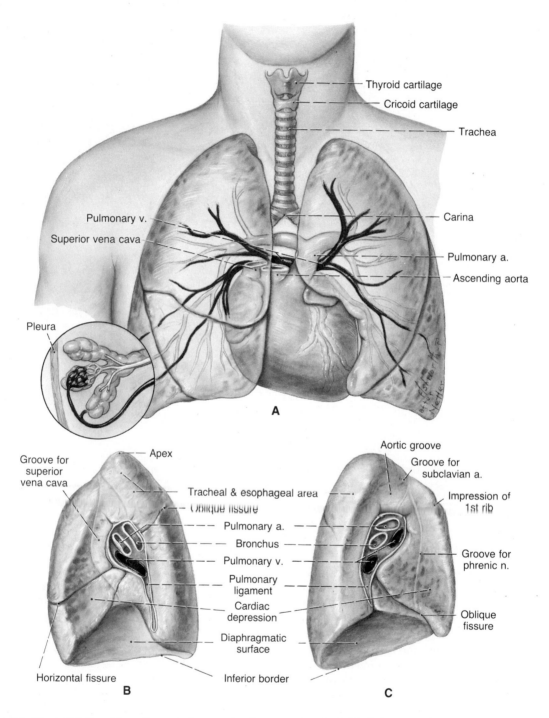

Thyroid cartilage

Cricoid cartilage

Trachea

Carina

Pulmonary a.

Ascending aorta

Pulmonary v.

Superior vena cava

Pleura

A

Apex

Aortic groove

Groove for subclavian a.

Groove for superior vena cava

Tracheal & esophageal area

Oblique fissure

Impression of 1st rib

Pulmonary a.

Bronchus

Pulmonary v.

Pulmonary ligament

Cardiac depression

Groove for phrenic n.

Diaphragmatic surface

Oblique fissure

Horizontal fissure

Inferior border

B

C

Figure 11–10   *A,* Relationships of lungs to heart and pulmonary vessels. *B,* Medial aspect of right lung. *C,* Medial aspect of left lung.

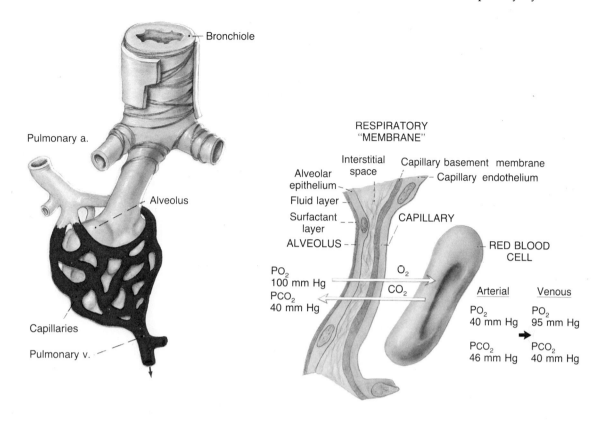

Figure 11-11   Basic microscopic functional unit of the lung. (Courtesy of Roche Laboratories.)

The total volume of air in the lungs upon maximal inhalation is called *total lung capacity.* The air remaining in the lungs even after maximal forced expiration is known as *residual volume.* The volume of air capable of being inspired at the end of a quiet respiration plus the tidal volume is called the *inspiratory capacity.* The *inspiratory reserve volume* is the volume capable of being inspired after quiet inspiration. The *expiratory reserve volume* is the volume of air capable of being expired at the end of a quiet expiration. *Functional residual capacity* is the expiratory reserve volume plus residual volume.

Clinically, respiratory volumes and capacities are measured by using a *spirometer* (from the Latin words *spirane,* meaning to breathe, and *metrum,* meaning to measure). Spirometric studies provide a graphic record of the volume that can be expelled from the lung after maximum inspiration (vital capacity) and of how fast the air can be expired. The spirometer can also be used to record the rate and depth of normal respiration and of activity-related respiration.

How Are the Gases Exchanged in the Lungs?

Upon entering the lungs, the venous blood moves through the thousands of tiny lung capillaries that surround the thousands of alveoli. During the passage through the capillaries, where the contact between the blood and the air in the lungs is closest, carbon dioxide is released from the blood into the alveolar space in exchange for oxygen, which is picked up (Fig. 11-13).

The most important mechanism in this exchange is simple diffusion. The concentration of carbon dioxide in the blood is much greater than in the alveolar spaces. As a result, there is a natural diffusion of carbon dioxide out of the blood into the air spaces. Similarly, the concentration of oxygen in the blood entering the lung capillaries is very low compared with the concentration of oxygen in the air spaces. So, again, oxygen diffuses from the lungs into the blood. Of course, if the air drawn into the

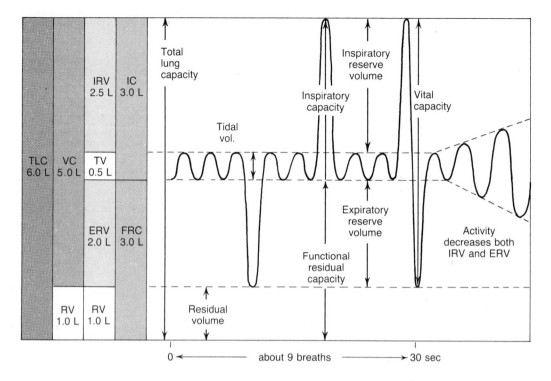

Figure 11–12 Spirometric graph showing respiratory capacities and volumes.

lungs is high in carbon dioxide and low in oxygen, there will be little or no difference between the blood entering and the blood leaving the lungs. Nature (primarily the green plants), however, provides us with an environment that has very little carbon dioxide and an adequate amount of oxygen to sustain life.

The natural process of diffusion of gases between the alveolar spaces and the blood in the capillaries of the lungs is greatly aided by the action of *hemoglobin.* Hemoglobin has the effect of "fooling" the diffusion process, because when oxygen enters the blood from the alveolar space, the hemoglobin combines with it and "hides" it. As a result, the diffusion process just keeps working, trying to even up the concentration of oxygen in the air and in the blood. This keeps happening until all the hemoglobin is used up in hiding oxygen molecules. Then the concentration of free oxygen in the blood rises until it equals the concentration in the alveolar air. By this rather ingenious process (of hiding oxygen molecules) the blood is able to absorb — by diffusion — about 60 times more oxygen than it would without hemoglobin.

The exchange mechanism for carbon dioxide is quite similar. Some of the carbon dioxide from the cells combines with a special amine molecule and then with hemoglobin in the blood. The large molecule, *carbaminohemoglobin* (kar-bam"i-no-he"-mo-glo'bin), quickly releases the carbon dioxide when it reaches the lungs, the hemoglobin then combining with an oxygen molecule. Some of the carbon dioxide, of course, just dissolves in the blood without being carried from the tissues by a hemoglobin combination. This dissolved carbon dioxide turns out to have much greater significance than the similarly dissolved oxygen because dissolved carbon dioxide is *acidic* (oxygen is neutral); the importance of this will be discussed in the following sections.

How Are the Gases Exchanged in the Tissues?

The exchange of gases in the tissues of the body is a very simple reverse of the exchange of gases in the lungs. Oxygen is released from the blood to the

EXCHANGE OF GASES

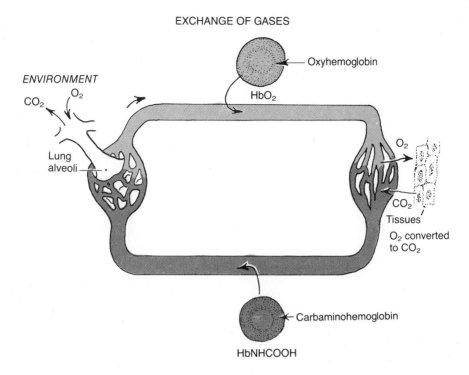

Figure 11–13 Oxygen combines with the hemoglobin of the red blood cell in the lungs to form oxyhemoglobin. Oxygen is carried to the tissues by the red blood cells in this form. When the red blood cell reaches the tissues, it releases the oxygen and picks up carbon dioxide. The carbon dioxide combines with the hemoglobin to form carbaminohemoglobin. The red blood cell carries the carbon dioxide to the lungs, where it releases it into the air in the lung. The lung operates to exchange gases with the environment.

tissue fluid, and carbon dioxide is picked up. The exchange occurs in the capillaries, and again the mechanism is simple diffusion, with the amplifying action of hemoglobin.

The concentration of carbon dioxide is normally high in the tissue fluid, and the concentration of oxygen is low; this is because the cells rapidly turn oxygen into carbon dioxide in their normal metabolic activities. Notice that these concentrations are the exact reverse of what is found in the air of the alveolar space (also environment). This simply serves to reverse the direction of diffusion.

What Are Acidosis and Alkalosis?

Acidosis (as"i-do'sis) is the condition in which there is too much acid in the blood. *Alkalosis* (al"kah-lo'sis) is the condition in which there is too little acid in the blood. The normal pH of the blood is 7.4.

Since carbon dioxide is acidic, a condition of acidosis will occur if there is too much carbon dioxide in the blood. This can occur when respiration is restricted and the carbon dioxide given off by the cells begins to build up.

Alkalosis occurs less frequently but can occur when respiration is overactive. For instance, in *hyperventilation* (too much breathing or ventilation) the exchange of gases occurs too rapidly, there is too little carbon dioxide in the blood, and the pH moves (increases to 7.5 or 7.6) toward alkaline. The chemistry of the blood is in a delicate balance in many complex ways, so that the acid-alkaline balance is very important. Most immediately, the acid level of the blood affects the concentration of sodium and potassium, so that an abnormal acid level can produce very serious side effects in a short period of time.

The respiratory system has the responsibility

for helping to maintain (homeostasis) the acid level of the blood at the normal pH 7.4. If for any reason the blood becomes too acidic, the respiratory system is stimulated to increase activity to give off more carbon dioxide and thereby to lower the acid level back to normal. If there is too little acid in the blood, respiration slows down, allowing carbon dioxide to build up until a normal acid level is reached again.

By holding your breath for a minute or so you can produce a mild acidosis, and by breathing rapidly (hyperventilation) you can produce a mild alkalosis. However, dangerous abnormalities in acid level of the blood cannot be brought about by these voluntary means because the automatic parts of the nervous system override the voluntary and "force" normalization.

What Factors Are Important in the Control of Respiration?

The parts of the nervous system that control respiration are located in the *medulla* (the bulb of the spinal cord) and *pons* in the brain. This general area is known as the *respiratory center.*

Several sets of sensory nerves bring different types of information into the respiratory center. For example, stretch receptors located in the pleura monitor the inspiration and expiration process. The underlying reflex arc, involving the stretch receptors, prevents overexpansion or collapse of the lungs as the extremes of inspiration and expiration are approached.

Several sensory receptors keep track of the CO_2, O_2, and pH levels in the blood. These receptors are known as *chemoreceptors.* If CO_2 concentration gets too high, it stimulates an increased rate of respiration. A similar action occurs if pH gets too low (acidity increase). When O_2 concentration gets too high, the rate and depth of respiration are decreased.

Age is another factor that influences respiratory rate. At birth the rate is rapid — from 40 to 70 times per minute. This decreases with age, so that at about 1 year, 35 to 40 times per minute is normal; at 5 years, about 25 times per minute is normal; at 10 years, a rate of 20; at 25 years, 16 to 18. With old age, however, the rate can increase again to more than 20 times per minute.

CLINICAL CONSIDERATIONS

The most important respiratory disorders are those in which the blood fails to become oxygenated. Nearly all respiratory problems tend toward *hypoxia* (decreased amount of oxygen in the tissues). Hypoxia (hi-pok'se-ah) sometimes results in *cyanosis* (si"ah-no'sis). Cyanosis refers to the fact that the skin, mucous membranes, and surfaces under the nails turn blue because of an increased presence of deoxygenated hemoglobin in the capillaries. The term "cyanosis" is from the Greek word meaning blue.

There are a number of generally recognized patterns of abnormal breathing. *Apnea* is a temporary stopping of breathing, commonly caused by an excess accumulation of oxygen or an insufficient amount of carbon dioxide in the circulation in the brain. Sleep-induced apnea results from the failure of the respiratory center to stimulate adequate respiration during sleep. *Dyspnea* is a shortness of breath and is experienced subjectively as a feeling of difficulty or distress in breathing. It is commonly associated with serious heart or lung disease. In healthy individuals it occurs with intense physical exertion or at high altitudes.

Orthopnea (or"thop-ne'ah; from the Greek, meaning straight and breathing) is the inability to breathe in a horizontal position, a condition that often arises in patients with pneumonia. *Hyperpnea* (hi"-perp-ne'ah) is an increased depth of breathing. *Tachypnea* (tak"ip-ne'ah) is excessively rapid and shallow breathing. Figure 11–14 explains the method of mouth-to-mouth respiration. Figure 11–15 shows a modern hospital artificial respirator.

What Is Emphysema?

Emphysema (em"fi-se'mah) is a condition in which the alveoli of the lungs are dilated (expanded) and the walls of the alveoli are thin and deteriorated. The condition may result from any factor producing repeated distention (stretching) of the lungs, particularly during expiration. This commonly occurs in patients with asthma or chronic bronchitis, which is an inflammation of the bronchial tubes. Heavy smokers have a high incidence of

ARTIFICIAL RESPIRATION
MOUTH-TO-MOUTH (MOUTH-TO-NOSE) METHOD

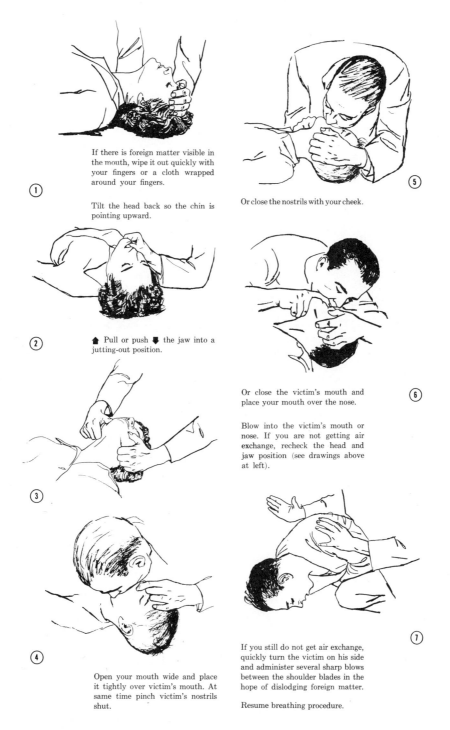

① If there is foreign matter visible in the mouth, wipe it out quickly with your fingers or a cloth wrapped around your fingers.

② Tilt the head back so the chin is pointing upward.

▲ Pull or push ▼ the jaw into a jutting-out position.

③

④ Open your mouth wide and place it tightly over victim's mouth. At same time pinch victim's nostrils shut.

⑤ Or close the nostrils with your cheek.

⑥ Or close the victim's mouth and place your mouth over the nose.

Blow into the victim's mouth or nose. If you are not getting air **ex**change, recheck the head and jaw position (see drawings above at left).

⑦ If you still do not get air exchange, quickly turn the victim on his side and administer several sharp blows between the shoulder blades in the hope of dislodging foreign matter.

Resume breathing procedure.

THE AMERICAN NATIONAL RED CROSS

Figure 11-14 Mouth-to-mouth respiration. (Courtesy of the American National Red Cross.)

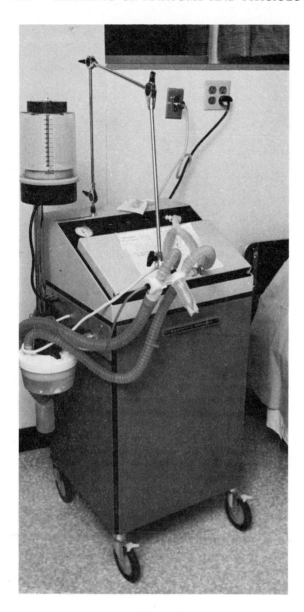

Figure 11–15 Artificial respirator.

emphysema. A patient with emphysema has a barrel-shaped chest, and in severe cases the patient exhibits *clubbing* (a broadening and thickening) of the ends of the fingers.

What Is Asthma?

Asthma is a condition of recurrent labored respiration caused by intermittent obstruction of the bronchi; it is characterized by wheezing and prolonged expiration. The outflow of air through the bronchioles is obstructed more than the inflow, permitting the asthmatic to inspire more easily than to expire. With long standing asthma, the chest becomes barrel shaped. In children, asthma is commonly caused by sensitivities to food; in adults it is frequently caused by sensitivities to pollen. Asthmatic attacks can result from emotional crises as well as from an allergen (substance causing an allergic reaction).

What Is Pneumonia?

Pneumonia is an inflammation of the lungs in which the alveoli are partially filled by fluid and white blood cells. The alveolar walls become inflamed, and there is generalized *edema* (collection of fluid in tissue spaces) of the lung tissue. As in many other pulmonary diseases, carbon dioxide is adequately excreted, but oxygenation of the blood is diminished. This is caused by the fact that carbon dioxide passes through the alveolar walls about 20 times as readily as does oxygen. Pneumonia occurs most frequently in young children and in the aged. In many cases, the disease is due to an organism, the *pneumococcus* (nu"mo-kok'us); the remainder are due to a variety of common viruses. The word pneumococcus derives from the Greek words, *pneumon,* meaning lung, and *kokkus,* meaning berry.

What Is Tuberculosis?

In tuberculosis (tu-ber"ku-lo'sis), the tubercle bacilli invade the lungs, producing a local tissue reaction. Initially, the area is invaded by macrophages and then becomes walled off by fibrous connective tissue. Thus, a characteristic "tubercle" (from the Latin word *tuber,* meaning a swelling) is produced. In the late stages, secondary infection by other bacilli is present, and more *fibrosis* (abnormal build-up of fibrous connective tissue) results. The fibrosis reduces the ability of the lung to expand and decreases the vital capacity. Fibrosis also decreases the working surface area of the lungs, thus decreasing the capacity for exchange of gases by diffusion.

What Is Pulmonary Edema?

Pulmonary edema, the collection of fluids in the tissue spaces of the lung, influences respiration in much the same way as pneumonia does. It is caused by an insufficiency of the left heart in pumping blood from the lungs to the rest of the body. Blood tends to collect in the lungs, and fluid leaks out of the capillaries into the tissue spaces, owing to the increased blood pressure in the lungs. The condition is generally the result of heart failure, in which the blood supply to the heart muscles is impaired, as in atherosclerosis.

SUMMARY

A. The respiratory system functions in the exchange of gases between the blood circulating through the lungs and the external environment.
   1. It serves to bring in oxygen and eliminate excess carbon dioxide.
   2. The respiratory system also functions to regulate the acid-base balance in the blood.
B. The upper respiratory tract forms an open passage between the lungs and the exterior environment.
   1. The nose and nasal cavity serve to warm and moisten the air on its way to the lungs.
      a. The mucous membrane lining also captures bacteria and dust particles.
      b. The olfactory cells, in the nasal cavity, function in the sense of smell.
      c. The sinuses are tiny spaces in the bony structures of the skull.
         i) They manufacture mucus for the cleansing of inspired air.
         ii) They also serve as sound chambers, giving us resonance.
   2. The pharynx, or throat, serves both the digestive and respiratory systems.
      a. Food passes from the pharynx into the esophagus.
      b. Air passes from the pharynx into the larynx.
      c. The epiglottis serves as gatekeeper.
      d. The eustachian tubes, tonsils, and adenoids are associated with the pharynx.
   3. The larynx, or "voice box," connects the pharynx and trachea.
      a. The chief function is sound production.
      b. Loose vocal cords produce low-pitched sounds, and tight cords produce high-pitched sounds.
   4. The trachea, or "windpipe," is a cylindrical passageway that reaches the lungs.
   5. The two primary bronchial tubes split from the trachea, each leading to one of the lungs.
C. The thoracic cavity is separated from the abdominal cavity by the diaphragm.
   1. The mediastinum is the middle compartment of the chest between the lungs.
   2. Each pleural cavity contains one lung.
D. The lungs are two cone-shaped organs extending from the diaphragm to just below the clavicle.
   1. The right lung has three lobes, and the left lung has two.
   2. The primary bronchi repeatedly branch to form thousands of air passages, like an upside-down tree.
   3. The smallest passages, the bronchioles, subdivide into very tiny twiglike passages called alveolar ducts.
   4. Each alveolar duct blossoms into a cluster of alveolar sacs—like clusters of grapes.
   5. Each sac, or alveolus, is surrounded by a rich network of capillaries, where the exchange of gases takes place.
   6. The interior surface area of the lungs is many times the surface area of the skin.
E. The process of breathing involves two phases: inspiration and expiration.
   1. Inspiration requires muscular expansion of chest volume drawing air into the lungs.
   2. Expiration is ordinarily passive; chest volume decreases, pushing air out.
   3. Costal breathing is shallow with an upward and outward movement of the chest.
      a. It is powered by the intercostal muscles.
      b. It is seen in runners at the end of a race.
   4. Diaphragmatic breathing is deep with movement of the abdominal wall.
      a. It is caused by contraction and descent of the diaphragm.
      b. It is usually seen during deep sleep.

F. Normal breathing moves the tidal volume back and forth.
   1. The vital capacity is the total of maximum inspiration plus maximum expiration.
   2. Total lung capacity is the volume at the point of maximal inhalation.
   3. Residual volume is the volume remaining after maximal expiration.
   4. Functional residual capacity is the expiratory reserve volume plus residual volume.
   5. The spirometer is used to measure respiratory volumes and capacities.
G. The most important mechanism in the exchange of gases is natural diffusion.
   1. Hemoglobin aids the diffusion process at the lungs by binding (or hiding) oxygen as it enters the blood.
   2. With hemoglobin the blood carries 60 times more oxygen than it could without it.
   3. Hemoglobin also increases the ability of the blood to carry carbon dioxide from the tissues to the lungs.
H. Acidosis, too much acid in the blood, and alkalosis, too little acid in the blood, are influenced by respiration.
   1. Carbon dioxide is acidic, so too much produces acidosis, and too little produces alkalosis.
   2. The normal pH of the blood is 7.4.
I. Respiration is controlled by the medulla (bulb of the spinal cord) and pons in the brain.
   1. Information is received from stretch receptors, chemoreceptors.
   2. Automatic parts of the nervous system override voluntary control when necessary for normalization.
J. The most serious respiratory disorders are those in which the blood fails to become oxygenated.
   1. Hypoxia is a decrease of oxygen in the tissues.
   2. Cyanosis refers to the bluish appearance of skin, mucous membranes, and surfaces under the nails due to an increased presence of deoxygenated blood.
K. There are several types of abnormal breathing.
   1. Apnea is a temporary stopping of breathing.
      a. It is usually caused by an excess accumulation of oxygen or an insufficient amount of carbon dioxide in the brain.
      b. Sleep-induced apnea results from failure of the respiratory center to stimulate adequate respiration during sleep.
   2. Dyspnea is a shortness of breath, a feeling of difficulty or distress in breathing.
      a. It is commonly associated with serious heart or lung disease.
      b. In healthy individuals it occurs with intense physical exertion or at high altitudes.
   3. Orthopnea is the inability to breath in a horizontal position; it is commonly associated with pneumonia.
   4. Hyperpnea is an increased depth of breathing.
   5. Tachypnea is excessively rapid and shallow breathing.
L. Emphysema involves a deterioration of the alveoli.
M. Asthma is a condition of recurrent labored respiration.
   1. It is caused by intermittent obstruction of the bronchi.
   2. It is characterized by wheezing and prolonged expiration.
N. Pneumonia is an inflammation of the lungs.
   1. The alveoli become inflamed and partially filled with fluid and white blood cells.
   2. There is a generalized edema—a collection of fluid in the lung tissue.
   3. Carbon dioxide is expelled, but oxygenation of the blood is more difficult.
   4. The pneumococcus organism is a common cause, although a variety of common viruses may also be responsible.
O. Tuberculosis is caused by infection with the tubercle bacilli.
P. Pulmonary edema is the collection of fluids in the tissue spaces of the lungs.
   1. It is generally associated with heart failure caused by an insufficiency of the left heart.
   2. Blood collects in the lungs, and fluid leaks out of the capillaries into the tissue spaces.

REVIEW QUESTIONS

1. What is the primary function of the respiratory system?

2. Identify an important secondary function of the respiratory system.

3. List the structures through which air passes from the nose to the alveoli.

4. What are the two sets of muscles that produce the mechanical force needed for breathing?

5. Explain the relation between the pleural cavities and the mediastinum within the thoracic cavity.

6. Where in the respiratory tract is the air filtered, warmed, and moistened?

7. What prevents food from entering the larynx during swallowing?

8. Foreign objects entering the trachea usually enter and potentially lodge in the right bronchus. Why?

9. Explain how the structure of the alveoli facilitates the exchange of gases.

10. There are two different mechanisms of breathing. Identify the muscles and other structures involved in each.

11. What is tidal volume? Vital capacity?

12. What is the most important mechanism in the exchange of gases?

13. How does hemoglobin aid the process of gas exchange?

14. Define acidosis and alkalosis.

15. How does respiration affect the pH of the blood? What is the effect of hyperventilation?

16. What are the two major brain areas constituting the respiratory center that are involved in the nervous control of breathing?

17. Several sets of sensory nerves bring information to the respiratory center. Give examples.

18. What two chemical factors modify respiratory rate and depth?

19. Explain how hypoxia usually results in cyanosis.

20. Define and distinguish apnea and dyspnea.

21. Define and distinguish orthopnea, hyperpnea, and tachypnea.

22. Characterize the following respiratory disorders: emphysema, asthma, pneumonia, tuberculosis, and pulmonary edema.

T W E L V E

The Digestive System

The aim of this chapter is to enable the student to do the following:

- Describe the overall functions of the digestive system.

- Construct and label a diagram of the gastrointestinal tract and its associated accessory organs showing their relative positions.

- Describe the specific function of each of the digestive system organs.

- Describe the main function of the peritoneal membrane system.

- List the sequence of events in swallowing.

- Describe the essential mechanical and chemical steps in the breakdown of foodstuffs as they move along the digestive tract.

- Explain how the structure of the villi

- aids the process of absorption in the small intestine.

- Explain the function of bile in the digestive process.

- Describe the role of the pancreas and the liver in glucose metabolism.

- List the end products of protein, fat, and carbohydrate metabolism.

- Explain what is meant by basal metabolic rate.

- Define and characterize dental caries, pyorrhea, ulcers, abnormal absorption, cirrhosis, cholecystitis, and jaundice.

- Explain the relation between saturated fats in the diet and cancer, stroke, and heart disease.

THE DIGESTIVE SYSTEM: AN OVERVIEW

What Does the Digestive System Do?

The digestive system has three primary functions: digestion, absorption, and elimination. *Diges-* *tion* (from the Latin word meaning to divide into parts) is the process of breaking down large food molecules into the simple nutrient molecules that can be used by the cells. *Absorption* is the process by which the simple nutrient molecules are transferred from the digestive tract into the blood stream for delivery to the cells. *Elimination* is the process of passing the leftover solid wastes of ingested foods from the body.

What is the Peritoneum?

The peritoneum (per"i-to-ne'um) is a lubricated, double-membrane system. One layer of the peritoneum, known as the *parietal* (pah-ri'e-tal) *peritoneum*, lines the abdominal cavity. The other layer, known as the *visceral* (vis'er-al) *peritoneum*, forms a covering that adheres to the surface of each abdominal organ. Between these two membrane layers is a small amount of lubricating serous fluid. The main function of the peritoneal membrane system is to allow the abdominal organs to slide freely and easily against each other during breathing and digestive movements. Without this system, frictional irritation would develop. Notice the similarity between the peritoneum and the pleural membrane system discussed in Chapter 11, The Respiratory System.

What Structures Make Up the Digestive System?

The digestive system consists of (1) a long, muscular *tube* beginning at the lips and mouth and ending at the anus and includes the pharynx, esophagus, stomach, and intestines; and (2) certain large accessory glands located outside the digestive tube, including the salivary glands, liver, gallbladder, and pancreas—each of which secretes its special digestive juice into the digestive tube (Fig. 12–1).

Other terms used frequently to refer to the digestive tube running from the mouth to the anus are the digestive tract and the gastrointestinal tract, or the GI tract for short. The term "gastro" or "gastric" is often used to refer to the stomach, its action, or its products. Alimentary (from the Latin word meaning to nourish) tract is another term referring to the digestive tract that you will encounter.

What Are the Digestive Functions of the Upper Portions of the Tract?

In the upper portions of the digestive tract, food is received into the *mouth* (Fig. 12–2), where the *tongue* functions to mix it with saliva from the salivary glands and to keep the mass pressed between

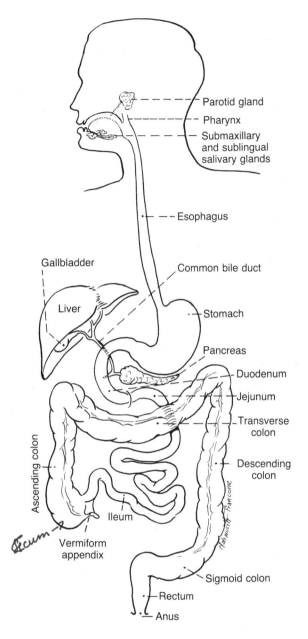

Figure 12–1 The digestive system and its associated structures.

the *teeth* for chewing (Figs. 12–3 and 12–4). In the process of swallowing, the tongue pushes the food back into the throat, initiating a wave of muscular contraction that propels the mixture to the stomach. The *pharynx* (far'inks) and *esophagus* are muscular tubes that convey the chewed food from the mouth

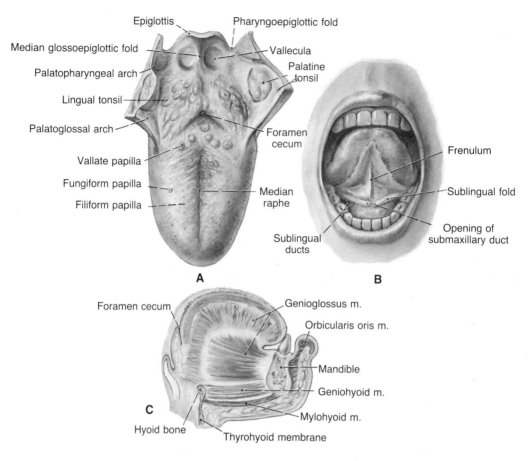

Figure 12-2 *A,* Dorsal view of the tongue. *B,* Anterior view of the oral cavity with tongue raised. *C,* Midsagittal section through the tongue.

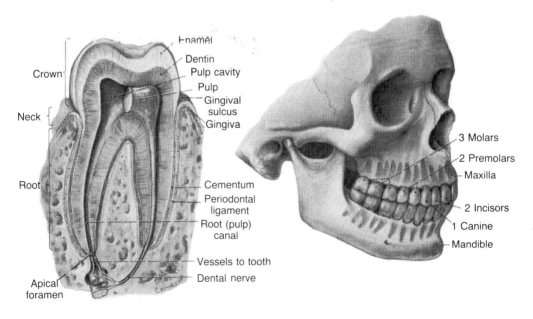

Figure 12-3 Midsagittal view of molar tooth, vertical position.

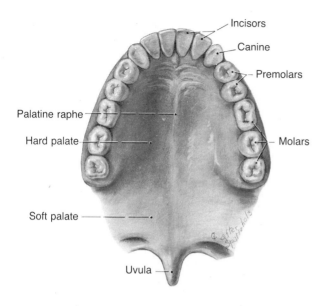

Incisors

Canine

Premolars

Palatine raphe

Hard palate

Molars

Soft palate

Uvula

Figure 12–4 Roof of mouth with adult teeth.

to the stomach. The passage of food from the upper portions of the digestive tract to the stomach is normally aided by gravitational forces; however, the type and arrangement of muscles in the pharynx and esophagus allow swallowing even in the weightless environment of outer space.

THE STOMACH

What Is the Nature of the Stomach?

The *stomach* is the most widened or enlarged portion of the digestive tube. It is located just below the diaphragm on the left side of the body (Fig. 12–5). Its three major functions are to store food; to mix food with gastric secretions until the semi-fluid mass of partly digested food called *chyme* (kime), the Greek word for juice, is formed; and to permit the chyme to slowly empty into the duodenum at a rate suitable for proper digestion and absorption by the small intestine.

When empty, the stomach is only about the size of a large sausage. After a meal, however, it expands considerably. There are three parts or sections to the stomach: the *fundus*, an upper portion ballooning to the left side of the body; the *body*, or central portion; and the *pylorus* (pi-lo′rus), a relatively narrowed

portion at the end of the stomach just before the entrance into the duodenum (small intestine). The term "pylorus" is from the Greek word for gatekeeper. At the very end of the pylorus is the *pyloric sphincter* (sfingk′ter), which opens and closes at appropriate times to allow the flow of chyme into the duodenum. The term "sphincter" always refers to a muscle that closes off some hollow tube or chamber.

The walls of the stomach have an extra layer of muscular tissue not found in other areas of the digestive tube. With its *three* layers of smooth muscle, the stomach is one of the strongest organs of the body. It is well suited to the task of mechanically breaking up food through its strong churning actions. This churning also serves to mix the tiny food particles thoroughly with the gastric juice. Recall that the term "gastric" is used to refer to anything directly related to the stomach.

The gastric juices, which begin the chemical breakdown of the food molecules, are secreted by the thousands of microscopic gland cells located in the inner lining of the stomach wall. Hydrochloric acid (HCl) is one of the more important and effective digestive substances making up the gastric juices.

What Is Peristalsis?

The muscular layers of the stomach, and of the intestines, take part in contractions that produce *peristalsis*, the circular, wavelike movement that propels food down the length of the digestive tract. Swallowing is actually an example of a very powerful peristaltic action. The term "peristalsis" is derived from the Greek words, *peri*, meaning around, and *stalsis*, meaning constriction. A peristaltic constriction narrows the digestive tube at the point of constriction and then travels down the tube, forcing the contents along.

THE SMALL INTESTINE

What Is the Nature of the Small Intestine?

The *small intestine* is about 18 feet long; however, it is noticeably smaller in diameter than the

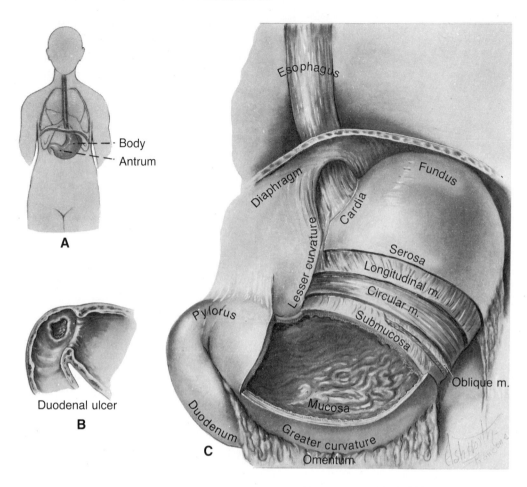

Figure 12–5 *A,* Anatomic position of esophagus and stomach. *B,* Duodenal ulcer. *C,* Anterior view of the stomach with portion of the anterior wall removed. Note the various layers that make up the stomach wall.

large intestine. This small diameter gives the small intestine its name. The small intestine has two primary functions: that of *chemical digestion* and that of *absorption* of nutrients into the blood. In other words, two of the three principle functions of the digestive system are carried out primarily by the small intestine. The upper digestive tract and the stomach function to prepare ingested food by mechanical digestion for the chemical digestive and absorptive processes of the small intestine.

The small intestine has three parts or sections; in the order in which food passes through them, they are the duodenum, the jejunum, and the ileum.

The *duodenum* (du"o-de'num) (from the Latin, *duodeni,* meaning twelve), named because it is about equal in length to the breadth of 12 fingers, is

the shortest, widest, and most fixed portion of the small intestine. The secretions of digestive juices from the liver and pancreas enter the digestive tube at the duodenum.

The inner, mucous lining of the small intestine is typical of the digestive tract as a whole but is distinguished by the thousands of microscopic *villi* or tiny fingerlike projections protruding into the *lumen* (the hollow interior) (Fig. 12–6). The villi absorb the simple, digested nutrients from the small intestine into the blood stream. Inside each villus is a rich network of blood and lymph capillaries. This system of thousands of villi creates a large surface area for contact between the digested nutrients and the blood. This arrangement is similar in function to the alveoli-capillary system in the lungs, which also

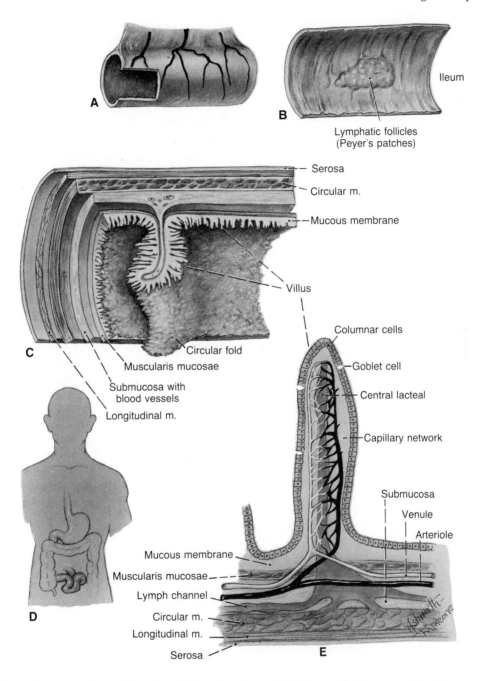

Figure 12-6 *A,* Segment of small intestine. *B,* Interior view of intestine with Peyer's patch. *C,* Layers composing intestinal wall. *D,* Anatomic position showing stomach and large and small intestines. *E,* Midsagittal section through villus.

creates a large surface area of contact for the exchange of gases. The large contact surface in the small intestine, owing to the many tiny villi, increases the rate and efficiency of the (one-way) absorption of nutrients into the blood.

Besides the villi, the inner lining of the small intestine also contains numerous tiny *intestinal glands* that secrete a major portion of the digestive enzymes into the intestinal contents. As will be discussed below under *digestion,* these digestive enzymes work to chemically break down the large food molecules into nutrients that can be easily used by the cells.

THE LARGE INTESTINE

What Is the Nature of the Large Intestine?

The *large intestine,* so named because of its large diameter, differs from the small intestine in several ways. The large intestine neither receives nor secretes digestive juices into its interior. There are no villi on its internal surface.

A considerable amount of fluid moves into the intestinal contents as they pass through the stomach and small intestine. Digestive juices are approximately 95 per cent water. Much of the water is reabsorbed through the walls of the large intestine. The remaining, increasingly solid waste, known as feces (fe'sez), is moved along by peristaltic waves to the *rectum,* where it is eliminated from the body through the *anal canal.*

The major areas of the large intestine in the order in which the contents pass through them are the cecum, the colon, the rectum, and the anal canal (Fig. 12–7).

The contents of the small intestine enter the large intestine at the *cecum* (se'kum), through the *ileocecal* (from *ileum* + *cecum*) *valve.* Attached to the base of the cecum is the *appendix.* In appendicitis, the appendix becomes damaged and inflamed because a solid obstruction (usually some piece of material) has lodged in its interior; in such cases removal of the appendix is usually indicated.

The *colon* is distinguished into three areas: the *ascending colon,* the *transverse colon,* and the *descending colon* (Fig. 12–7). The *rectum* begins at the end of the descending colon and terminates in the narrow *anal canal.* Vertical folds of muscular tissue called rectal columns line the wall of the rectum. These columns are subject to abnormal enlargements known as *hemorrhoids.* Hemorrhoids are either internal (in the anal canal) or external (at the mouth of the anus) and can cause bleeding and pain (Fig. 12–8).

ACCESSORY ORGANS OF DIGESTION

What Is the Digestive Function of the Pancreas?

The *pancreas* (pan'kre-as) is a large, lobulated (having lobes) gland resembling the salivary glands in structural appearance (Fig. 12–9). It is a dual purpose gland, having both exocrine and endocrine functions. *Exocrine* glands secrete into ducts, and in its exocrine function the pancreas secretes *pancreatic juice* (a digestive juice) by way of the pancreatic duct into the duodenum. This pancreatic juice is produced and secreted into the duct by the *acinar* (as'i-nar) *tissue* of the pancreas. The term "acinar" is derived from the Latin word for grape and is appropriate because the acinar tissue looks like tiny clumps of grapes. The pancreatic juices are very important in the chemical breakdown of proteins.

Endocrine glands secrete directly into the blood, and the endocrine portion of the pancreas secretes *insulin* and *glucagon* (gloo'kah-gon), two hormones that are important in controlling the metabolism of glucose. This endocrine portion of the pancreas will be discussed in Chapter 7, The Endocrine System.

What Are the Digestive Functions of the Liver and Gallbladder?

The *liver,* which is the largest organ in the body, is located in the upper part of the abdominal cavity under the dome of the diaphragm. The liver is composed of four major *lobes.* Each lobe is divided into numerous lobules (little lobes), which are the functional units of the liver (Fig. 12–10).

One of the main functions of the liver is to secrete *bile,* a light brown to greenish-yellow alkaline fluid that acts to emulsify fats, neutralize intestinal acid, and remove toxins from the liver. Fats (oils) do not dissolve in water, as do salts. In an emulsion very tiny globules of fat are dispersed and suspended in water; for instance, milk is an emulsion of fats suspended in water. Some of the bile drains out of the liver by way of the *hepatic ducts.* (The term "hepatic" refers to anything concerning the liver

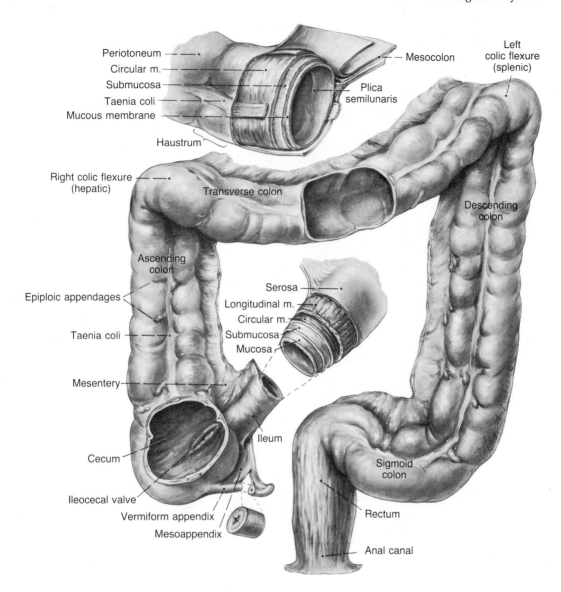

Figure 12-7 Position and structure of the large intestine. The walls of both the large and small intestine have been enlarged and dissected to show their various layers.

and is used similarly to the term "renal," which refers to anything concerning the kidneys.) Between meals, however, bile goes up the *cystic duct* into the *gallbladder* (Fig. 12-11) for concentration and storage. "Gall" is the old word for bile. After meals, when fats are prevalent in the duodenum, bile drains from both the gallbladder and the liver proper, joining in the *common bile duct* and entering

the duodenum. Bile is very important in the digestive breakdown of fats and is essential for the absorption of fat-soluble vitamins.

Notice all the previous discussion of ducts; the production and secretion of substances into a duct is the defining characteristic of exocrine glands. The liver, then, is an exocrine gland in this functional relation to the digestive system.

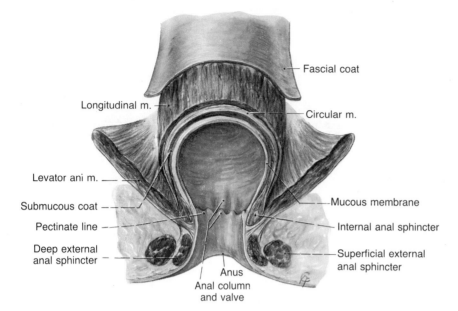

Fascial coat

Longitudinal m.

Circular m.

Levator ani m.

Submucous coat

Pectinate line

Deep external anal sphincter

Mucous membrane

Internal anal sphincter

Superficial external anal sphincter

Anus

Anal column and valve

Figure 12–8 The anal canal and the various layers of the rectum.

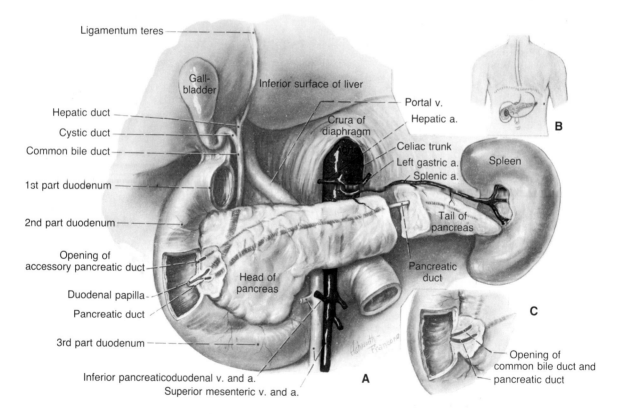

Ligamentum teres

Gall-bladder

Inferior surface of liver

Hepatic duct

Cystic duct

Common bile duct

1st part duodenum

2nd part duodenum

Opening of accessory pancreatic duct

Duodenal papilla

Pancreatic duct

3rd part duodenum

Inferior pancreaticoduodenal v. and a.

Superior mesenteric v. and a.

Portal v.

Crura of diaphragm

Hepatic a.

Celiac trunk

Left gastric a.

Splenic a.

Spleen

Tail of pancreas

Head of pancreas

Pancreatic duct

Opening of common bile duct and pancreatic duct

B

C

A

Figure 12–9 *A,* Relationship of the pancreas to the duodenum, showing the pancreatic and bile ducts joining at the duodenal papilla. A section has been removed from the pancreas to expose the pancreatic duct. *B,* Anatomic position of the pancreas. *C,* Common variation.

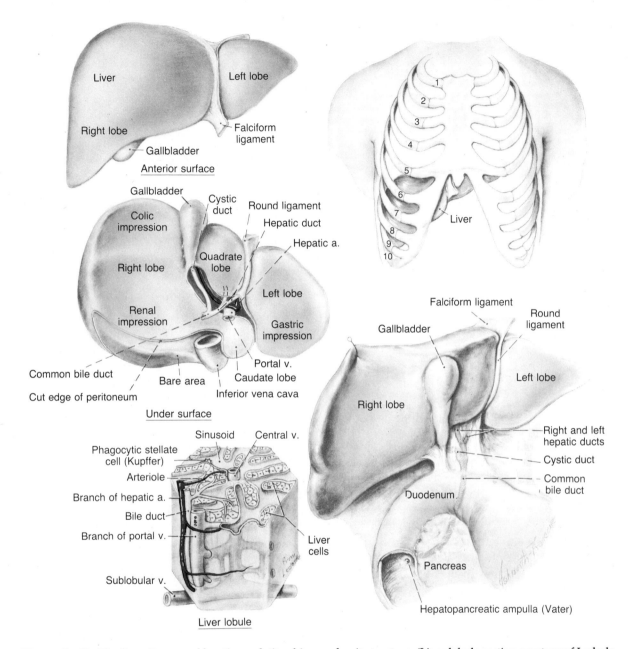

Figure 12–10 The liver, its normal location, relationships, and unit structure. (Liver lobule section courtesy of Lederle Laboratories.)

What Is the Role of the Liver in Glucose Metabolism?

It has already been mentioned that parts of the pancreas are important in glucose metabolism (production of the hormones insulin and glucagon). The liver cells play a different role in glucose metabolism but one of great, and perhaps equal, importance.

Since glucose is easily absorbed into the blood from the small intestine, its concentration in the blood increases after a meal. As its level in the blood begins to rise, the liver cells take up the glucose and

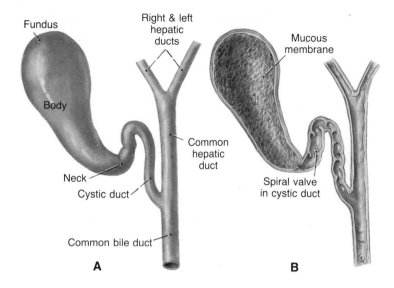

Figure 12-11 *A,* External view of the gallbladder. *B,* Sagittal section through the gallbladder.

combine it into the large molecules of *glycogen* (gli'ko-jen); in this manner glucose is stored for later use. This process is known as *glycogenesis* (*glyco* for glycogen + *genesis,* to make). Later, between meals, the liver cells will reverse the process, in a regulated way, to supply glucose to the blood as the body needs it. This reverse process is known as *glycogenolysis* (*glycogen* + *olysis,* to dissolve into parts).

One other important process occurring in liver cells that is related to glucose metabolism is known as *gluconeogenesis* (*gluco-se* + *neo,* new, + *genesis,* to make), which means literally "making new glucose." It consists of a series of chemical reactions performed by the liver cells to produce glucose molecules from proteins and fats. The process involves breaking down the proteins or fats into molecular pieces and then building up glucose molecules from some of the parts.

The liver cells also store vitamins A, D, E, and K as well as B_{12} and certain other water-soluble vitamins. Table 12-1 lists the major vitamins, their source, function, and the results of deficiencies.

DIGESTION

What Is Involved in the Process of Digestion?

Digestion is the process by which ingested foods are broken down both mechanically and chemically into simple nutrient molecules, which can later be most easily used by the cells.

The first stage of the process of digestion involves chewing, swallowing, and the mixing of substances in the stomach to produce chyme. This is the stage of mechanical breakdown of the food, although even during this period some chemical breakdown of large food molecules has begun. Special digestive enzymes that begin this chemical breakdown are secreted into the mouth by the salivary glands and into the stomach by the glands in the stomach lining.

The final tasks of chemical digestion take place in the small intestine, where the digestive juices from the pancreas and the intestinal lining, and bile from the liver, are delivered into the duodenum. Figure 12-12 illustrates the time required for food substances to reach various portions of the digestive tract.

How Are Proteins Digested?

Protein digestion is accomplished by the digestive enzymes from the pancreas and intestinal walls (Fig. 12-13). Protein molecules are broken down by stages into amino acids. *Amino acids* are sometimes called the "building blocks of proteins." These small, nutritive molecules are then transported to the cells, where they are used to make new proteins that serve specific human body functions. Amino acids are the same in all organisms. Many protein

Table 12–1   VITAMINS

VITAMIN	SOURCE	FUNCTION	DEFICIENCY
Fat Soluble			
A	Yellow vegetables, fish liver oils, milk, butter, eggs	Essential for maintenance of normal epithelium; synthesis of visual purple for night vision	Faulty keratinization of epithelium; susceptibility to night blindness
D	Egg yolk, fish liver oils, whole milk, butter	Facilitates absorption of calcium and phosphorus from the intestine; utilization of calcium and phosphorus in bone development	Rickets in children; osteomalacia in adults
E	Lettuce, whole wheat, spinach	Essential for reproduction in rats; no definite function has been determined in humans	Sterility in rats; no known effects on humans
K	Liver, cabbage, spinach, tomatoes	Synthesis by the liver of prothrombin; necessary for coagulation	Impaired mechanism of blood coagulation
Water Soluble			
B complex:			
B_1 (thiamine)	Whole grain cereals, eggs, bananas, apples, pork	Coenzyme in metabolism of carbohydrate as thiamine pyrophosphate (cocarboxylase); maintains normal appetite and normal absorption	Beriberi, polyneuritis
B_2 (riboflavin)	Liver, meat, milk, eggs, fruit	Coenzyme in metabolism (as flavoprotein)	Glossitis, dermatitis
B_6 (pyridoxine)	Whole grain cereal, yeast, milk, eggs, fish, liver	Coenzyme (as pyridoxal phosphate) in amino acid metabolism	Dermatitis
Niacin	Liver, milk, tomatoes, leafy vegetables, peanut butter	Niacinamide in metabolic processes, especially energy release	Pellagra
B_{12}	Liver, kidney, milk, egg, cheese	Maturation of erythrocytes	Pernicious anemia
Pantothenic acid	Egg yolk, lean meat, skim milk	Necessary for synthesis of acetyl coenzyme A, metabolism of fats, synthesis of cholesterol, and antibody formation	Neurologic defects
Folic acid	Fresh, leafy green vegetables, liver	Production of mature erythrocytes	Macrocytic anemia
Biotin	Liver, egg, milk; synthesized by bacteria in the intestinal tract	Coenzyme in amino acid and lipid metabolism	Not defined in humans, since a large excess is produced by intestinal flora
C (ascorbic acid)	Citrus fruits, tomatoes, green vegetables, potatoes	Production of collagen and formation of cartilage	Scurvy; susceptibility to infection; retardation of growth, tender, swollen gums, pyorrhea, poor wound healing

molecules contain 1000 or more amino acids in very specific sequences and arrangements.

In other words, the proteins of one species are almost never identical to those of another species, so that it is necessary for the human body to break down the ingested proteins from meat, fish, eggs, and cheese into constituent amino acids, and then build up new proteins from the amino acids. These new proteins will work in the human body but would not work in the body of another species.

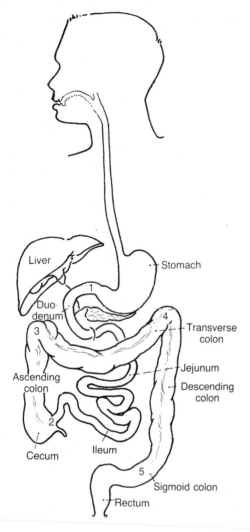

1—1–5 min.
2—4½ hrs.
3—6½ hrs.
4—9½ hrs.
5—12–24 hrs.

Figure 12–12 The time required for food substances to reach various portions of the digestive tract.

How Are Carbohydrates and Fats Digested?

Digestion of *carbohydrates,* such as sugars and starches, occurs mainly in the small intestine (Fig. 12–14). The chemical breakdown is effected by the enzymes of the pancreatic juice and those of the intestine. The main end product of carbohydrate digestion is *glucose* (from the Greek word for sweet). Glucose is the principal source of energy for the cells—it is the "energy molecule." Other end products of carbohydrate digestion are galactose and fructose.

Digestion of *fats* is slow until *bile* from the liver and gallbladder is introduced into the duodenum (Fig. 12–15). Bile breaks down the large fat globules into tiny particles; then the pancreatic enzymes split the fat molecules into glycerol and fatty acids. These two substances are the end products of fat digestion. They can be easily absorbed into the blood and picked up and utilized by the cells.

ABSORPTION OF NUTRIENTS

How Are the Nutrient Molecules Absorbed into the Blood?

Absorption is the process by which the end products of digestion are transferred from the interior of the digestive tract into the blood stream. The mechanism of absorption is mostly by *passive diffusion,* but *active transport* of substances into the blood is not uncommon.

Absorption through the wall of the stomach is limited, but small amounts of water, simple salts, glucose, and alcohol can be absorbed to some extent.

The small intestine, with its large number of *villi,* is the site of most absorption from the digestive tract. The major absorption of carbohydrate, protein, and fat occurs through the capillaries of the villi in the small intestine (Fig. 12–16).

If absorption of substances from the digestive tube into the blood did not occur, the cells would never get any of the substances that pass down through the digestive tract.

How Are the Specific Nutrients Utilized?

Figures 12–17 to 12–19 summarize the specific metabolism of carbohydrates, proteins, and lipids.

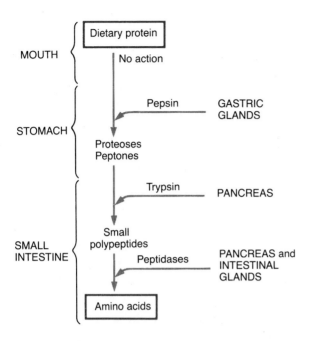

Figure 12–13 Digestion of protein. Note that protein is broken down to proteoses and peptones in the stomach and to small polypeptides and amino acids in the small intestine.

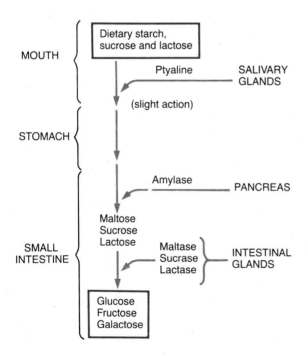

Figure 12–14 Digestion of carbohydrate. Note that the major digestion of carbohydrate occurs in the small intestine, with the end products being glucose, fructose, and galactose.

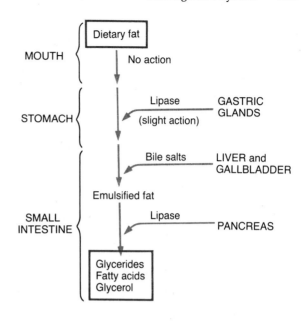

Figure 12–15 Digestion of neutral fat, with the end products being glycerides, fatty acids, and glycerol.

The illustrations show how, or from what source, the specific substance enters the blood stream, and then (on the right) when it is utilized in the body. All nutrients originally enter the blood through the intestine, but many are stored in the liver or tissues, from where they can be released more slowly into the blood as needed.

What is Basal Metabolic Rate?

Recall that the term *metabolism* refers to all the chemical reactions of the body. When biologists and physiologists speak generally of metabolic rate, however, they are normally referring to the rate of energy metabolism. The standard measure of the rate of energy metabolism is called *basal metabolic rate* or *BMR*. The word "basal" derives from the same root as the word "basic."

Basal metabolic rate, then, refers to the rate of utilization of energy (how much energy is used) by an individual who has not eaten for 12 to 24 hours —this time interval being the standard for comparison between individuals. The units of BMR are usually given in calories per hour. This measure is arrived at by determining the amount of oxygen consumed per minute in normal activity.

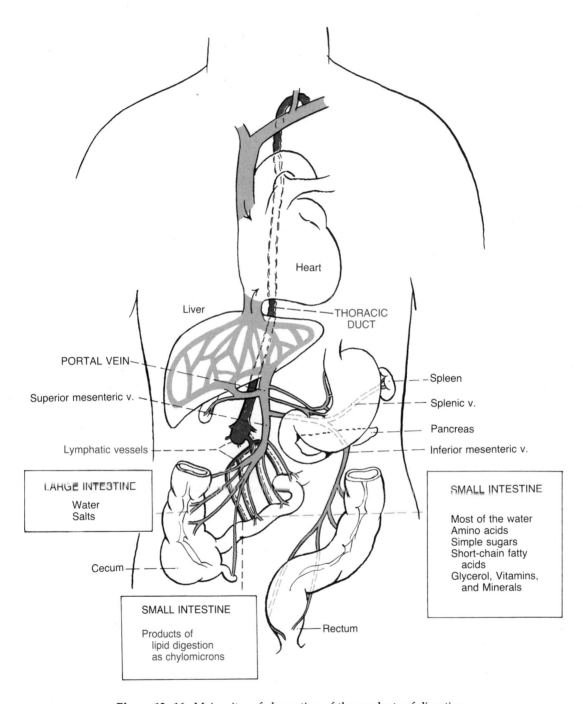

Figure 12–16   Major sites of absorption of the products of digestion.

CARBOHYDRATE METABOLISM

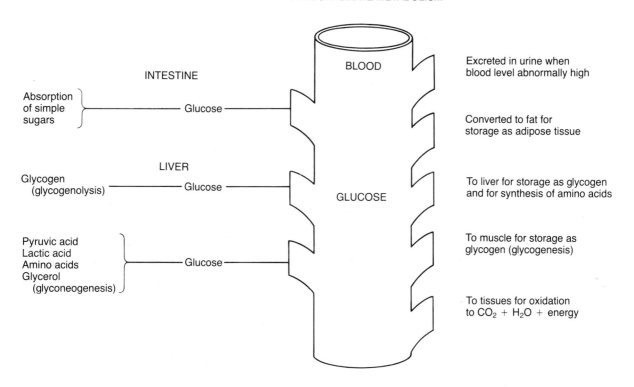

Figure 12-17 Metabolism of carbohydrate.

CLINICAL CONSIDERATIONS

The Teeth and Gums

Dental Caries Caries (ka're-ez) is a progressive disease of the teeth that destroys the enamel and causes *cavities*. The term "caries" is from the Latin word meaning dry rot. Dental caries is largely preventable by ingesting fluoride. When proper amounts of fluoride are ingested during dental development, a reduction in caries of about 60 per cent has been demonstrated.

Fluoridation of water is a widely accepted method of supplying dental fluoride.

Pyorrhea (pi"o-re'ah) This is an inflammatory process of the gums in which the teeth become loose and fall out. Bacteria from dental infection can spread through the blood to the heart, causing inflammation of the lining membrane of the heart (bacterial endocarditis).

The Stomach and Duodenum

Ulcer An ulcer is a sore or lesion on the surface of the skin of a mucous membrane. A peptic ulcer is an ulcer that occurs in either the stomach or duodenum. This relatively frequent condition results from an oversecretion of gastric juices, particularly hydrochloric acid (HCl). The major goal of treatment is to reduce this oversecretion of HCl through dietary control and ingestion of antacids or by inhibiting nerve stimulation of the stomach. Occasionally,

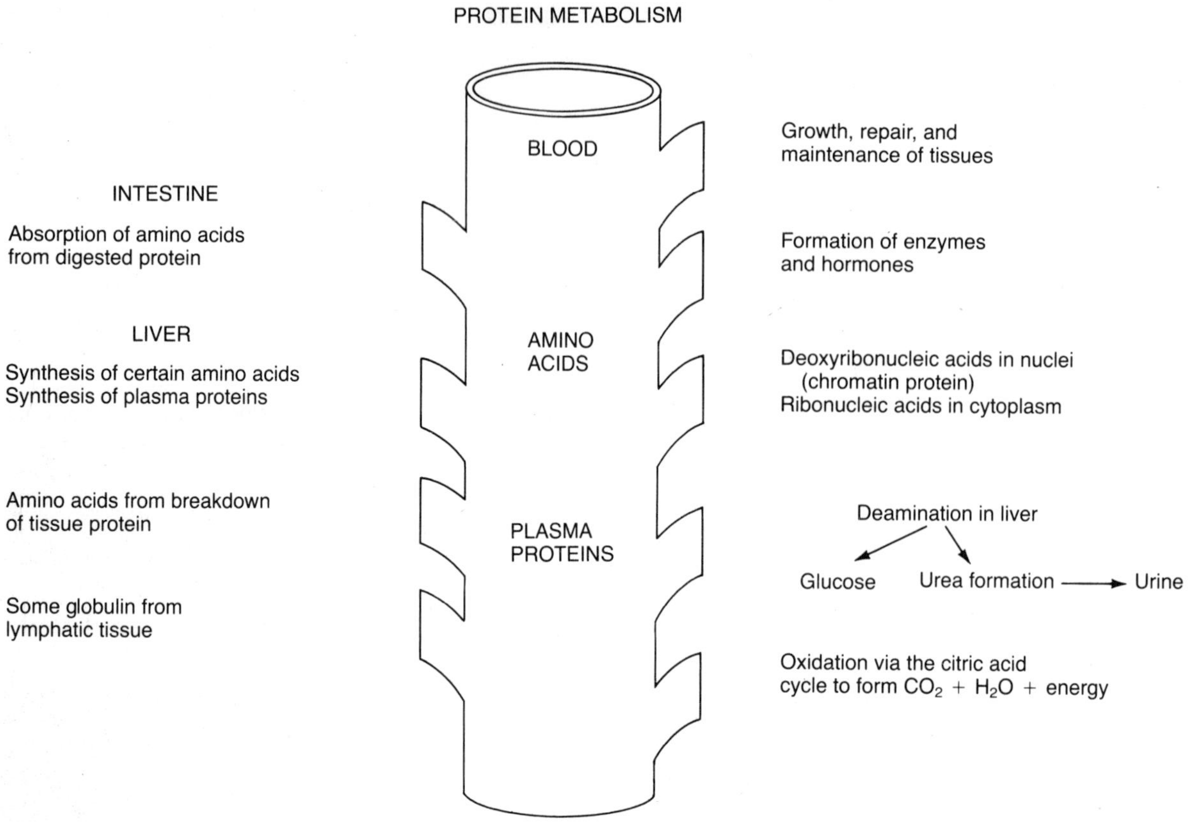

PROTEIN METABOLISM

INTESTINE

Absorption of amino acids
from digested protein

LIVER

Synthesis of certain amino acids
Synthesis of plasma proteins

Amino acids from breakdown
of tissue protein

Some globulin from
lymphatic tissue

BLOOD

AMINO
ACIDS

PLASMA
PROTEINS

Growth, repair, and
maintenance of tissues

Formation of enzymes
and hormones

Deoxyribonucleic acids in nuclei
(chromatin protein)
Ribonucleic acids in cytoplasm

Deamination in liver

Glucose   Urea formation ———→ Urine

Oxidation via the citric acid
cycle to form $CO_2 + H_2O$ + energy

Figure 12-18   Metabolism of protein.

surgical removal of part of the stomach or duode
num is necessary.

Abnormal Absorption

Several conditions can lead to abnormal absorption of digested nutrients from the small intestine. A number of diseases and disorders of the
small intestine itself will inhibit proper absorption.

Disorders of the accessory glands, such as the
liver and pancreas, can cause inadequate absorption
because of incomplete digestion.

A balanced diet is necessary for proper absorption to take place; the necessity of having vitamin D
in the diet in order for calcium absorption to occur is

an example of this. Some researchers have argued
that arteriosclerosis, the cholesterol (lipid) disorder,
can be prevented by proper diet. Modern nutrition
research has turned up many cases where absorption of one nutrient is either increased or inhibited
by the presence of some other substance in the diet.

The Liver and Gallbladder

Cirrhosis (sir-ro'sis)   This is a disease of the
liver leading to a progressive degeneration of liver
cells. It is characterized anatomically by an increase
in connective tissue (scar tissue) throughout the
liver. In alcoholic cirrhosis, its most common form,
the disease is preceded by a dietary deficiency. The
alcoholic person tends to have a reduced intake of

LIPID METABOLISM

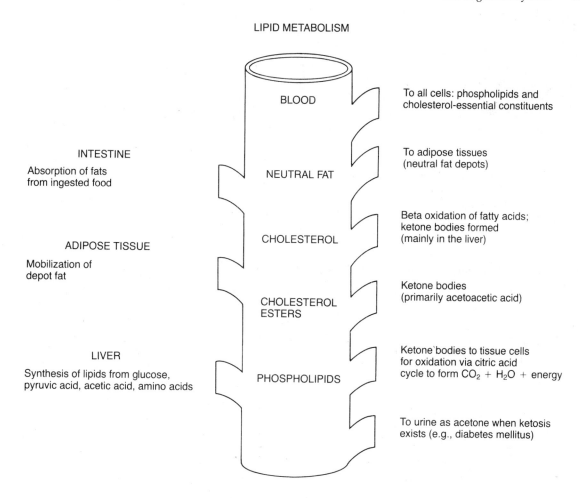

Figure 12–19   Metabolism of lipids.

fat, protein, and carbohydrate as well as of vitamins, especially B_{12}.

Cholecystitis (ko"le-sisti'tis)   This is an inflammation of the gallbladder. The term derives from the Greek roots, *chole,* meaning bile, and *kystis,* meaning bladder, + *itis,* meaning inflammation. *Cholelithiasis* (ko"le-li-thi'ah-sis), stones in the gallbladder, is associated with a chronic inflammation of the bladder wall, giving rise to a loss of normal capacity to absorb and concentrate. The term

derives from the Greek roots, *chole,* meaning bile, + *lithos,* meaning stone.

Jaundice (jawn'dis)   A term derived from the French word for yellow, jaundice is a yellow discoloration of the skin, mucous membranes, and body fluids because of an excess of bile pigment. The most common type is obstructive jaundice, which is caused by internal blockage of the bile duct by gallstones or by a growth such as a tumor. Hepatic jaundice is a result of hepatitis, an inflammation of the liver, usually due to an *acute infection.*

Fat in the Diet

Since the 1940s there has been demographic evidence—through comparison of diets and the incidence of disease in various countries—suggesting a direct link between the amount of saturated (animal) fats in a person's diet and his or her likelihood of cancer, heart disease, and stroke. For instance, in communities in which the diets are based on vegetables, grains, and fruits, with smaller amounts of animal fat, the incidence of cancer and circulatory diseases is extremely low.

This early evidence alone, although compelling, did not clearly rule out a genetic explanation. Recently, more careful follow-up studies have established beyond a reasonable doubt the link between a high intake of saturated (animal) fats and the incidence of cancer, stroke, and heart disease.

The later studies compared people from the same genetic pool as they moved to other countries with different diets. They also watched the consequences of affluence in some oil-rich African countries where there was a shift among a portion of the population to Western lifestyles and diets. In these latter cases, those who shifted to the Western diets displayed the higher incidence of cancer and circulatory disease characteristic of Western countries, while those remaining on the traditional diet showed no increase in the incidence of these diseases.

The common culprit suspected in the diets of most industrialized nations is the high intake of saturated fats, particularly animal fats: eggs, dairy products (including butter and cheese), and fats of meats (primarily red meat). Another source of problematic saturated fats is altered vegetable fats, which may become saturated incidentally through cooking (frying) or deliberately by hydrogenation in processing. The introduction of some highly saturated vegetable oils such as palm and coconut oils has been a particular problem in the last 2 decades.

The later research also showed that the negative effects of overconsumption of animal fats were partially offset (reduced) in those countries where there was also a high consumption of fiber in the diet. Another line of research has discovered that balancing the intake of animal fats with a greater intake of another type of fat (omega-3 fatty acids from fish) can offset some of the effects of the overconsumption of animal (saturated) fats.

Currently, in most industrialized countries the average diet is nearly 40 per cent fat, with about half that being saturated fats.

Based on this more recent evidence, in 1985 the National Cancer Institute (NCI) of the National Institutes of Health concluded that at least 35 per cent of all cancers are traceable to this dietary factor. (They mention, as many less conservative groups believe, that the correct figure could be as high as 60 per cent.)

NCI has since changed its official recommendation on fats in the diet, recommending cutting the percentage of total fats to 25 per cent, and saturated fats to 10 per cent, of total intake of calories.

NCI proposes through a change in diet, quitting smoking (half the current smokers), and a conservative cancer screening program that the death rate from cancer in the United States could be lowered by 50 per cent by the year 2000. They state that the likelihood of finding a cure for 50 per cent of the cancers by then is much lower.

Stroke and heart disease appear to be two diseases that are almost totally preventable. In communities with balanced low fat diets, stroke and heart disease are almost unknown.

The American Heart Association (AHA), recognizing the overwhelming evidence of a link between dietary fats and the incidence of stroke and heart disease, has made a new dietary recommendation (1986) of total fat intake of less than 30 per cent of calories, and saturated fat intake of less than 10 per cent.

The AHA further recommends a specific restriction of dietary cholesterol to less than 300 mg/day. Dietary as well as other measures, such as exercise and relaxation, to reduce blood cholesterol are strongly recommended. In a somewhat surprising finding, no lower limit (or threshold) has been found to the relationship: the lower the concentration of blood cholesterol, the lower the risk of heart disease.

SUMMARY

A. The digestive system digests foodstuffs, facilitates their absorption into the blood, and eliminates solid wastes.
   1. Digestion breaks down large foodstuffs into simple nutrient molecules.
   2. The simple nutrients are absorbed into the blood for delivery to the cells.
   3. Leftover solid wastes are eliminated from the body.
B. The peritoneal membrane system functions to allow the abdominal organs, including major portions of the digestive system, to slide freely against each other.
   1. This double membrane system lines the abdominal cavity and covers the abdominal organs.
   2. Without the lubricating function of this system, the process of digestion would create friction and damaging irritation.
C. The digestive system consists of the gastrointestinal tract and the accessory organs.
   1. The gastrointestinal (alimentary) tract is a long muscular tube.
      a. It runs continuously from the mouth to the anus.
      b. It includes the pharynx, esophagus, stomach, and intestines.
   2. The accessory organs are located outside the tube.
      a. These include the salivary glands, liver, gallbladder, and pancreas.
      b. Each secretes its special digestive juice into the digestive tube.
D. The upper GI tract consists of the mouth, tongue, teeth, pharynx, and esophagus.

   1. The mouth receives and holds the food during chewing.
   2. The tongue mixes the food with saliva from the salivary glands and positions it for chewing.
   3. The tongue pushes the chewed food back into the pharynx, initiating a wave of muscular contraction.
   4. This peristaltic wave propels the mixture down the esophagus to the stomach.
E. The stomach is the most widened portion of the digestive tube.
   1. The three main portions are the fundus (upper), body, and the pylorus (lower).
   2. Three layers of smooth muscle allow for powerful churning action to break down food mechanically.
   3. Microscopic gland cells located in the inner lining of the stomach wall secrete gastric juices, including hydrochloric acid.
   4. Chyme is the semifluid mix of food with gastric secretions.
   5. The pyloric sphincter regulates the flow of chyme into the duodenum.
F. Peristalsis is the circular, wavelike movement that propels food down the length of the digestive tract.
   1. The muscular layers produce a constriction, which then travels down the tube, forcing the contents along.
   2. Swallowing is a very powerful peristaltic action.
G. The small intestine is the primary site of chemical digestion and absorption of nutrients into the blood.
   1. The first portion to receive food (chyme) from the stomach is the duodenum, next the jejunum, and finally the ileum.
   2. The digestive juices from the liver and pan-

creas enter the GI tract at the short, wide duodenum.

3. The inner, mucous lining of the small intestine is made up of thousands of microscopic villi protruding into the lumen.
   a. The villi absorb the simple nutrients into the blood stream.
   b. Inside each villus is a rich network of blood and lymph capillaries.
   c. The villi create an enormous surface area that is similar in arrangement to the alveoli-capillary system in the lungs.
   d. The large surface area increases the rate and efficiency of the (one-way) absorption of nutrients.
4. Numerous tiny intestinal glands line the inner surfaces of the small intestine.
   a. These glands secrete digestive enzymes into the lumen.
   b. These digestive enzymes operate in chemical digestion of large food molecules.

H. The large intestine reabsorbs water from the intestinal contents as it moves them along toward elimination from the body.
1. The areas of the large intestine are the cecum, colon, rectum, and anal canal.
2. The contents of the small intestine enter at the cecum through the ileocecal valve.
   a. The appendix is attached to the base of the cecum.
   b. The colon is composed of the ascending colon, transverse colon, and descending colon.
3. The rectum begins at the end of the descending colon and terminates at the anal canal.
   a. Vertical folds of muscular tissue line the wall of the rectum.
   b. Hemorrhoids are enlargements of these rectal columns and can cause pain and bleeding.
      i. Internal hemorrhoids are within the anal canal.
      ii. External hemorrhoids occur at the mouth of the anus.

I. The pancreas is a large lobulated gland with both exocrine and endocrine functions.
1. In its exocrine function it secretes pancreatic juice into the duodenum.
   a. The pancreatic juice is produced by the grapelike clumps of acinar tissue.
   b. The pancreatic juice enters the duodenum by way of the pancreatic duct.
   c. The pancreatic juice is very important in the chemical breakdown of proteins.
2. In its endocrine function it secretes hormones directly into the blood.
   a. The pancreas secretes both insulin and glucagon.
   b. These endocrine hormones help control glucose metabolism.

J. The liver, the largest organ in the body, is located in the upper part of the abdominal cavity under the dome of the diaphragm.
1. The liver is composed of four major lobes, each divided into numerous lobules.
2. The lobules are the functional units.
3. One of the main functions of the liver, as an exocrine gland, is to secrete bile.
   a. Bile is a light brown to greenish-yellow alkaline fluid.
   b. Bile acts to emulsify fats, neutralize intestinal acid, and remove toxins from the liver.
   c. In an emulsion fats are broken down into very tiny globules and suspended in water.
      i. Fats (oils) do not dissolve in water.
      ii. Milk is an emulsion.
   d. Some bile drains directly out of the liver through the hepatic ducts.
   e. Between meals the bile goes up the cystic duct into the gallbladder for concentration and storage.
   f. Bile is essential for the absorption of fat-soluble vitamins.
4. There are three aspects to the important role of the liver in glucose metabolism.
   a. In glycogenesis, liver cells take up glucose from the blood and store it within large molecules of glycogen.
   b. The reverse process, glycogenolysis, releases the stored glucose into the blood in a regulated way.
   c. Gluconeogenesis consists of breaking down proteins and fats into molecular pieces in order to build up glucose molecules from the pieces.
5. The liver also serves to store vitamins A, D, E,

and K as well as B_{12} and certain other water-soluble vitamins.

K. Digestion is the process of breaking down ingested food, both mechanically and chemically, into simple nutrient molecules.

1. The first stage is mechanical breakdown by chewing, swallowing, and the mixing in the stomach to produce chyme.
2. Chemical breakdown begins with the secretion of digestive enzymes by the salivary and stomach glands.
3. The final stages of chemical digestion occur when digestive juices and bile enter the duodenum.

L. Proteins are digested, in stages, into amino acids—the building blocks of proteins.

1. Chemical digestion is accomplished by digestive enzymes from the pancreas and the glands of the intestinal walls.
2. Amino acids are the same in all organisms, with many proteins containing 1000 or more amino acids.
3. Proteins of one species are almost never identical to the proteins of another species.
4. The amino acids are transported to the cells, where they are used to build new, specifically human, proteins.

M. Carbohydrates, such as sugars and starches, are digested into glucose, galactose, and fructose.

1. Chemical digestion of carbohydrates is accomplished by digestive enzymes from the pancreas and the glands of the intestinal walls.
2. Glucose is the main end product of carbohydrate digestion and the principal source of energy for the cells.

N. Fats are digested in two stages.

1. Bile from the liver and gallbladder breaks down large fat globules into tiny particles (molecules).
2. Pancreatic enzymes split the fat molecules into glycerol and fatty acids, which are absorbed into the blood and utilized by the cells.

O. In absorption, the end products of digestion are transferred from the interior of the digestive tract to the blood stream.

1. Absorption occurs primarily by passive diffusion, although there is some active transport.
2. Small amounts of water, simple salts, glucose, and alcohol are absorbed through the stomach wall.
3. Most absorption of digested nutrients occurs through the villi in the small intestine.

P. Basal metabolic rate refers to a standard measure of the rate of energy metabolism, or the rate of utilization of energy.

1. To achieve a standard comparison, the individual must not eat for 12 to 24 hours before the measurement.
2. The measure is arrived at by determining the amount of oxygen consumed per minute at rest.
3. The results are expressed as calories per hour consumed.

Q. There are a variety of disorders of the digestive system.

1. Caries is a disease of the teeth that destroys enamel, causing cavities; it is largely preventable by ingesting fluoride.
2. Pyorrhea is an inflammatory disease of the gums.
3. A peptic ulcer is a sore or lesion on the surface of the mucous membrane in either the stomach or duodenum.
4. Several conditions can lead to abnormal absorption of digested nutrients from the small intestine.
   a. Disorders of the accessory glands can cause inadequate absorption because of incomplete digestion.
   b. A balanced diet is essential for proper absorption of many nutrients.
   c. The common, high fat, high cholesterol diet is believed to be a major factor in the development of cancer, stroke, and heart disease.
5. Cirrhosis of the liver is characterized by progressive degeneration of liver cells and an increase in scar tissue throughout the liver; it is common in alcoholics.
6. Cholecystitis (meaning stones in the gallbladder) is an inflammation of the gallbladder.
7. Jaundice is a yellow discoloration of the skin, mucous membranes, and body fluids caused by excess bile.

a. Most commonly, obstructive jaundice, is caused by internal blockage of the bile duct by stones or a tumor.

b. Hepatic jaundice is a result of hepatitis, an inflammation of the liver, usually due to acute infection.

R. Diets high in saturated fats appear to be one of the primary causes of cancer, heart disease, and stroke.

1. This effect is partially offset in diets that are also high in fiber and/or fish.

2. About 40 per cent of the calories in the average American's diet consist of fat, with about half this being saturated fat.

a. The National Cancer Institute recommends 25 per cent of total calories as fats, with only 10 per cent saturated.

b. The American Heart Association recommends 30 per cent of total calories as fats, with only 10 per cent saturated.

3. There is strong evidence to support the claim that the lower blood the concentration of cholesterol, the lower the risk of heart disease.

REVIEW QUESTIONS

1. Identify and label on a simple line drawing the specialized sections, organs, that make up the continuous gastrointestinal tract.

2. In the proper locations on the drawing, add the liver, pancreas, and the salivary glands, indicating the point at which each empties its secretions into the GI tract.

3. Describe two functions of the tongue in the initial mixing of food with saliva.

4. Astronauts report that it is not only possible to swallow in outer space but also that the contents of the digestive tract continue to move in the same mouth-to-anus direction even without gravity. How is this possible?

5. What special feature of the stomach facilitates its role in the mechanical breakdown of food?

6. What is the primary gastric juice secreted by the microscopic gland cells in the stomach lining?

7. Where does most nutrient absorption occur?

8. Describe the structure and function of the villi.

9. What is the action of the large intestine that leads to the feces being solid?

10. Explain the movement of bile during and between meals.

11. Define glycogenesis, glyconeogenesis, and glycogenolysis.

12. Where does protein digestion take place? What are the sources of the main enzymes responsible for protein digestion? What are the end products of protein digestion?

13. If proteins of all species are made up of the same few amino acids, why is it necessary to breakdown the proteins and make new ones? Why not just utilize appropriate proteins directly?

14. Where does carbohydrate digestion take place? What are the sources of the main enzymes responsible for carbohydrate digestion? What are the end products of carbohydrate digestion?

15. Where does fat digestion take place? What are the sources of the main enzymes responsible for fat digestion? What are the end products of fat digestion?

16. What nutrient is the primary source of food for individual cells? What food group is most important for building cell structures?

17. Define BMR. What factor needs to be controlled for standardization between individuals?

18. Name and characterize the common digestive system disorders, starting with the mouth and moving down the GI tract.

19. Aside from smoking, what is the single main cause of cancer, heart disease, and stroke? What measures have been recommended by the National Institutes of Health and the American Heart Association to reduce cancer, stroke, and heart disease dramatically?

T H I R T E E N

The Urinary System

The aim of this chapter is to enable the student to do the following:

- Construct and label a diagram of the organs of the urinary system showing their relative positions.

- Identify the large scale regions and structures of the kidney.

- Describe the structural and functional characteristics of the nephron.

- Explain the process of urine formation, including the role of antidiuretic hormone and aldosterone.

- Describe the normal composition of urine and the typical substances in abnormal urine.

- Describe the structure and function of the ureters, urinary bladder, and urethra.

- Define polyuria, anuria, and oliguria.

- Identify the major urinary tract disorders.

- Explain hemodialysis and the role of transplantation.

FUNCTION OF THE URINARY SYSTEM

What Does the Urinary System Do?

The *urinary system* functions to *eliminate* the wastes of protein metabolism (mostly urea) and to *regulate* the amount of water in the body and the concentrations of a variety of salts in the blood, including sodium, potassium, calcium, phosphate, and chloride. These tasks are accomplished through the formation and elimination of urine. Urine is mostly water—about 90 per cent—however, the precise make-up depends on what substances are in excess in the blood at the time.

The organs responsible for the formation of urine are the two *kidneys*. The *urinary bladder* receives and holds the urine from the kidneys and periodically eliminates it from the body. The term *renal* is from the Latin word *renalis,* meaning kidney; it is a very common term used normally to refer to anything directly associated with the kidneys.

STRUCTURES OF THE URINARY SYSTEM

What Are the Kidneys?

The *kidneys* are two large bean-shaped organs lying behind the abdominal organs against the muscles of the back (Fig. 13–1). A renal artery, vein, and nerves as well as lymphatic vessels enter and leave the concave (inward curving) surface of each kidney through a notch called the *hilus* (hi'lus). The cavity located at the hilus is a urine-collecting portion called the *renal pelvis.* The renal pelvis also forms the expanded upper portion of the *ureter.* The ureter is a long tube that carries the urine from the kidney to the urinary bladder.

What Is the Internal Structure of the Kidney?

In cross section, the kidney is seen to have an inner darkened area called the *medulla* and an outer pale area called the *cortex* (Fig. 13–2). (The word "cortex" comes from the Latin word for bark [of a tree] or rind [of an orange], so the cortex of an organ — whether it be the kidney, the brain, or the adrenal glands — is its outer layer. Similarly, the medulla of an organ is always its inner portion.)

The *cortex* contains the working parts of the kidney, the *nephrons,* each of which is a tiny urine producing factory. Nephrons have three main parts: a glomerulus, a Bowman's capsule, and a tubule, or renal tubule (Fig. 13–3).

The *glomerulus* (the Latin word *glomero* means to wind into a ball) is a tightly interwoven network (or tuft) of blood capillaries fitted inside a cuplike structure called *Bowman's capsule.* Extending from Bowman's capsule is a long *renal tubule.* The term "tubule," pronounced too'byool, means little tube.

The first segment of each renal tubule is called the *proximal convoluted tubule* — proximal (next to) because it lies nearest the tubule's origin from Bowman's capsule and *convoluted* (Latin meaning, rolled together) because it twists around to form several coils. Next, the tubule forms a loop called the *loop of Henle* (hen'le), after its discoverer. After the loop of Henle comes a larger collecting tube serving many nephrons (Fig. 13–4).

In the *renal medulla* one finds a branching out of the renal artery that feeds into the (outer) cortex. Separately, the urine collecting tubes from the cortex come together in the medulla, finally forming the renal pelvis, which extends to form the ureter.

How Does the Nephron Work?

Three processes are involved in the formation of urine by the nephron. The simplest to understand is the first step, glomerular filtration. But the real magic of the nephron occurs in the next two processes, which take place in the renal tubules, tubular reabsorption and tubular secretion (Fig. 13–5).

Glomerular Filtration   The thin walls of the capillaries of the glomerulus act like a semipermeable membrane. They permit a *protein-free plasma filtrate* to pass out of the blood in the capillaries into Bowman's capsule. The mechanisms underlying the process of glomerular filtration are essentially passive and can be explained mostly in terms of simple diffusion under pressure.

The specific rate of glomerular filtration varies directly with filtration pressure, which is dependent on blood pressure. If blood pressure falls too low, glomerular filtration will stop; the kidneys will shut down. Normally, approximately 1200 ml of blood or about one fourth of the total cardiac output is filtered through the kidneys each minute. Of this, the outflow of protein-free plasma from all the glomerate of both kidneys is about 125 ml, or about 1 ml of filtrate for every 10 ml of blood filtered per minute. If all this became urine, your bladder would be completely filled every 3 to 5 minutes. Surely most of this must be reabsorbed back into the blood stream. But how?

Tubular Reabsorption   Of the 125 ml of glomerular filtrate normally formed each minute, approximately 124 ml is reabsorbed by the cells of the renal tubules and transported back into the blood capillaries surrounding the tubules (see Fig. 13–4). Only 1 ml eventually passes on to the bladder as urine. Different parts of the renal tubule specialize in reabsorbing different substances from the filtrate. Also, the rate at which reabsorption of specific substances takes place can be increased or decreased, depending on various factors. For example, when the amount of water in the body is low (dehydra-

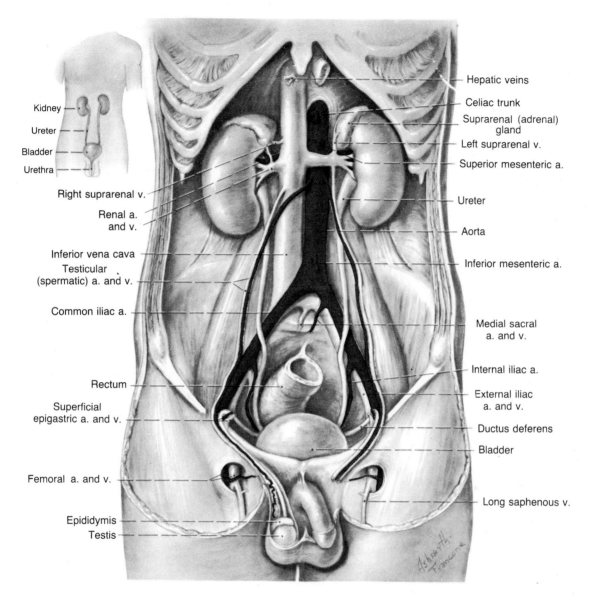

Kidney

Ureter

Bladder

Urethra

Right suprarenal v.

Renal a. and v.

Inferior vena cava

Testicular (spermatic) a. and v.

Common iliac a.

Rectum

Superficial epigastric a. and v.

Femoral a. and v.

Epididymis

Testis

Hepatic veins

Celiac trunk

Suprarenal (adrenal) gland

Left suprarenal v.

Superior mesenteric a.

Ureter

Aorta

Inferior mesenteric a.

Medial sacral a. and v.

Internal iliac a.

External iliac a. and v.

Ductus deferens

Bladder

Long saphenous v.

Figure 13–1 Posterior abdominal wall, showing relationship of urinary system, genital system, and great vessels.

tion), antidiuretic hormone (ADH) is secreted by a gland in the mid-brain (the pituitary), which stimulates the cells of the distal tubule to reabsorb even more water than normal from the filtrate. More water then flows back from the nephron (more specifically, from the tubular filtrate) into the blood, and less urine, or more concentrated urine, is formed. In this way the body prevents further loss of water (and further dehydration) through the urine.

Tubular Secretion Tubular secretion is the reverse of tubular reabsorption. However, the substances secreted are most often different from those that are reabsorbed. In the process of tubular secretion the renal tubular cells — that is, the cells forming the tubules — take substances from the surrounding capillaries and add them to the filtrate inside the tubules. This increases the concentration of these particular substances in the filtrate (soon to be urine). One of the most important substances

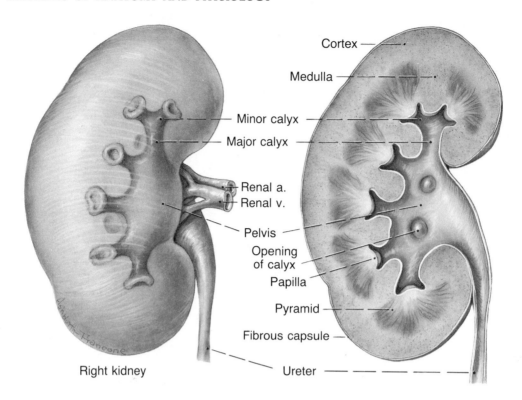

Cortex

Medulla

Minor calyx

Major calyx

Renal a.

Renal v.

Pelvis

Opening
of calyx

Papilla

Pyramid

Fibrous capsule

Right kidney   Ureter

Figure 13–2 Entire and sagittal views showing relation of calyces to kidney as a whole.

secreted into the filtrate by the tubular cells is *hydrogen ion.* This is the active part of all acid substances. When the blood becomes too acidic, the proximal tubules are very active in increasing the elimination of hydrogen ion (the ion of acid) from the blood. The filtration of the blood at the glomerulus, of course, captures many hydrogen ions, but the cells of the renal tubules go even farther by actually drawing these ions out of the blood capillaries in the area and then secreting them into the filtrate fluid. This process can make the urine very acid, but this is much better than having acidic blood.

The renal elimination of acid from the blood is slower to respond to quick increases in blood activity than is the respiratory system. Recall that the respiratory system can increase its activity to eliminate carbon dioxide through the lungs, and since carbon dioxide has an acidic effect while in the blood ($CO_2 + H_2O \rightarrow H^+ + HCO_3$), this helps to reduce the acidity. Over a period of time the kidneys can eliminate a larger amount of acid than can the respiratory system, since the respiratory system is limited by the amount of carbon dioxide that can be safely eliminated. (Table 13–1 summarizes the function of different parts of the nephron. Table 13–2 summarizes the composition of the urine.)

What Controls Kidney Function?

Since it is the function of the kidneys to regulate the concentration of many substances in the blood, it is necessary for the tubules to be highly selective in what they reabsorb and what they secrete. Some of the selective elimination by the nephrons is simply passive. For instance, when there is an excess of phosphate in the blood, more phosphate is naturally eliminated, and when there is too little, a correspondingly smaller amount is found in the urine. This occurs naturally through the general filtering action of the glomerulus.

The body also has ways of actively influencing both the amount and composition of the urine that

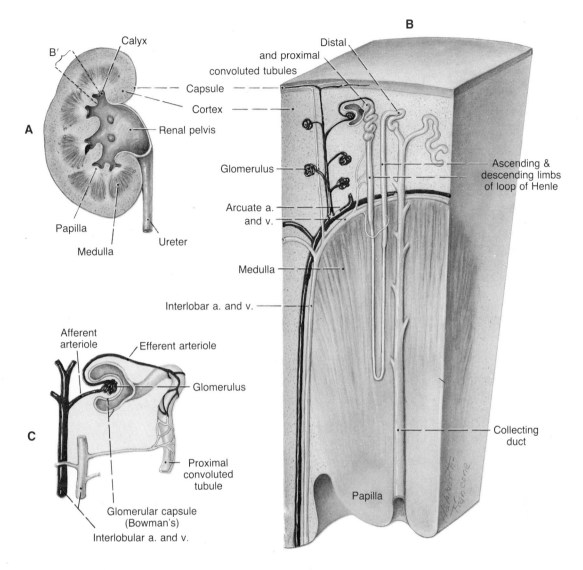

Figure 13–3 *A,* Sagittal section through kidney showing gross structure (note pelvis, calyces, medulla, cortex). *B,* Nephron and its relationship to medulla and cortex. The dotted lines in *A* show the area of the kidney from which this section was taken. *C,* Magnified view of nephron.

is produced by the kidneys. This active influencing occurs primarily with the control of the amount of water and sodium that are reabsorbed (from filtrate back to the blood) by the renal tubules. For instance, as mentioned before, when the body needs to retain water more than it needs to form urine (as in dehydration), the pituitary gland (see Chapter 7, The Endocrine System) secretes a chemical stimulant or *hormone* (specifically, antidiuretic hormone, or

ADH). This hormone stimulates the cells of the renal tubules to reabsorb even more water than normal. ADH is sometimes referred to as the "water-retaining hormone."

Another hormone, *aldosterone,* is secreted by the adrenal gland when sodium concentration in the blood is low; for example, when a person drinks a lot of water without taking salt after perspiring all day. Aldosterone stimulates the cells of the renal

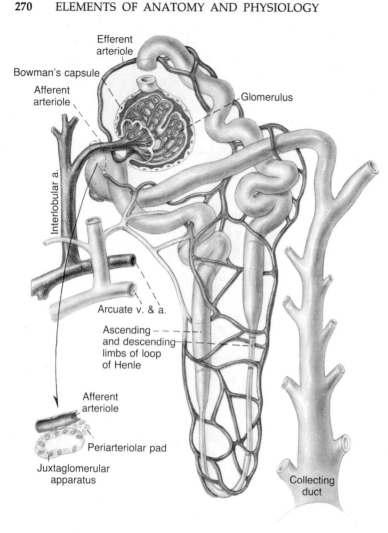

Figure 13–4 Detail of nephron showing vascular supply and juxtaglomerular apparatus.

tubules to reabsorb almost all sodium from the glomerular filtrate. This prevents any further loss of sodium by passage into the urine. Aldosterone is sometimes referred to as the "sodium-retaining hormone."

A *diuretic* (from *dia*, meaning intensive, and *uresis*, meaning urination) is any substance that causes a significant increase in the amount of urine formed. Diuretics also have the opposite effect of ADH, since in order to form more urine you need more water. Diuretics are often used to treat patients who have abnormal water retention. For example, *edema* (from the Greek word meaning swelling) is a condition in which abnormal blood pressure and/or osmotic forces lead to a build-up of water in the tissue spaces between cells. Administration of a di-

uretic can help to restore a more proper water distribution. In such a case, however, it is important to understand that the diuretic does not cure whatever caused the edema in the first place but rather only helps to alleviate the serious resulting symptom.

What Are the Ureters?

The *ureters* are two tubes that function to convey urine from the kidneys to the urinary bladder. Urine first drains out of the renal tubules into the larger, collecting tubes and finally into the *renal pelvis*. The renal pelvis forms the funnel-shaped upper end of the ureter. The ureter proper passes

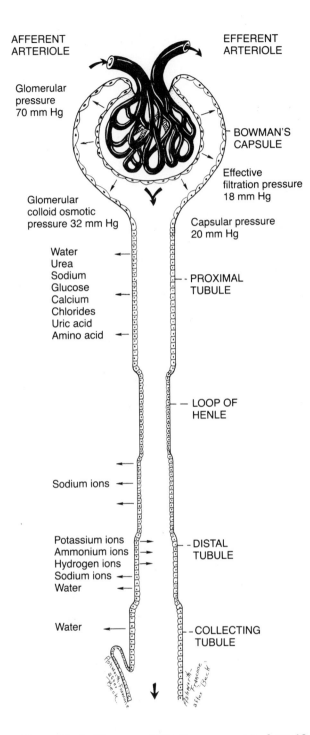

AFFERENT ARTERIOLE

EFFERENT ARTERIOLE

Glomerular pressure 70 mm Hg

BOWMAN'S CAPSULE

Effective filtration pressure 18 mm Hg

Glomerular colloid osmotic pressure 32 mm Hg

Capsular pressure 20 mm Hg

Water
Urea
Sodium
Glucose
Calcium
Chlorides
Uric acid
Amino acid

PROXIMAL TUBULE

LOOP OF HENLE

Sodium ions

Potassium ions
Ammonium ions
Hydrogen ions
Sodium ions
Water

DISTAL TUBULE

Water

COLLECTING TUBULE

Figure 13-5 The normal filtration pressure is about 18 mm Hg. Glomerular hydrostatic pressure (70 mm Hg) minus glomerular colloid osmotic pressure (32 mm Hg) minus capsular pressure (20 mm Hg) equals filtration pressure, 18 mm Hg. The passage of substances in and out of the tubule varies in different portions of the tubule and collecting duct.

Table 13-1   FUNCTIONS OF DIFFERENT PARTS OF NEPHRON

PART OF NEPHRON	FUNCTION
Glomerulus	Produces filtrate of protein-free plasma
Proximal convoluted tubule and loop of Henle	Absorption of Na^+, K^+, and glucose by active transport. Absorption of Cl^- by diffusion. Obligatory water absorption by osmosis. Secretion of certain drugs such as penicillin and iodopyracet by active transport
Distal convoluted tubule	Absorption of Na by active transport. Secretion of H^+, K^+
Collecting tubule	Water absorption by osmosis. ADH-controlled absorption of water

from the renal pelvis to the backside of the urinary bladder. Each ureter is about ¼ inch in diameter and is 10 to 12 inches long—the distance between the kidneys and the bladder—and consists of outer fibrous, middle muscular, and inner mucous layers. Contractions of the muscular layer produce *peristaltic* (from the Latin words meaning around and constriction) waves that carry urine from the renal pelvis to the urinary bladder.

Table 13-2   COMPOSITION OF URINE

Solutes 60 gm daily	Organic wastes 35 gm	Urea	30 gm
		Creatinine	1-2 gm
		Ammonia	1-2 gm
		Uric acid	1 gm
		Others	1 gm
	Inorganic salts* 25 gm	Chloride	Sodium
		Sulfate	Potassium
		Phosphorus	Magnesium

* Sodium chloride is the chief inorganic salt in urine.

What Is the Urinary Bladder?

The *urinary bladder* serves as a holding reservoir and organ of elimination for the urine produced by the kidneys (Fig. 13–6). As the bladder gradually fills, its elastic, muscular walls become *distended* (stretched). In the distended state, the muscular wall partially contracts, and the pressure within the bladder increases. The normal capacity of the bladder is slightly more than ½ pint (300 to 350 ml).

As the volume gradually increases, the tension continues to rise. Finally, stretch and tension receptors are stimulated, producing a desire to urinate. Voluntary control can be exerted until the bladder pressure increases to the point at which involuntary voiding occurs. Normal *micturition* (urination) is under voluntary control. Pressure sufficient to accomplish voiding is created by contraction of the *detrusor muscles* (bladder muscles), the abdominal wall, fixation of the chest wall and diaphragm, and relaxation of the urethral musculature.

What Is the Urethra?

The *urethra* is the tube leading from the bladder to the exterior of the body. It is currently believed that the entire urethra in the female, and the prostate and urethra in the male, function as the *sphincter* (muscle that closes off) of the bladder (Fig. 13–7). When urination begins, the musculature of the urethra relaxes and urine is forced down the narrow urethral tube.

In the female, the urethra is 1½ inches in length and serves only a urinary function. The male urethra is about 8 inches long and also serves in the reproductive system as a passageway for semen.

The mucous membrane that lines the renal pelvis, ureters, and bladder also lines the urethra — it is one continuous cellular sheet. This helps to explain the fact that an infection in the urethra may spread upward throughout the urinary tract to the kidneys.

CLINICAL CONSIDERATIONS

The clinical terms used to describe the production, or lack of production, of urine by a patient during a specified period are *anuria*, meaning literally the absence of urine, *oliguria*, meaning very little urine, and *polyuria*, meaning unusually large amounts of urine.

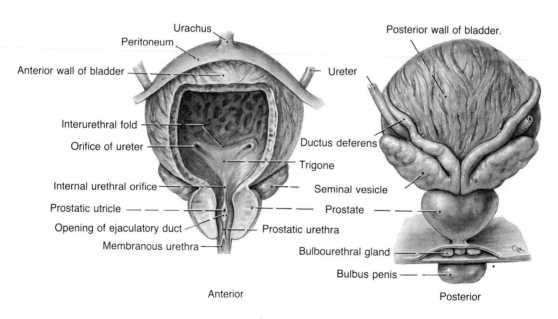

Figure 13–6 Internal and external aspects of the urinary bladder and related structures.

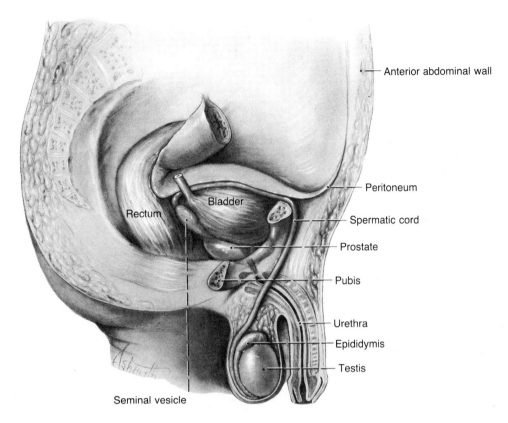

Figure 13–7   Sagittal section through the male pelvis.

Uremia, which literally means "urea in the blood," is a symptom of renal insufficiency. One of the characteristic signs of uremia is a "uremic" odor of the breath caused by ammonia (NH_3) produced by the breakdown of urea.

What Are Some Common Disorders of the Kidneys?

Nephritis refers to any inflammation of the kidneys and is relatively common. *Glomerulonephritis* (glo-mer"u-lo-ne-fri'tis), an inflammation that specifically involves the glomeruli, generally develops in persons under 20 years of age 10 to 20 days after an acute infection. Most patients recover spontaneously (without treatment). Chronic (or recurrent) glomerulonephritis can in later life result in hypertension and uremia. *Pyelonephritis* (pi"e-lo-ne-fri'tis) is an inflammation of the kidney with special involvement of the renal pelvis (*pyelo* is the Greek word for trough or pelvis).

Nephrosis is a degenerative disease of the renal tubules. A *degenerative disease* is one that tends to bring about the gradual destruction of the structures involved.

Cystitis is an inflammation of the mucous lining of the urinary bladder.

What Is Hemodialysis?

Hemodialysis (from the Latin, meaning to separate the blood) or dialysis, for short, is an increasingly common therapy used to maintain patients whose kidneys either have stopped working altogether or are not functioning adequately. It works by the simple principle of diffusion. The dialysis machine uses a semipermeable membrane between

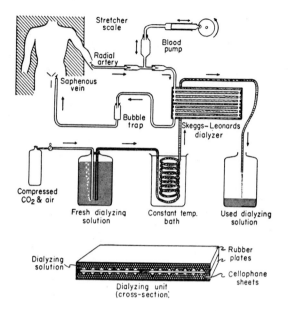

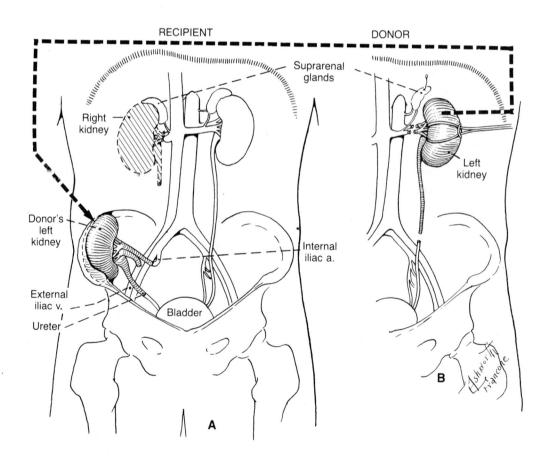

Figure 13-8 Schematic diagram of the Skeggs-Leonards artificial kidney.

the blood from the patient and a wash solution (Fig. 13-8).

If there is a relatively high level of any substance in the blood of a patient, and none in the wash solution, that substance will diffuse from the patient's blood into the wash solution. Urea, potassium, phosphate, and other molecules present in toxic (poisonous) quantities in the uremic patient can thus be removed by hemodialysis. It is now possible by hemodialysis to keep patients alive without any functioning kidney tissue for many years.

What About Kidney Transplantation?

During the past decade, homologous kidney transplantation has become increasingly common for patients suffering from kidney failure. "Homol-

Figure 13-9 *A,* Kidney transplanted to right pelvis. *B,* Kidney of donor.

ogous transplants" are those done between individuals of the same species who are not identical twins. A system of tissue typing, similar to the ABO blood type system, has been developed to increase the likelihood of a "take." The use of drugs to suppress the immune response — "rejection" of the inevitable foreign proteins of the transplanted kidney — has allowed excellent long-term function in a majority of these patients. The best results in homotransplantation occur when the donor is closely related to the recipient; better than 90 per cent of the kidneys survive for 1 year or longer. Kidney transplants between identical twins may function almost indefinitely (Fig. 13–9).

SUMMARY

A. The urinary system accomplishes its functions through the formation and elimination of urine.
  1. The urinary system functions to eliminate the wastes of protein metabolism, which mostly consist of urea.
  2. The urinary system functions to regulate the composition of the blood.
    a. It regulates the amount of water in the body.
    b. It regulates the concentrations of a variety of salts in the blood, including sodium, potassium, calcium, phosphate, and chloride.
B. The kidneys are two large bean-shaped organs lying behind the abdominal organs against the muscles of the back.
  1. The renal artery, vein, nerves, and lymphatic vessels enter and leave the concave surface through the hilus.
  2. The renal pelvis is the urine-collecting portion.
  3. The renal pelvis also forms the upper portion of the ureter.
  4. The inner area of the kidney is called the medulla.
  5. The outer area of the kidney, called the cortex, contains millions of nephrons.

C. Nephrons have three main parts: glomerulus, Bowman's capsule, and renal tubule.
  1. The glomerulus is a tightly woven network of blood capillaries.
  2. The glomerulus is fitted inside a cuplike structure called Bowman's capsule.
  3. Extending from Bowman's capsule is a long renal tubule.
    a. The first segment is called the proximal convoluted tubule.
    b. Next, the tubule forms a loop called the loop of Henle.
    c. Finally, the distal tubule joins a larger collecting tube serving many nephrons.
D. There are three processes involved in the formation of urine by the nephron.
  1. In glomerular filtration, protein-free plasma filtrate passes from the capillary blood and into Bowman's capsule.
    a. Filtration is by passive diffusion under pressure.
    b. The rate of filtration varies with blood pressure.
    c. About 125 ml of filtrate is created every minute.
  2. The renal tubule reabsorbs 124 ml of filtrate per minute, returning it to the surrounding blood capillaries.
    a. Reabsorption rate of specific substances can be increased or decreased.
    b. Different parts of the tubule specialize in reabsorbing different substances.
    c. ADH stimulates the distal tubule to reabsorb even more water.
  3. The renal tubule secretes substances (reverse of reabsorption), moving them from the capillaries to the filtrate.
    a. When the blood becomes too acidic, the proximal tubule is very active, secreting hydrogen ion.
    b. This acid reduction system is slower than that of the respiratory system but can eliminate a larger amount.
E. Kidney function is controlled by natural concentrations and hormones.
  1. Passive filtering increases the amount of substances in high concentration that pass into the urine.
  2. Antidiuretic hormone (ADH), "water-retaining hormone," stimulates reabsorption of even more water than normal.

3. Aldosterone, the "sodium-retaining hormone," can stimulate reabsorption of almost all sodium.

4. A diuretic is any substance that increases the amount of urine formed.

F. The urine collecting tubes from the cortex come together in the medulla.

1. The medulla is formed around the renal pelvis.

2. The renal pelvis extends to form the ureter.

G. The ureters are two tubes that function to convey urine from the kidneys to the urinary bladder.

H. The urinary bladder serves as a holding reservoir and organ of elimination for the urine.

1. Its elastic muscular walls distend, and partially contract, as it fills.

2. As volume increases, tension receptors are stimulated, producing the desire to urinate.

3. Normal micturition (urination) is under voluntary control.

4. Several factors combine to accomplish voiding.

a. The urethral musculature relaxes.

b. Pressure is created by the actions of the detrusor muscles, the abdominal wall, and fixation of the chest wall and diaphragm.

I. The urethra is the tube leading from the bladder to the exterior.

1. The urethra serves as the sphincter in the female.

2. The urethra and the prostate serve as the sphincter in the male.

3. In the male the urethra also serves as part of the reproductive system as a passageway for semen.

4. An infection in the urethra may spread up the internal mucous membrane lining to bladder and kidneys.

J. Anuria means absence of urine, oliguria means very little urine, and polyuria means unusually large amounts of urine.

K. Uremia refers to an abnormal amount of urea in the blood.

1. Uremia is a symptom of renal insufficiency.

2. Uremia produces a characteristic odor caused by ammonia, a breakdown product of urea.

L. There are several common disorders of the kidneys.

1. Nephritis is an inflammation of the kidneys.

a. Glomerulonephritis is a specific inflammation of the glomeruli.

b. Pyelonephritis is an inflammation of the renal pelvis.

2. Nephrosis is a degenerative disease of the renal tubules.

3. Cystitis is an inflammation of the mucous lining of the bladder.

M. Hemodialysis, or dialysis, is provided by an artificial kidney machine.

1. It uses diffusion across a semipermeable membrane between the blood and a wash solution.

2. It serves to cleanse the blood of a person without kidney function.

N. Kidney transplantation has become an increasingly common therapeutic option.

1. Homologous transplants are those between people of the same species who are not identical twins.

2. A system of tissue typing increases the likelihood of success, but greatest success is still with a relative.

REVIEW QUESTIONS

1. List the organs of the urinary system and describe the general function of each.

2. Describe the gross structure and location of the organs of the urinary system.

3. Draw a longitudinal cross section of the kidney and identify the cortex, medulla, and pelvis.

4. Name the structural and functional unit of the kidney.

5. Draw a structural and functional diagram of the nephron, labeling the parts and briefly describing their function.

6. Describe the orientation and distribution of the nephrons in the kidney.

7. Explain the phases and processes involved in the formation of urine by the individual nephron. What is the function of the glomerulus? What two functions are performed by the tubules?

8. How does the glomerular filtrate differ from plasma?

9. Explain the differences between filtrate and urine.

10. Explain the actions of the aldosterone and antidiuretic hormone.

11. What is a diuretic and how does it work?

12. Define micturition. What produces the desire to urinate.

13. Why is it that an infection in the urethra has a tendency to spread upward throughout the urinary tract to the kidneys?

14. How is the female urethra different from that of the male in structure and function?

15. Define anuria, oliguria, and polyuria.

16. What is uremia? What is its common symptom? What does uremia indicate?

17. Distinguish and characterize nephritis, glomerulonephritis, pyelonephritis, and nephrosis.

18. Define cystitis.

19. How does hemodialysis work?

F O U R T E E N

The Reproductive System

O B J E C T I V E S

The aim of this chapter is to enable the student to do the following:

- Discuss the function of the reproductive system.

- Construct and label a diagram identifying the organs of the male reproductive system and discuss the general function of each.

- Distinguish the endocrine and exocrine products of the testes.

- Define erection, ejaculation, and circumcision.

- Construct and label a diagram identifying the organs of the female reproductive system and discuss the general function of each.

- Describe the functions of the graafian follicles and corpus luteum of the ovary.

- Define myometrium, endometrium, and ovulation.

- Describe the process of spermatogenesis and oogenesis.

- Describe the phases and control of the menstrual cycle.

- Discuss the functions of the placenta.

- Explain the biochemistry of pregnancy testing.

- List the principle methods of contraception and outline how each works.

- Define and describe the most common sexually transmitted diseases.

The function of the reproductive systems is to bring about the formation of a new member or members of the species. In one-cell organisms, reproduction is accomplished through simple mitotic division, resulting in two "new" daughter cells. Higher species, such as the human, have evolved into a two-sex (male and female) system of reproduction.

Formation of a human offspring occurs through the growth of a single egg cell (from the female) fertilized by a single sperm (from the male) (Fig. 14–1). This fertilized egg grows and matures within the reproductive system by means of billions of individual cell divisions to produce the offspring at birth.

All the structures of the male and female repro-

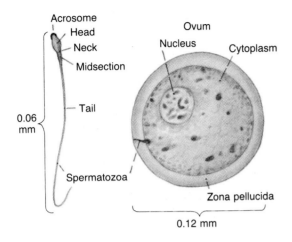

Figure 14-1 Size relationships of sperm and ovum.

ductive systems are designed to bring about *fertilization* and the subsequent *development* and *nourishment* of the new offspring (Fig. 14-2).

THE MALE REPRODUCTIVE SYSTEM

What Are the Scrotum and Penis?

The scrotum and penis are the visible external male organs of reproduction. The testes are also external but are contained in the scrotum (Figs. 14-3 and 14-4).

The *scrotum* is a pouch that hangs behind the penis. It is a continuation of the abdominal wall and is divided into two sacs by a septum (Latin for wall). Each sac contains one of the testes, with its epididymis or connecting tube leading up into the abdominal cavity.

The *penis* contains the male *urethra*, which functions to carry both urine from the bladder and *semen* (Latin for seed) from the ejaculatory duct. The penis is composed primarily of erectile tissue surrounding many small compartments, or spaces, that are normally collapsed (Fig. 14-5). During periods of sexual stimulation, the arteries that supply the penis dilate, and a large quantity of blood under pressure enters the erectile-tissue compartment.

This causes the penis to become fixed and erect and facilitates its penetration into the female vagina during intercourse. During intercourse, semen passes into the vagina, setting the stage for fertilization of the female egg.

The end of the penis is covered by a loose skin that is folded inward and then backward upon itself; this is called the *prepuce* (from the Latin, *praeputium,* meaning foreskin). This foreskin covering the end of the penis protects the opening from infective agents. The common belief that removal of the foreskin serves to keep this area cleaner is not supported by scientific evidence. The traditional, ritualistic removal of the foreskin in newborn boys is accomplished by a surgical procedure known as circumcision (Fig. 14-6) and is no longer considered medically justified. Although over 80 per cent of the males in the United States are still circumcised, over 80 per cent of the males in Europe are not.

What Are the Internal Male Organs of Reproduction?

The internal organs of reproduction in the male can be divided into *three groups.*

First, there are the male *gonads,* or *testes.* These function to produce sperm and secrete the male sex hormone, *testosterone.*

The second group consists of a series of ducts, including the *epididymis* (ep"i-did'i-mis), *ductus deferens,* and *urethra.* These carry the sperm and semen from the testes and accessory organs into the vagina during intercourse.

The third group of internal organs is the accessory glands; the *seminal vesicles,* the *prostate,* and the *bulbourethral* (Cowper's) *glands.* These glands secrete fluid that carries the sperm through the penile urethra into the female vagina during intercourse.

What Are the Functions of the Testes?

The male *gonads* (Latin for seed) are called the *testes* or *testicles* (singular testis or testicle). They correspond to the ovaries in the female. The two testes are the organs that produce the male repro-

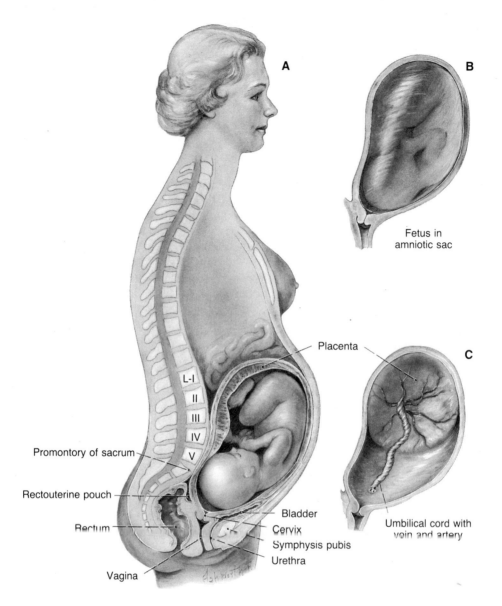

Figure 14-2   *A,* Midsagittal section of a pregnant woman showing fetal position. *B,* Amniotic sac with fetus. *C,* Placenta in uterus with fetus removed.

ductive cells—the *sperm* (Greek for seed), or *spermatozoa* (Greek, *sperma* = seed + zoon = animal). The testes also contain glandular tissue that secretes the male sex hormone, *testosterone,* into the blood. The testes, therefore, are endocrine glands as well (Fig. 14-7).

Each testis is an oval organ about 2 inches in length and is located in the pouch-like scrotum.

Each testis is divided into about 250 wedge-shaped lobes. Each lobe contains one to three narrow, coiled tubes known as *seminiferous tubules* (the term "seminiferous" derives from the Latin words, "semen," meaning seed, and "fero," meaning to carry). Male reproductive cells, known as *sperm* or *spermatozoa,* are found within these tubules at different stages of development. If uncoiled, a tubule

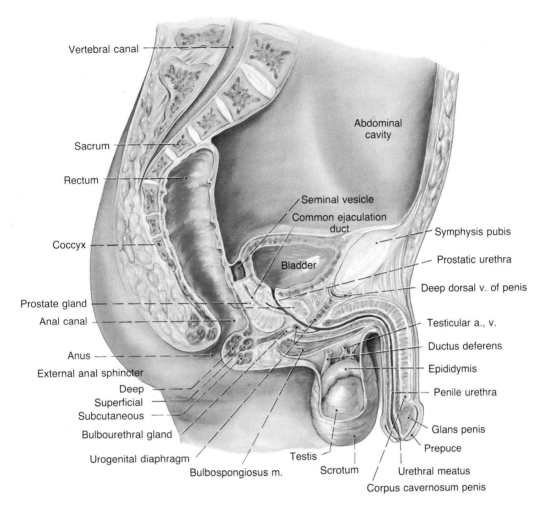

Vertebral canal

Sacrum

Rectum

Coccyx

Prostate gland

Anal canal

Anus

External anal sphincter

Deep

Superficial

Subcutaneous

Bulbourethral gland

Urogenital diaphragm

Bulbospongiosus m.

Abdominal cavity

Seminal vesicle

Common ejaculation duct

Bladder

Testis

Scrotum

Symphysis pubis

Prostatic urethra

Deep dorsal v. of penis

Testicular a., v.

Ductus deferens

Epididymis

Penile urethra

Glans penis

Prepuce

Urethral meatus

Corpus cavernosum penis

Figure 14-3 Midsagittal section of the male pelvis and external genitalia. (The course of the ductus deferens is shown in Fig. 13-7).

would measure about 2 feet in length. Any one of the millions of sperm cells formed by each testis may join with a female reproductive cell (the egg or ovum) to eventually become a new human being.

Scattered among the tubules are the *interstitial cells*, which produce and secrete testosterone. These cells perform the endocrine activities of the testes. The increase in secretion of testosterone during puberty produces dramatic changes, transforming a little boy into a man. Testosterone lowers the pitch of the voice, increases the muscular development, promotes beard growth, and influences changes in the size and shape of the bones. Testosterone is known as the "masculinizing" hormone. The secre-

tion of testosterone by the interstitial cells is controlled by the anterior pituitary gland secretions of FSH, which is referred to as interstitial cell–stimulating hormone, ICSH, when discussing the male. FSH and ICSH are the same substance.

What Are the Functions of the Epididymis, Ductus Deferens, and Urethra?

The *epididymis* (Greek, *epi* = upon + *didymous* = the two or twins) extends from the upper

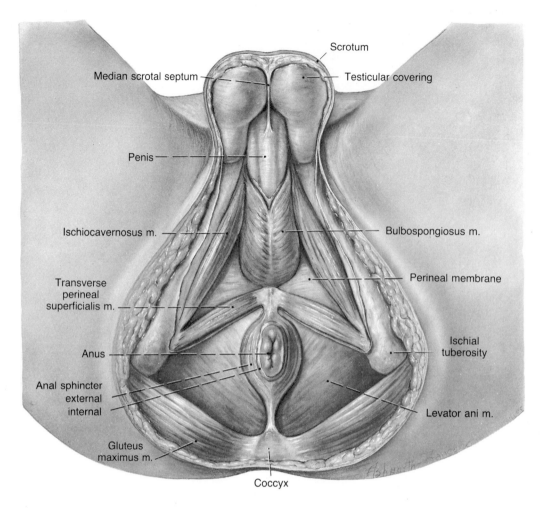

Figure 14–4 Male perineum with skin and superficial fascia removed.

end of each testis downward along the posterior side for about 1½ inches. About 16 feet of tube are coiled within this short distance. The epididymis is the first part of the duct system leading from the testes (Fig. 14–8).

The *ductus deferens* (Latin, *ductus* = duct + *defero* = carry down) can be considered a continuation of the epididymis and has been described as "the excretory duct of the testis." It is also called the *vas deferens* (Latin, *vas* = vessel). It extends from the testis about 18 inches, up into the abdomen, where it contacts and forms a common duct (the ejaculatory duct) with one of the seminal vesicles. The ejaculatory duct opens into the *urethra*, which carries both semen and urine out of the body.

A *vasectomy* (removal of a segment of the vas deferens) is a minor surgical operation wherein the ductus deferens is either tied off or severed or sewn closed. This achieves artificial sterility by stopping the normal passage of sperm.

What Are the Functions of the Seminal Vesicles, Prostate, and Cowper's Glands?

There are two *seminal vesicles*. They are membranous pouches lying behind the urinary bladder near its base, each consisting of a single tube coiled

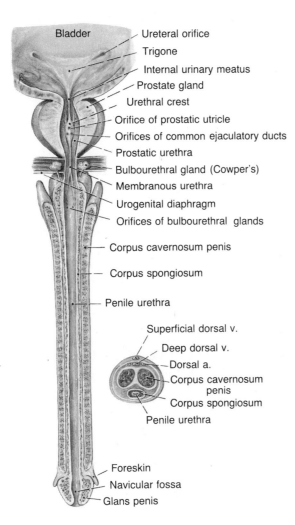

Bladder
Ureteral orifice
Trigone
Internal urinary meatus
Prostate gland
Urethral crest
Orifice of prostatic utricle
Orifices of common ejaculatory ducts
Prostatic urethra
Bulbourethral gland (Cowper's)
Membranous urethra
Urogenital diaphragm
Orifices of bulbourethral glands

Corpus cavernosum penis

Corpus spongiosum

Penile urethra

Superficial dorsal v.
Deep dorsal v.
Dorsal a.
Corpus cavernosum penis
Corpus spongiosum
Penile urethra

Foreskin
Navicular fossa
Glans penis

Figure 14-5 Section through the bladder, prostate gland, and penis.

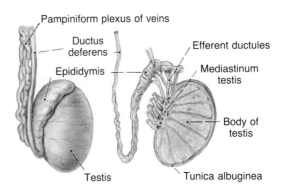

Pampiniform plexus of veins
Ductus deferens
Epididymis
Efferent ductules
Mediastinum testis
Body of testis
Testis
Tunica albuginea

Figure 14-7 Male testis, entire and sectioned views.

upon itself (Fig. 14-9). The seminal vesicles secrete a fluid that is one of the components of semen. *Semen,* which is the thick, whitish fluid that carries the sperm, leaves through the urethra and enters the vagina during intercourse. The seminal vesicle fluid serves to give the sperm motility (ability to move). The tube of each seminal vesicle ends in a straight, narrow duct joining the ductus deferens to form the ejaculatory duct. The ejaculatory duct actually ejects the spermatozoa-containing fluid from the seminal vesicle into the urethra.

The *prostate gland* is a cone-shaped body about the size of a chestnut lying under the urinary bladder. It surrounds the first inch of the urethra and secretes an alkaline (high pH, low acidity) fluid,

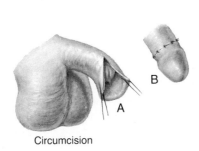

Circumcision

Figure 14-6 In *circumcision* the prepuce is removed. *A,* Incision in the prepuce. *B,* Closure of the wound after removal of the prepuce.

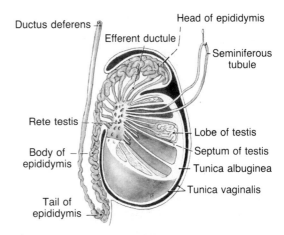

Ductus deferens
Head of epididymis
Efferent ductule
Seminiferous tubule
Rete testis
Lobe of testis
Body of epididymis
Septum of testis
Tunica albuginea
Tunica vaginalis
Tail of epididymis

Figure 14-8 Diagram of a section of the male testis showing detail of a seminiferous tubule.

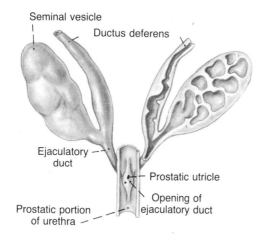

Seminal vesicle

Ductus deferens

Ejaculatory duct

Prostatic utricle

Opening of ejaculatory duct

Prostatic portion of urethra

Figure 14–9 Seminal vesicle and related parts. On the left the vesicle and duct are intact; the right side is sectioned to show internal detail.

which also aids the motility of the sperm cells. In older men, a progressive enlargement of the prostate commonly obstructs the urethra and interferes with the passage of urine. This condition calls for the surgical removal of part of the prostate gland. The prostate is also a frequent site of cancer in elderly men.

The *bulbourethral glands,* also called *Cowper's glands,* are two glandular bodies about the size of a pea located below the prostate on either side of the urethra. These also secrete alkaline fluid as a part of the semen.

THE FEMALE REPRODUCTIVE SYSTEM

What Are the External Reproductive Structures of the Female?

The external female reproductive organs are collectively known as the *vulva* (Figs. 14–10 and 14–11). "Vulva" is a Latin word meaning a wrapper, covering, or seed covering. The structures of the vulva are as follows. The *labia majora* (major lips) are two longitudinal rounded folds of skin that are similar in structure to the scrotum in the male. Two

smaller folds of skin, the *labia minora,* lie between the labia majora. The *clitoris* is a small, rounded projection of erectile tissue, nerves, and blood vessels; it occupies the apex that is formed by the anterior meeting of the labia minora. The clitoris is partially hooded by a *prepuce.*

The *vestibule* (from the Latin word for outer chamber) of the vagina lies between the labia minora. Situated within the cleft of the vestibule are the *hymen,* the *vaginal orifice* (opening), the *urethral orifice* and the openings of the *vestibular glands.*

The *hymen* (Greek for membrane) is a thin fold of vascularized mucous membrane separating the vagina from the vestibule. It may be entirely absent, or it may cover the vaginal orifice partly or completely. Anatomically, neither its absence nor presence can be considered a criterion of virginity.

INTERNAL FEMALE ORGANS OF REPRODUCTION (Figs. 14–12 and 14–13).

What are the Ovaries?

The female *gonads* are called *ovaries* (singular, ovary; from the Latin word *ovum,* meaning egg). They correspond to the testes in the male. The ovaries are the organs that produce the female reproductive cells—the *ova* (plural of ovum). The cells of the ovaries also contain glandular tissue, which secretes the female sex hormones, the *estrogens* and *progesterone.*

The *ovaries* are two oval-shaped structures about 1½ inches in length. They are located in the upper part of the pelvic cavity, one on each side of the uterus, and are anchored to the uterus by the *ovarian ligament.*

The inner structure of the ovary consists of a meshwork of several thousand sacs, too small to be seen without a microscope. These are the *graafian* (graf'e-an) *follicles* (sacs); they are found at different stages of development within each ovary. "Graafian" derives from DeGraaf, the Dutch anatomist who first identified the follicles some 300 years ago. The term "follicle" derives from the Latin word meaning a small sac. Within each follicle is an

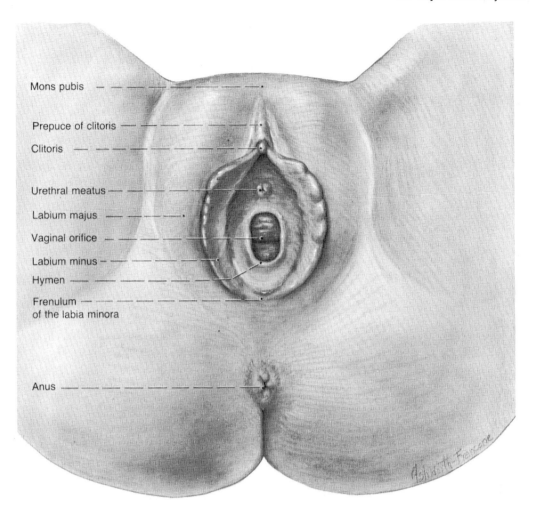

Mons pubis

Prepuce of clitoris

Clitoris

Urethral meatus

Labium majus

Vaginal orifice

Labium minus

Hymen

Frenulum
of the labia minora

Anus

Figure 14-10   Female external genitalia.

ovum, which matures as the follicle grows. At the point of maturity the follicle bursts open, releasing the ovum for possible later fertilization.

After the ovum is released, the ruptured follicle develops into the *corpus luteum* under the stimulation of luteinizing hormone (LH) from the anterior pituitary. The corpus luteum (corpus = body, *luteum* = yellowish or golden), or "golden body," is a secretory body that produces and secretes estrogens and progesterone during the second half of the menstrual cycle and during pregnancy if fertilization occurs.

The two major functions of the ovaries, then, are development and expulsion of the female ova

and production and secretion of female sex hormones, the estrogens and progesterone.

What Are the Uterine Tubes?

The *uterine,* or *fallopian* (after the Italian anatomist Fallopius), *tubes* serve as the ducts to carry the ova from the ovaries to the uterus. The uterine tubes differ from the corresponding ducts for the male testes in that the uterine tubes are *not actually connected* to the ovaries. Rather, when an ovum is expelled from the ovary, the fingerlike projections

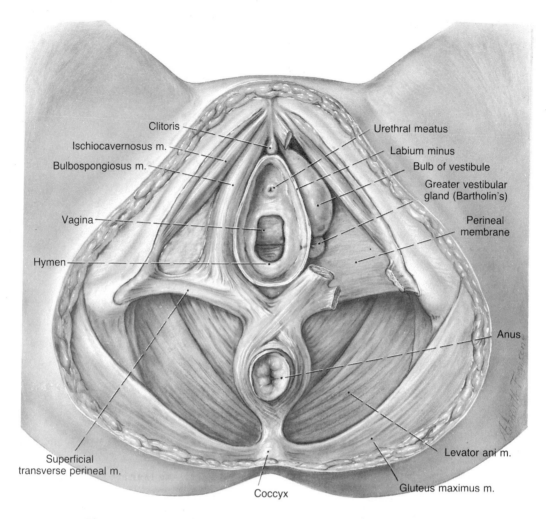

Clitoris

Ischiocavernosus m.

Bulbospongiosus m.

Vagina

Hymen

Urethral meatus

Labium minus

Bulb of vestibule

Greater vestibular gland (Bartholin's)

Perineal membrane

Anus

Levator ani m.

Superficial transverse perineal m.

Coccyx

Gluteus maximus m.

Figure 14-11 Female perineum with skin and superficial fascia removed.

from the ends of the uterine tubes draw the ovum into the tube, and then transport it to the uterus.

Occasionally, an ovum becomes fertilized without entering the uterine tube. The term *ectopic pregnancy* means a pregnancy that develops outside of its proper place in the cavity of the uterus. The term "ectopic" is from the Greek *ek*, meaning out of, and *topos*, meaning place; together they mean, literally, out of place.

What Is the Uterus?

The *uterus* is a pear-shaped, thick-walled, muscular organ suspended in the pelvic cavity above the bladder and in front of the rectum. In its normal state it measures about 3 inches in length and 2 inches in width. The uterine tubes enter into its upper end, one into each side, and the lower end projects into the vagina. The lower portion, called the *cervix* (Latin for neck), corresponds to the neck of an inverted pear. The upper main portion of the uterus is known as the *fundus* (Latin for bottom, or portion farthest from the opening).

The wall of the uterus consists of three layers. The outer layer, called the peritoneal layer, is continuous with the broad ligaments that suspend the uterus. The middle layer, the *myometrium* (Greek, *myo* = muscle, and *metra* = uterus), is a thick muscular layer that greatly increases in thickness during pregnancy.

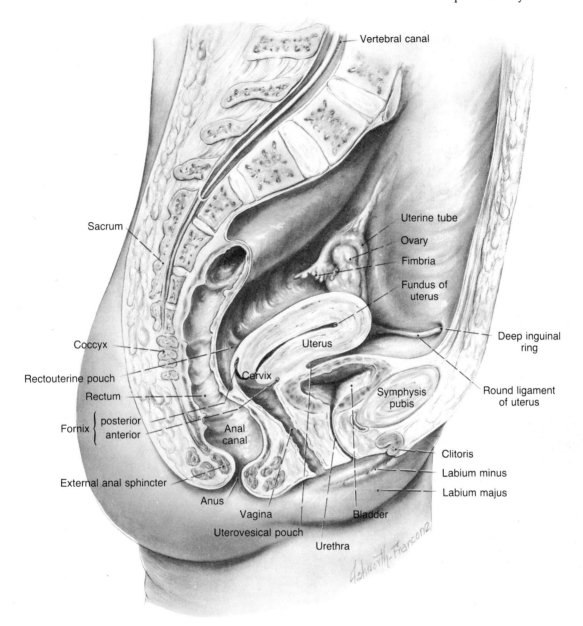

Figure 14–12 Midsagittal section of the female pelvis.

The inner coat of the uterine wall is the mucous membrane, or *endometrium* (Greek, *endo* = inside + *metra* = uterus). It consists of an epithelial lining and connective tissue. In *menstruation* (from the Latin word for monthly), the superficial portion of the endometrium pulls loose, leaving torn blood vessels underneath. Blood and bits of endometrium trickle out of the uterus into the vagina and out of the body. Regeneration of a new endometrial lining begins immediately after menstruation.

What Is the Vagina?

The *vagina* is a tubular canal 4 to 6 inches in length, directed upward and backward and extend-

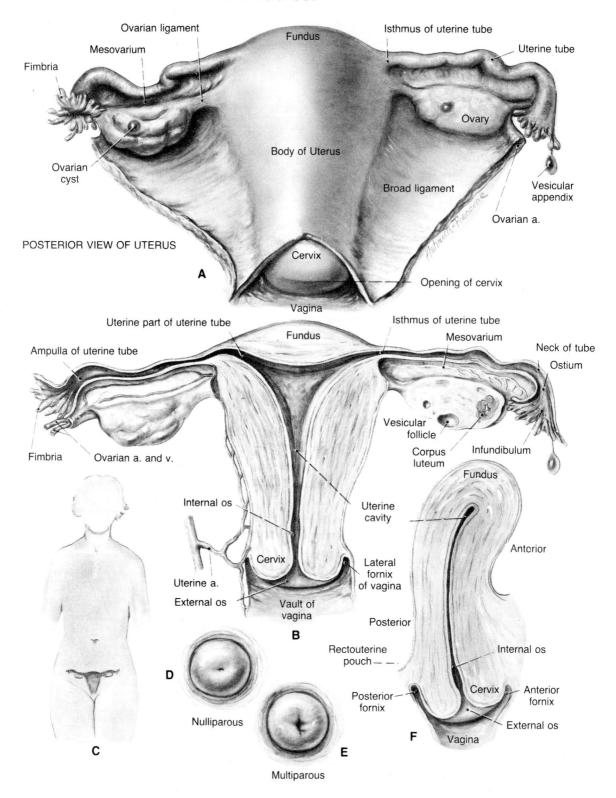

Figure 14–13 Female organs of reproduction. *A*, Uterus, posterior view. *B*, Uterus sectioned to show internal structure. *C*, Position in body. *D* and *E*, Shape of cervix before and after childbirth. *F*, Right lateral sagittal view.

ing from the external vestibule to the uterus. It is situated between the bladder and the rectum. The vaginal wall consists of an internal membranous lining and a muscular layer capable of constriction and enormous dilation (enlargement). They are separated by a layer of erectile tissue. The mucous membrane forms thick transverse folds and is kept moist by cervical secretions (the cervix is the lower part of the uterus).

The vagina serves as part of the birth canal and represents the female organ of copulation.

THE MAMMARY GLANDS

What Are the Mammary Glands?

The two *mammary* (from the Latin word for breast) *glands,* or *breasts,* are accessory reproductive organs. The breasts of pregnant women secrete milk for nourishment of the newborn. The *nipples,* con-taining the openings of the milk ducts, are located near the center of the breasts. A wider, circular area of pigmented skin, known as the *areola* (ah-re'o-lah), surrounds each nipple. There are from 15 to 20 lobes of glandular tissue arranged radially within the breast (Fig. 14–14).

What Are Some Factors That Affect Milk Production?

Ovarian hormones exert specific control over growth and development of the breast. Estrogen stimulates the development of the ducts; progester-one influences the growth of the milk-producing, glandular tissue.

Lactation, the production of milk, is a complex process requiring the interplay of various hormonal and nervous factors. *Prolactin,* which is secreted by the anterior pituitary, appears to be the prime fac-tor. Suckling of the newborn stimulates release of *oxytocin* from the posterior pituitary, which stimu-lates release of milk from the glandular cells into the ducts, making it available to the infant.

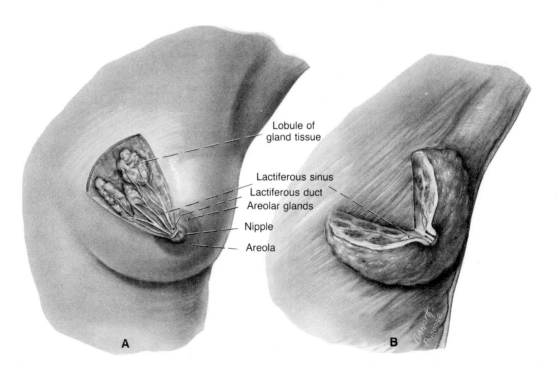

Lobule of gland tissue
Lactiferous sinus
Lactiferous duct
Areolar glands
Nipple
Areola

A   **B**

Figure 14–14   The female breast. *A,* The skin has been partly removed to show the underlying structures. *B,* A section has been removed to show the internal structures in relation to the muscles.

THE OVARIAN HORMONES

What Are Estrogens? What Is Progesterone?

Estrogens and progesterone are essential ovarian hormones. Estrogens (Greek, *oistros* = mad desire + *gen* = to beget) are secreted by the maturing graafian follicles, the sacs in the ovary that contain the ova. Progesterone is secreted by the *corpus luteum*, the "golden body" that forms each month from the follicle that has matured and discharged its ovum.

The secretion of the estrogens and progesterone occurs in response to two specific hormones produced by the anterior pituitary gland — the follicle-stimulating hormone (FSH) and the luteinizing hormone (LH).

Estrogens are responsible for the development of female characteristics at puberty. They stimulate the growth of the uterus and the vagina; they also assist in the development of secondary sex characteristics, such as breast development, including the formation of ducts in the mammary glands.

During the menstrual cycle, estrogens cause thickening of the endometrium of the uterine wall in preparation for implantation of the fertilized egg. They also stimulate repair of the endometrium following menstruation.

Progesterone is secreted by the corpus luteum and also by the *placenta* during pregnancy. It helps to prepare the uterine wall for implantation of the fertilized ovum and is necessary for the process of implantation.

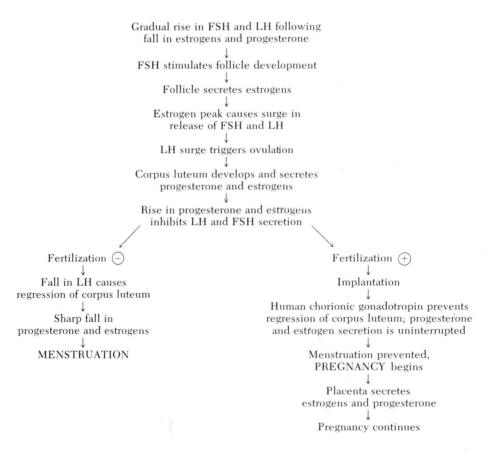

Figure 14–15 Hormonal interrelations during the menstrual cycle and hormonal changes following prevention of the initiation of a new cycle by implantation.

Progesterone maintains the development of the placenta and prevents the ovary from producing ova during pregnancy. It is responsible for enlargement of the breasts during pregnancy and for development of the milk-secreting cells of the mammary gland.

Diminished secretion of progesterone leads to menstrual irregularities in nonpregnant women and spontaneous abortion in pregnant women.

THE MENSTRUAL CYCLE

What Is Menarche? What Is Menopause?

The first menstrual cycle, or *menses* (from the Latin word meaning monthly), initiates the age of puberty. This now occurs around 10 to 11 years of age in Western industrialized nations, a significant decline from the age of around 14 years of age half a century ago. (See the section Tumors of the Breast under Clinical Considerations.) This beginning is known as *menarche* (me-nar'ke) (from the Greek, *men,* meaning monthly + *arche,* meaning the beginning). From this beginning the menstrual cycle continues on a fairly regular basis, every 28 days, for about 35 years until *menopause* (Greek, *meno* = monthly + *pausis* = cessation).

The day of onset of the menstrual flow is considered the *first day* of the cycle. The cycle ends on the last day prior to the next menstrual flow. Typically, the cycle is 28 days in duration, but it can vary from 22 to 35 days.

What Are the Three Phases of the Menstrual Cycle?

Three phases of the menstrual cycle will be discussed in the following sections — the menstrual phase, the proliferative phase, and the secretory phase (Figs. 14–15 and 14–16).

Menstrual Phase The menstrual phase lasts from the first to the fourth day of the cycle. When the ovum is not fertilized, the corpus luteum re-

gresses. This leads to a decrease in the ovarian (corpus luteum portion) secretion of both estrogen and progesterone, which leads to the disintegration of the endometrial lining of the uterus. With some resultant bleeding, the endometrium drains out of the uterus, through the vagina, and out of the body.

Proliferative Phase This phase, characterized by estrogen stimulation, begins about the fifth day of the cycle and extends through the ovulation, which occurs near the midpoint of the cycle — around day 14. This stimulation of estrogen secretion by the ovaries is begun by the secretion of FSH from the anterior pituitary. If synthetic estrogen is introduced at the beginning of this phase, FSH secretion is inhibited. As a result, the ovaries are not stimulated to grow, and no ovum will be produced. This is a simplified version of how oral contraceptives work.

Secretory Phase The normal *secretory phase* begins at ovulation. The rupture of the mature follicle and release of the ovum are stimulated by a rapid increase in the secretion of LH — sometimes called the "ovulation hormone." LH continues to act on the ruptured follicle, transforming (luteinizing) it into the secreting body, the *corpus luteum.* The corpus luteum secretes estrogens and, for the first time during the menstrual cycle, begins a significant secretion of progesterone. The secretions of the corpus luteum also further prepare the uterine wall for implantation, should the ovum become fertilized.

If implantation does not occur, the corpus luteum decreases its activity, which leads to disintegration of the endometrium and menstruation — the beginning of the menstrual cycle again.

At this point, you should reread the description of the menstrual phase.

FSH and LH

For summary purposes, one can consider the function of FSH to be stimulation of growth of the graafian follicles until one follicle matures and releases its ovum, which occurs on about the fourteenth day of the menstrual cycle.

The actual ovulation (release of the ovum from the mature follicle) is stimulated by a large secretion of LH. Subsequent LH secretions develop and maintain the corpus luteum.

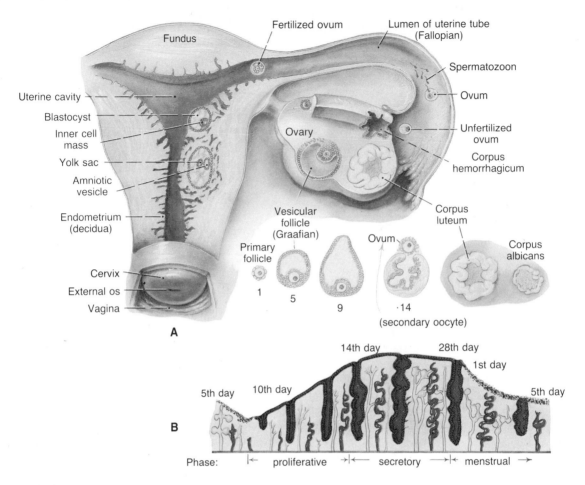

Figure 14-16   *A,* Physiologic processes of the ovary and uterus, showing ovulation, transportation of the ovum, and implantation. *B,* Cyclic menstrual changes in the uterine endometrium.

CLINICAL CONSIDERATIONS

Pregnancy Testing

In the early diagnosis of pregnancy, attention has recently been concentrated on tests designed to detect the presence of a substance peculiar to the pregnant state, human chorionic gonadotropin hormone, HCG. This hormone is secreted by the developing placenta in large amounts beginning on about day 26 of pregnancy.

Previously, the most widely used tests for the presence of HCG by examination of the patient's urine involved injecting the urine into mice or other experimental animals. After 5 days the animal was examined for stimulation of its ovaries, which HCG affects. If the animal's ovaries had been stimulated, this indicated that HCG was present in the patient's urine and that the patient was in fact pregnant. The accuracy of this test has been relatively good, although it is time-consuming and expensive.

More recent procedures for detection of HCG involve blood reaction tests and various procedures to detect it chemically in the urine. These procedures are fast, inexpensive, and over 99 per cent accurate when performed by trained laboratory personnel. The test is most accurate during the second and third months of pregnancy.

Symptoms and signs indicating that a pregnancy test should be given are largely subjective, and are appreciated by the patient herself. The signs include cessation of menses, changes in the breasts, alteration of the color of the mucous membranes, and increased pigmentation. The early symptoms include nausea, with or without vomiting, and frequency in urination.

Contraception and Abortion

There are many and varied methods utilized in the prevention of pregnancy. The mechanical means by which contraception is achieved with varying degrees of success include the use of the condom, the diaphragm, and the intrauterine device (IUD). This latter device is simply a coil, or loop, placed within the uterus.

Physiologic or chemical means of contraception include the rhythm method, douching, suppositories, foams, and the contraceptive pill.

Oral contraceptives rely upon the hormone balance of the menstrual cycle for their effectiveness. Most birth control pills are taken 20 or 21 consecutive days of each cycle. Beginning on the fifth day after the initiation of the menstrual flow, a pill containing both estrogen and progesterone is taken. (Some contraceptives vary this protocol slightly.) As long as these two hormones are taken orally, secretion of FSH does not begin, and the follicles of the ovaries are not stimulated to grow. Otherwise, the normal menstrual cycle proceeds, and menstrual flow will begin a few days after the pill is discontinued. The pill must be taken for each cycle, but its efficacy as a contraceptive is ensured even on the days that dosage is omitted and the menstrual flow permitted.

An *abortion* is any interruption of pregnancy prior to the period when the fetus is viable. (When infection occurs, the process is known as a septic abortion.) The fetus is considered viable when it weighs 500 grams (just over one pound) or more and the pregnancy is over 20 weeks in duration. The term *miscarriage* is used when spontaneous loss occurs after 20 weeks.

Tumors of the Breast

Fibrocystic breast disease is characterized by fibrous growth in the breast tissue. It is quite common but does not occur before adolescence and rarely, if ever, develops after menopause. A breast biopsy (removal and examination of tissue for diagnosis) is needed to distinguish between benign fibrous tumors and cancerous tumors.

When a malignant tumor is found in the breast, one of three surgical procedures is usually employed: a *lumpectomy* (-ec-tomy means removal), removing the tumor but leaving the breast intact; a *simple mastectomy,* or removal of the whole breast; or a *radical mastectomy,* removal of the breast, the associated lymph node chains, and any potentially involved muscles.

Radio- and chemotherapy following surgery have been shown to improve significantly the long-term survival rate of patients with breast cancer.

The relatively rapid decline in menarche in Western industrialized nations (from approximately 14 years of age to 10 years of age) appears to be linked to an increase in dietary fat intake, particularly saturated fats, in the diets of children in these Western nations. Furthermore, the lower average age of onset of puberty in a community appears to be strongly correlated with a later higher rate of breast cancer. Independent studies indicate that reducing dietary fat intake could have a very significant effect in reducing the incidence of breast cancer.

Sexually Transmitted Diseases

Gonorrhea (gon"o-re'ah) This is a contagious inflammation of the genital mucous membrane transmitted chiefly by sexual intercourse and caused by the bacteria *Neisseria gonorrhoeae.* The disease is marked by pain, difficulty in urinating, and a discharge of mucus and pus. Complications can occur, such as infection of other tissues and organs in the genital area. It may also produce arthritis and endocarditis (inflammation of the endothelial lining of the heart). This disease has reached nearly epidemic proportions in many areas of the United States and occurs primarily in persons between 14 and 20 years of age.

Syphilis Another disease that is almost invariably transmitted by sexual contact is syphilis. This disease is of particular clinical importance because the initial lesion and later widespread invasion are often not accompanied by disturbing signs or symptoms. The initial, *primary*, stage consists of the development of a local chancre (sore) in the male — frequently not detected in the female — between the end of the first week and the subsequent 3 months following contact. In 2 to 12 weeks the secondary stage becomes manifest in the form of a generalized skin rash, sometimes accompanied by involvement of the mucous membranes. An asymptomatic period lasting up to several decades follows the secondary stage. A final tertiary stage may develop in later life, involving primarily the tissues of the brain and heart. The development of the disease process beyond the secondary stage is quite unpredictable; medical treatment is indicated in all cases.

Genital Herpes This is a localized viral infection caused by a virus called herpes simplex, type 2. It produces sores (lesions) on the penis in the male or on the cervix, vagina, or vulva in the female. (Herpes simplex, type 1 is a common cause of "cold sores" around the mouth but is neither caused by, nor a cause of, genital herpes.) Hervesvirus type 2 infection can be transmitted to the newborn infant during passage through an infected birth canal. Transmission to the newborn is serious, and although the infection in infants is often mild, it may also be fatal. Premature infants are more susceptible than others.

AIDS Acquired immunodeficiency syndrome (AIDS) is a sexually transmitted disease caused by human immune virus (HIV). The virus attacks and disables some parts of the immune system so that the body becomes vulnerable to invasion by a host of other microorganisms. Refer to Chapter 10, The Immune System, for more details.

SUMMARY

A. The function of the reproductive system is to bring about the fertilization, development, and nourishment of offspring.

B. The external male organs of reproduction are the penis and the scrotum, which contains the testes.

1. The penis functions to carry both urine and semen.
    a. The prepuce, or foreskin, covering the end of the penis protects the opening from infective agents.
    b. Circumcision, the removal of the foreskin, is no longer considered medically justified.
    c. The penis is composed of erectile tissue and many, normally collapsed spaces.
    d. Erection occurs when the arteries to the penis dilate, filling the spaces with blood.

2. The two testes, contained in the scrotum, function to produce sperm and secrete testosterone into the blood.
    a. The scrotum is a divided pouch that hangs behind the penis.
    b. Each of the two testes is an oval organ divided into about 250 wedge-shaped lobes.
        i. Each lobe contains seminiferous tubules.
        ii. Sperm reproduce and develop to maturity in the tubules.
    c. Interstitial cells, between the tubules, produce and secrete testosterone.
        i. Testosterone secretion during puberty matures a boy into a man.
        ii. Secretion is controlled by FSH, referred to in the male as interstitial cell–stimulating hormone.

C. The internal male reproductive organs include the duct system and the semen-producing accessory glands.

1. The epididymis, ductus deferens, and the urethra form a duct system that carries sperm and semen into the vagina during intercourse.
    a. The coiled epididymis leads from the testes.
    b. The ductus, or vas deferens, is the excretory duct of the testes.
        i. It extends up into the abdomen.
        ii. It contacts and forms, with the seminal vesicles, the ejaculatory duct.
    c. The ejaculatory duct opens into the urethra, which carries both semen and urine out of the body.
    d. A vasectomy achieves artificial sterility by closing the vas deferens.

2. Semen is a thick whitish fluid, composed of a mixture of secretions of the testes, the seminal vesicles, the prostate gland, and the bulbourethral glands.

a. The two seminal vesicles, located behind the urinary bladder, secrete a fluid that is one of the components of semen.

b. The prostate gland surrounds the first inch of the urethra.

   i. It secretes an alkaline fluid that promotes sperm motility.

   ii. In older men, enlargement of the prostate causing obstruction of the urethra is common, requiring partial removal.

   iii. The prostate is a frequent site of cancer in the elderly male.

c. The bulbourethral glands (Cowper's glands) below the prostate on either side of the urethra secrete an alkaline fluid as a part of the semen.

D. The external female reproductive structures are collectively known as the vulva.

  1. The labia majora are two folds of skin similar to the scrotum.

  2. The labia minora, two smaller folds of skin, lie between the labia majora.

  3. The clitoris is a small rounded projection of erectile tissue, nerves, and blood vessels at the apex of the labia minora.

  4. The vaginal vestibule contains the hymen, vaginal orifice, urethral orifice, and openings of the vestibular glands.

    a. The hymen is a thin membrane separating the vagina from the vestibule.

    b. Neither the presence nor the absence of the hymen can be considered criterion of virginity.

E. The internal organs of female reproduction include the ovaries, the uterine tubes, the uterus, and the vagina.

  1. The two ovaries produce ova—female reproductive cells (eggs)—and the female sex hormones.

    a. The ovaries are small, oval-shaped structures above and to either side of the uterus.

    b. Internally they consist of thousands of graafian follicles.

     i. Each follicle contains an ovum that matures as the follicle grows.

     ii. At maturity, the follicle bursts and releases the ovum for possible fertilization.

    c. The ruptured follicle develops into the corpus luteum under stimulation of LH.

     i. The corpus luteum, or golden body, produces and secretes estrogens and progesterone during the second half of the menstrual cycle.

     ii. If fertilization occurs, it continues to produce and secrete hormones throughout pregnancy.

  2. The fallopian tubes serve as ducts to transport the ova from the ovaries to the uterus.

    a. The tubes are not connected to the ovaries.

    b. The fingerlike projections from the ends of the tubes draw the ovum into the tube.

    c. An ectopic pregnancy is a condition in which a fertilized ovum develops outside the cavity of the uterus.

  3. The uterus is a pear-shaped muscular organ located above the bladder in front of the rectum.

    a. The uterine tubes enter into its upper end.

    b. The lower end, the cervix, projects into the vagina.

    c. The upper main portion is known as the fundus.

    d. The wall of the uterus consists of three layers.

     i. The outer, peritoneal layer is continuous with the broad ligament.

     ii. The middle layer, the myometrium, is a thick muscular layer that greatly enlarges during pregnancy.

     iii. The inner coat of the mucous membrane, the endometrium, consists of epithelial and connective tissue.

    e. In menstruation portions of the endometrium pull loose, exposing blood vessels.

     i. Blood and bits of endometrium trickle into the vagina and out of the body.

     ii. Regeneration of a new endometrial lining begins almost immediately.

  4. The vagina, the female organ of copulation, is a tubular canal directed upward from the vestibule to the uterus.

    a. It is located between the bladder and the rectum.

    b. The vaginal wall consists of an inner, moist mucous membrane and an outer muscular layer; they are separated by a layer of erectile tissue.

    c. The vagina serves as part of the birth canal.

F. The two mammary glands, or breasts, secrete milk for nourishment of the newborn.
  1. The nipples contain the openings of the milk ducts.
    a. A wider circular area of pigmented skin, the areola, surrounds each nipple.
    b. There are 15 to 20 lobes of glandular tissue arranged radially in each breast.
  2. Estrogen stimulates the development of the ducts.
  3. Progesterone influences the growth of the milk-producing glandular tissue.
  4. Lactation, the production of milk, is complex, involving both nervous and hormonal factors.
    a. Suckling of the newborn stimulates production and release of prolactin and oxytocin.
    b. Prolactin, which comes from the anterior pituitary gland, stimulates milk production by glandular tissue.
    c. Oxytocin, which comes from the posterior pituitary, stimulates release of milk into the ducts.
G. Estrogens and progesterone are essential ovarian hormones.
  1. Production and secretion of estrogens and progesterone occur in response to FSH and LH.
  2. Estrogens are secreted by the maturing graafian follicles.
    a. Estrogens produce feminization at puberty.
    b. In the menstrual cycle they cause early thickening, and later regeneration, of the endometrium.
  3. Progesterone is secreted by the corpus luteum and by the placenta during pregnancy.
    a. It helps prepare the uterine wall for implantation and is necessary for implantation.
    b. It maintains development of the placenta.
    c. It prevents the ovary from producing ova during pregnancy.
    d. It is responsible for breast enlargement during pregnancy.
    e. It is responsible for development of milk-secreting cells.
    f. Lack of progesterone leads to menstrual irregularities and spontaneous abortions.

H. The menstrual cycle begins with menarche and ends with menopause.
  1. First menses (menarche) is at about 10 to 11 years of age in Western industrialized nations.
    a. The cycle takes from 22 to 35 days, with an average of 28.
    b. Menopause, the cessation of the cycle, occurs about 35 years later.
  2. The menstrual cycle consists of three phases.
    a. The menstrual phase lasts from the first to the fourth day.
      i. When the ovum is not fertilized, the corpus luteum regresses.
      ii. Regression of the corpus luteum decreases estrogen and progesterone secretion and disintegration of the endometrial lining.
    b. The proliferative phase begins on the fifth day with FSH stimulation of estrogen secretion.
    c. The secretory phase begins on about the fourteenth day at ovulation.
      i. Ovulation is the rupture of the mature follicle and release of the ovum.
      ii. The ovulation event is marked by a rapid increase in the secretion of LH.
      iii. LH continues to work on the ruptured follicle, transforming it into the corpus luteum.
      iv. The corpus luteum continues estrogen secretion and begins to secrete progesterone.
      v. Secretions of the corpus luteum prepare the uterus wall for implantation.
    d. If implantation does not occur, the corpus luteum decreases its activity, the endometrium disintegrates, and the new cycle begins.
I. Modern pregnancy testing is based on the detection of HCG.
J. There are numerous methods of contraception: condoms, diaphragm, IUD, the rhythm method, douching, suppositories, foams, and the contraceptive pill.
K. Fibrocystic breast disease is characterized by fibrous growth in the breast tissue.
  1. Biopsies are usually necessary to distinguish between benign and malignant fibrous tumors.

2. Cancerous tumors are treated with surgery, irradiation, and chemotherapy.

L. Several sexually transmitted diseases are of common clinical importance.

   1. Gonorrhea is a contagious inflammatory disease caused by the bacteria *Neisseria gonorrhoeae*.
   2. Syphilis is a sexually transmitted disease with three phases of long-term development.
   3. AIDS is a sexually transmitted viral disease that attacks the immune system.
   4. Genital herpes is a localized viral infection.
      a. It produces sores (lesions) on the penis in the male or on the cervix, vagina, or vulva in the female.
      b. The virus involved is herpes simplex, type 2.

REVIEW QUESTIONS

1. What are the primary sex organs, or gonads, of the male? What are their two major functions?

2. In which structure of the testes does spermatogenesis take place?

3. Name the series of ducts through which the sperm pass to reach the urethra.

4. Name the accessory glands that contribute to the formation of semen.

5. How does erection and ejaculation occur?

6. Name three male secondary sexual characteristics that occur at puberty as a result of the secretion of testosterone.

7. Explain how the enlargement of the prostate gland in older men can interfere with urinary function.

8. List and describe the external organs of the female reproductive system.

9. Name the female gonads and identify their two major functions.

10. Name the structures of the female duct system and describe the functions of each.

11. Explain how the mature ovum released from the ovary reaches the uterus.

12. What is a follicle? What is ovulation? Explain how anterior pituitary hormones cause follicle development and ovulation.

13. Describe the principal changes occurring in the uterus in the phase before and after ovulation. How does implantation prevent the initiation of a new cycle?

14. Name three female secondary sexual characteristics that occur at puberty as a result of the secretion of estrogens.

15. Identify the source and explain the function of progesterone during the normal menstrual cycle. What are its functions during pregnancy?

16. List and describe the three phases of the menstrual cycle.

17. Define menarche and menopause. Explain their significance to women.

18. Outline the changes in the mammary glands at puberty and during and following pregnancy as a result of estrogens and progesterone. What is the role of infant suckling?

19. Explain the basis of the modern pregnancy test.

20. List and describe the basis of several alternative methods of contraception.

21. Define abortion.

22. Characterize fibrocystic breast disease and explain how its growths are distinguished from cancer.

23. Discuss the relationship between dietary fat intake and the incidence of breast cancer.

24. Describe four common sexually transmitted diseases.

Glossary

Abdomen (ab-do′men) The portion of the body between the diaphragm and the pelvis.

Abduct (ab-dukt′) To draw or move away from the midline of the body; opposite of adduct.

Abortion (ah-bor′shun) Termination of pregnancy before embryo/fetus is viable outside the uterus.

Absorption (ab-sorp′shun) The taking in of fluids or other substances, for instance, by the skin or across a membrane.

Acetabulum (as″e-tab′u-lum) The large cup-shaped cavity with which the head of the femur articulates.

Acetylcholine (as″e-til-ko′len) One of several chemical transmitter substances released at nerve endings.

Achilles tendon (ah-kil′ez ten′dun) Tendon at the back of the heal; attaches to the calf muscles and is inserted on calcaneus. So named from Greek myth, wherein Achilles′ mother held him by this tendon as she dipped him in the river Styx, thereby making him invulnerable except in this area.

Acidosis (as″i-do′sis) Excessive accumulation of acid in the blood.

Acromegaly (ak″ro-meg′ah-le) Disorder caused by overproduction of growth hormone after puberty.

Addison′s disease (ad′i-sonz di-zez′) Disorder resulting from hyposecretion of adrenal cortical hormones.

Adduct (ah-dukt′) To move toward the midline of the body; opposite of abduct.

Adenohypophysis (ad″e-no-hi-pof′i-sis) The anterior portion of the hypophysis; anterior pituitary gland.

Adenoid (ad′e-noid) Literally, glandlike; adenoids (plural) refers to nasopharyngeal tonsils.

Adipose (ad′i-pos) Of a fatty nature; fat.

Adrenal glands (ah-dre′nal) Endocrine glands located on top of the kidneys; functionally distinguished into cortex and medulla.

Adrenalin (ah-dren′ah-lin) Brand name for epinephrine.

Aerobic (a-er-o′bik) Requiring oxygen; to live or grow.

Aldosterone (al′do-ster-on) Hormone from the adrenal cortex, important in sodium retention and reabsorption by kidney tubules.

Alkalosis (al″kah-lo′sis) The hormone secreted from the cortex of the adrenal glands; principal mineralo-corticoid.

Allergy (al′er-je) A condition in which there is a hypersensitivity to a particular foreign substance.

Alveolus (al-ve′o-lus) Literally, a small cavity; in the lungs, saclike dilations of the terminal bronchioles.

Amino acid (ah-me′no as′id) Organic compound; building blocks of proteins.

Anaerobic (an″a-er-o′bik) Not requiring oxygen; to live or grow.

Anatomy (ah-nat′o-me) The science of the structure of living organisms.

Androgen (an′dro-jen) The masculinizing hormone; male sex hormone.

Anemia (ah-ne′me-ah) Condition in which oxygen transport by red blood cells is deficient.

Aneurysm (an′u-rizm) Abnormal saclike dilation of the artery wall.

Angina pectoris (an-ji′nah pek′to-rus) A severe suffocating chest pain caused by lack of oxygen to the heart.

Anorexia (an″o-rek′se-ah) Lack or loss of appetite for food.

Anoxia (ah-nok′se-ah) deficient oxygen supply to tissues.

Anterior (an-ter′e-or) The front or ventral portion of a part or organ; opposite of posterior or dorsal.

Antibody (an″ti-bod″e) Any of a range of specific proteins produced by the B cells of the immune system in response to specific antigens.

Antidiuretic hormone (ADH) (an″ti-di″u-ret′ik hor′mon) From the posterior pituitary; promotes reabsorption of water by the kidney.

Antigen (an′ti-jen) Any substance that, when introduced into the body, causes formation of an antibody against it.

Anus (a′nus) The distal end of the digestive tract and the outlet of the rectum.

Aorta (a-or′tah) The main vessel rising from the left ventricle of the heart; provides arterial circulation for most of the body.

Apnea (ap-ne′ah) A transient cessation of breathing.

Arachnoid (ah-rak′noid) The middle of the three coverings (meninges) of the brain; weblike.

Areola (ah-re′o-lah) The pigmented ring around the nipple.

Arteriole (ar-te're-ol)   A very small branch of an artery.

Arteriosclerosis (ar-te"re-o-skle-ro'sis)   Degenerative changes in the arteries leading to decreased elasticity; hardening.

Artery (ar'ter-e)   Vessel carrying blood away from the heart.

Articulation (ar-tik"u-la'shun)   The site of union or juncture between two or more bones in the skeleton.

Asphyxia (as-fik'se-ah)   Loss of consciousness due to deficient oxygen supply.

Atherosclerosis (ath"er-o"skle-ro'sis)   Changes in large arteries due to fatty deposits in their walls; early arteriosclerosis.

Atrium (a'tre-um)   One of the upper chambers of the heart receiving blood from the veins.

Atrophy (at'ro-fe)   A wasting away of tissue; decreasing in size.

Auricle (aw're-kl)   The flap of the ear.

Autoimmune response (aw"to-im-mun' re-spons')   A condition in which antibodies or T cells attack the body's own tissues.

Autonomic (aw"to-nom'ik)   Self-controlling, functionally independent.

Axilla (ak-sil'ah)   Armpit.

Axon (ak'son)   Elongated portion (nerve) of neuron carrying impulses away from the body of the neuron.

B cells   Lymphoctyes that produce and secrete antibodies into the blood and lymph to combat infection.

Bacteria (bak-te're-ah)   Any of a wide range of diverse, one-celled microorganisms found in humans, animals, plants, soil, air, and water.

Basal metabolic rate (BMR) (ba'sal met-ah-bol-ik rat)   A measure of the rate of energy consumption by the body per unit time; measured under controlled (basal) conditions: at rest, 12 hours after a meal.

Benign (be-nin')   Not malignant; not life threatening.

Biceps (bi'seps)   A muscle having two heads.

Bicuspid (bi-kus'pid)   Having two points or cusps.

Bile (bil)   A fluid produced by the liver, stored in the gallbladder, and released into the small intestine; aids in the digestion of fats.

Bowman's capsule (bo'manz kap'sul)   Cuplike portion of the nephron; the glomerular capsule.

Brachial (bra'ke-al)   Pertaining to the arm.

Bradycardia (brad"e-kar'de-ah)   Abnormal slowness of the heartbeat, below 60 beats per minute.

Bronchiole (brong'ke-ol)   Small branch of the bronchial tree.

Buccal (buk'al)   Pertaining to the cheek.

Buffer (buf'er)   Substance or substances that stabilize the pH of a solution.

Bursa (ber'sah)   Sac or saclike cavity filled with fluid located at points of friction, especially near joints.

Calcitonin (kal"si-to'nin)   A hormone from the thyroid gland that increases calcium levels in the blood.

Calculus (kal'ku-lus)   A stone formed in various parts of the body, typically in ducts, hollow organs, or cysts.

Calorie (kal'o-re)   A unit of heat (energy); the large calorie (1000 times the small calorie) is the heat required to raise 1 kg of water 1 °C.

Calyx (ka'liks)   A cup-shaped organ or cavity.

Capillary (kap'i-lar"e)   Microscopic blood vessel that connects the venules and the arterioles.

Carbohydrate (kar"bo-hi'drat)   An organic compound containing carbon, hydrogen, and oxygen; includes starches, sugars, and cellulose.

Carcinogen (kar-sin'o-jen)   Cancer-causing agent.

Carcinoma (kar"si-no'mah)   Cancer; a malignant tumor.

Cardiac (kar'de-ak)   Pertaining to the heart.

Carotid (kah-rot'id)   Principal artery on each side of the neck.

Carpal (kar'pal)   Of or pertaining to the wrist.

Cartilage (kar'ti-lij)   Elastic, semihard connective tissue.

Cataract (kat'ah-rakt)   Partial or complete opacity of the eye lens.

Cecum (se'kum)   A dilated pouch that is the first portion of the large intestine.

Cellulose (sel'u-los)   The main structural carbohydrate in plants.

Centriole (sen'tri-ol)   A microscopic body found near the nucleus in cell division.

Cerebellum (ser"e-bel'um)   Portion of the brain that coordinates movement; located behind the cerebrum.

Cerebrospinal fluid (ser"e-bro-spi'nal floo'id)   The clear, colorless fluid that surrounds the central nervous system.

Cerebrum (ser'e-brum)   The higher brain cells; the largest portion of the brain; controlling conscious thought.

Cervix (ser'viks)   The lower neckline portion of the uterus.

Chemoreceptor (ke"mo-re-sep'tor)   Receptors sensitive to specific chemical substances.

Cholecystectomy (ko"le-sis-tek'to-me)   Removal of the gallbladder.

Cholesterol (ko-les'ter-ol)   A chemical component of animal fats and oils; excessive amounts are deposited in blood vessels and may be a factor in causing hardening of the arteries.

Choroid (ko'roid)   The pigmented layer of the eye.

Chromosome (kro'mo-som)   The body within a cell that contains the genes.

Chyme (kim)   The partially digested contents of the stomach just prior to passage into the small intestine.

Cilia (sil'e-ah)   Minute, hairlike projections on cell surfaces that move in a wavelike manner.

Circumcision (ser"kum-sizh'un)   Removal of the foreskin of the penis.

Cirrhosis (sir-ro'sis)   Inflammatory disease of the liver marked by replacement of liver cell by fibrous scar tissue.

Clitoris (klit'o-ris)   A small, erectile structure; part of the external female genitals; homologous to the penis in the male.

Cochlea (kok'le-ah)   Spiral cavity portion of the inner ear.

Coitus (ko'i-tus) Sexual intercourse.

Coma (ko'mah) Unconsciousness from which the person cannot be aroused.

Condom (kon'dum) A covering for the penis used during sexual intercourse to prevent infection or pregnancy.

Congenital (kon-jen'i-tal) Existing at birth.

Contraception (kon"trah-sep'shun) The prevention of conception; birth control.

Cornea (kor'ne-ah) The transparent membrane on the anterior surface of the eyeball; pupil in the center.

Cortex (kor'teks) Outer surface portion of an internal organ.

Corticosteroids (kor"ti-ko-ste'roidz) Hormones from the adrenal cortex.

Cortisol (kor'ti-sol) Hormone of the adrenal cortex; glucocorticoid.

Cranial (kra'ne-al) Pertaining to the skull.

Cretinism (kre'tin-izm) Condition caused by thyroid deficiency; dwarfism.

Cushing's syndrome (koosh'ingz sin'drom) Condition caused by excessive secretion of adrenocortical hormone (ACTH).

Cutaneous (ku-ta'ne-us) Pertaining to the skin.

Cyanosis (si"ah-no'sis) Bluish appearance to the skin and mucous membranes due to oxygen deficiency.

Cystitis (sis-ti'tis) Inflammatory disease of the urinary bladder.

Cytoplasm (si'to-plasmz") Main portion of a cell; distinct from the nucleus, contained by the cell membrane.

Cytotoxic (si"to-tok'sik) Poisonous to cells.

Defecation (def"e-ka'shun) The elimination of the contents of the bowels (feces).

Dehydration (de"hi-dra'shun) A condition resulting from excessive loss of water.

Dendrite (den'drit) A branched and treelike process of a neuron that conducts impulses toward the cell body.

Dentin (den'tin) The chief tissue of the teeth; surrounds the tooth pulp.

Deoxyribonucleic acid (DNA) (de-ok"se-ri"bo-nu'kle-ic as'id) A large molecule found in the nucleus that carries the genetic code of the organism.

Dermis (der'mis) The main, connective tissue layer of skin; beneath the epidermis.

Diabetes insipidus (di"ah-be'tez in-sip'i-dus) A disease characterized by discharge of large quantities of dilute urine and abnormal thirst and dehydration; a hypothalmic disorder.

Diabetes mellitus (di"ah-be'tez mel-li'tus) A disease characterized by a deficient release of insulin, resulting in the inability of cells to utilize glucose.

Dialysis (di-al'i-sis) Separation in solution of smaller particles from larger particles through a semipermeable membrane.

Diapedesis (di"ah-pe-de'sis) The migration of blood cells through the intact walls of blood vessels.

Diaphragm (di'ah-fram) Membrane of partition separating two areas; the muscular partition between the thorax and abdomen.

Diaphysis (di-af'i-sis) The shaft of a long bone.

Diarthrosis (di"ar-thro'sis) Freely moveable joint.

Diastole (di-as'to-le) The relaxation and dilation of the ventricles of the heart; opposite of systole.

Diastolic Pressure Blood pressure in the arteries during diastole.

Diffusion (di-fu'zhun) The random movement of particles in solution toward a uniform distribution.

Digestion (di-jest'yun) The breakdown of food, both mechanically and chemically.

Distal (dis'tal) Toward the end of a structure; opposite of proximal.

Diuresis (di"u-re'sis) Increased urine production.

Dorsal (dor'sal) Pertaining to the back; posterior; opposite of ventral.

Dura mater (du'rah ma'ter) The outermost, toughest of the three meninges covering the brain.

Dysfunction (dis-funk'shun) Abnormality of function.

Dyspnea (disp'ne-ah) Difficult or labored breathing.

Dystrophy (dis'tro-fe) Faulty nutrition.

Ectopic (ek-top'ik) Not in the normal place; for instance, an ectopic pregnancy occurs outside the uterus.

Edema (e-de'mah) Excessive fluid in the tissues, causing swelling.

Effector (ef-fek'tor) Responding organ; activated by nerve endings.

Efferent (ef'er-ent) Carrying away from, especially a nerve fiber that carries impulses away from the central nervous system.

Electrocardiogram (ECG) (e-lek"tro-kar'de-o-gram") A graphic record of the electric current produced by the excitation of heart muscle.

Electroencephalogram (EEG) (e-lek"tro-en-sef'ah-lo-gram") A graphic record of the electrical activity of the brain.

Elimination (e-lim"i-na'shun) Expulsion of the wastes from the body.

Embolism (em'bo-lizm) The obstruction of a blood vessel by a clot carried in the blood stream.

Emesis (em'e-sis) Vomiting.

Emphysema (em"fi-se'mah) A condition caused by the enlargement of the pulmonary alveoli; makes breathing more difficult and may eventually damage the heart.

Emulsion (e-mul'shun) Particles of one fluid suspended in another fluid; as oil (fat) in water.

Endocardium (en"do-kar'de-um) The endothelial membrane lining the interior of the heart.

Endocrine (en'do-crin) Secreting internally, directly into the blood and lymph; as in endocrine glands.

Endometrium (en-do-me'tre-um) The mucous membrane lining of the uterus.

Endoplasmic reticulum (en"do-plas'mik re-tik'u-lum) Network of tubules and vesicles in the cytoplasm.

Enzyme (en'zim) A protein produced by cells capable of accelerating biochemical reactions.

Epicardium (ep″i-kar′de-um)   External layer of the heart.

Epidermis (ep″i-der′mis)   Outermost, superficial layer of the skin.

Epinephrine (ep″i-nef′rin)   Adrenaline; hormone from the adrenal medulla.

Epiphysis (e-pif′i-sis)   Ends of the long bone.

Epithelium (ep″i-the′le-um)   One of the four primary types of tissue; covers and lines internal and external surfaces of the body.

Equilibrium (e″kwi-lib′re-um)   Balance of opposite reactions or forces; the result is often homeostasis.

Erythrocyte (e-rith′ro-sit)   Red blood cell.

Estrogen (es′tro-jen)   Female sex hormone; stimulates female secondary sex characteristics.

Eupnea (up-ne′ah)   Easy, normal respiration.

Excretion (eks-kre′shun)   The elimination of waste products from the body.

Exocrine (ek′so-krin)   Secretion through ducts onto an endothelial surface; as in exocrine glands.

Expiration (eks″pi-ra′shun)   Expelling air from the lungs.

Fallopian tubes (fal-lo′pe-an tub)   Pair of tubes that conduct ovum from ovary to uterus.

Fascia (fash′e-ah)   Sheet of connective tissue; typically covering and separating muscles.

Feces (fe′sez)   Waste materials from the intestines; composed of food residues, secretions, and bacteria.

Fetus (fe′tus)   The unborn young; from the third month until birth.

Fibrin (fi′brin)   Insoluble protein formed from fibrinogen; important in blood clotting.

Fibrinogen (fi-brin′o-jen)   A soluble protein in the blood plasma; converted to fibrin by thrombin.

Fissure (fish′ur)   Any cleft or groove; normal or otherwise.

Follicle-stimulating hormone (FSH) (fol′li-kl stim′u-lat-ing hor′mon)   Hormone from the anterior pituitary that stimulates ovarian follicles in females and sperm production in males.

Foramen (fo-ra′men)   A natural hole or passage, especially one into or through bone.

Fundus (fun′dus)   The base of an organ most remote from the entrance.

Gallbladder (gawl′blad-der)   The sac beneath the right lobe of the liver used for bile storage.

Gallstones (gawl′stonz)   Particles of hardened cholesterol or calcium salts that occasionally form in the gallbladder.

Ganglion (gang′gle-on)   A collection or mass of nerve cell bodies in the peripheral nervous system.

Gastric (gas′trik)   Pertaining to the stomach.

Gene (jen)   The biologic unit of heredity; located on chromosome; composed of DNA.

Genitals (jen′i-talz)   The external sex organs; genitalia.

Gland (gland)   An organ specialized to secrete or excrete substances.

Glomerulus (glo-mer′u-lus)   A coil or cluster of capillaries in Bowman's capsule; part of the nephron.

Glucagon (gloo′kah-gon)   A hormone from the pancreas released in response to low blood levels of glucose; raises blood levels of glucose.

Glucocorticoid (gloo″ko-kor′ti-koid)   A hormone from the adrenal cortex having many metabolic actions.

Gluconeogenesis (gloo″ko-ne″o-jen′e-sis)   The synthesis of new glucose from protein and fat compounds.

Glucose (gloo′kos)   The principal sugar in the blood.

Glycogen (gli′ko-jen)   The chief carbohydrate storage material in animals.

Glycogenesis (gli″ko-jen′e-sis)   Formation of glycogen.

Goiter (goi′ter)   Enlargement of thyroid gland.

Gonad (gon′ad)   Sex gland in which reproductive cells are formed.

Gonorrhea (gon″o-re′ah)   Sexually transmitted disease caused by bacteria.

Graafian follicle (graf′e-an fol′i-kl)   Small sac in ovary containing a developing ovum.

Growth hormone   A hormone from the anterior pituitary that stimulates growth in general; somatotropin (STH).

Gustatory (gus′tah-to″re)   The act of tasting; the sense of taste.

Heart block   An impaired transmission of impulses from atrium to ventricle.

Hematocrit (he-mat′o-krit)   The ratio (or percentage) of erythrocytes to total blood volume.

Hematopoiesis (hem″ah-to-poi-e′sis)   The formation of red blood cells.

Hemoglobin (he″mo-glo′bin)   The oxygen-carrying protein molecule contained in the erythrocytes.

Hemolysis (he-mol′i-sis)   The destruction of red blood cells.

Hemorrhage (hem′or-ij)   Bleeding; usually a major loss of blood from a ruptured vessel.

Heparin (hep′ah-rin)   A substance that prevents clotting of blood.

Heredity (he-red′i-te)   Transmission of genetic characteristics from parents to children.

Hernia (her′ne-ah)   Protrusion of a loop of an organ through an abnormal opening.

Homeostasis (ho″me-o-sta′sis)   An active tendency toward uniformity or stability of temperature and composition of an organism.

Hormone (hor′mon)   The secretions of the endocrine glands; exert regulatory effects throughout the body or on specific target organs.

Human immunodeficiency virus   (HIV) Virus that causes acquired immunodeficiency syndrome.

Hydrocortisone (hi″dro-kor′ti-son)   A hormone secreted by the adrenal cortex; also referred to as cortisol.

Hymen (hi′men)   Mucous membrane that may partially or entirely occlude the vaginal opening.

Hyoid (hi′oid)   U-shaped bone between the root of the tongue and the larynx.

Hyperkalemia (hi″per-kah-le′me-ah) Higher than normal concentration of potassium in the blood.

Hypernatremia (hy″per-na-tre′me-ah) Higher than normal concentration of sodium in the blood.

Hyperopia (hi″per-o′pe-ah) Farsightedness.

Hyperplasia (hi″per-pla′ze-ah) Overgrowth of a tissue or organ.

Hyperpnea (hi″perp-ne′ah) Abnormal increase in the depth and rate of respiratory movements.

Hypertension (hi″per-ten′shun) High blood pressure.

Hyperthermia (hi″per-ther′me-ah) Fever; elevated body temperature above 37°C.

Hypertrophy (hi-per′tro-fe) Increase in the size of an organ.

Hypoglycemia (hi″po-gli-se′me-ah) Lower than normal concentration of sugar in the blood.

Hypokalemia (hi″po-kah-le′me-ah) Lower than normal concentration of potassium in the blood.

Hyponatremia (hi″po-nah-tre′me-ah) Lower than normal concentration of sodium in the blood.

Hypophysis (hi-pof′i-sis) The pituitary gland.

Hypothalamus (hi″po-thal′ah-mus) A part of the brain below the cerebrum.

Hypothermia (hi″po-ther′me-ah) Subnormal body temperature.

Hypoxia (hi-pox′se-ah) Reduced oxygen level in the tissues.

Hysterectomy (his″te-rek′to-me) Surgical removal of the uterus.

Immunity (i-mu′ni-te) The body's ability to resist many organisms and chemicals that can damage the body.

Infarct (in′farkt) A region of dead, deteriorating tissue; typically, resulting from a lack of blood supply.

Inferior (in-fer′e-or) situated below; caudal.

Inflammation (in″flah-ma′shun) The reaction of the tissues to injury; marked by pain, heat, swelling, and redness.

Inguinal (ing′gwi-nal) Pertaining to the groin region.

Insertion (in-ser′shun) Place of attachment of a muscle to the bone that it moves.

Inspiration (in″spi-ra′shun) The drawing of air into the lungs.

Insulin (in′su-lin) Hormone from the pancreas affecting blood glucose levels and other aspects of energy metabolism.

Intercellular (in″ter-sel′u-lar) Between the bodies of the cells.

Interferon (in″ter-fer′on) Small proteins produced by the immune system that inhibit virus multiplication.

Interstitial (in″ter-stish′al) Pertaining to or situated in the gaps or spaces of a tissue.

Intracellular (in″trah-sel′u-lar) The region within a cell; bounded by the cell membrane.

Ion (i′on) An atom or group of atoms having a positive or negative electrical charge.

Ipsilateral (ip″si-lat′er-al) Pertaining to the same side.

Irritability (ir″i-tah-bil′i-te) Ability to react to a stimulus; excitability.

Ischemia (is-ke′me-ah) Local and temporary deficiency of blood to an area.

Isometric (i″so-met′rik) Of the same length; refers commonly to isometric exercise, in which the muscles remain the same length as they encounter a load.

Isotonic (i″so-ton′ik) Having the same tone or tension; refers to exercise with constant load; also used to refer to any solution with the same osmotic pressure as normal body fluids.

Jaundice (jawn′dis) A disorder in which there is an accumulation of bile pigments in the blood, producing a yellow color to the skin.

Jejunum (je-joo′num) The part of the small intestine between the duodenum and ileum.

Joint (joint) The junction of two or more bones; articulation.

Keratin (ker′ah-tin) An insoluble protein found in tissues such as hair, nails, and the epidermis of the skin.

Ketones (ke′tonz) Acid waste products from fat metabolism.

Ketosis (ke-to′sis) Excess amounts of ketone bodies in the blood.

Labium (la′be-um) A lip or lip-shaped organ.

Lacrimal (lak′ri-mal) Pertaining to tears.

Lactation (lak-ta′shun) The production of milk by the mammary glands.

Lactose (lak′tos) Milk sugar; a disaccharide.

Lacuna (lah-ku′nah) A small pit, hollow, or depression; lacunae in bone contain bone cells.

Lateral (lat′er-al) A position toward the side; farther away from the median line.

Leukemia (loo-ke′me-ah) Cancer of the blood characterized by an abnormal increase in white blood cells.

Leukocyte (loo′ko-cit) A white blood cell.

Leukocytosis (loo″ko-si-to′sis) Abnormally high white blood cell numbers in the blood.

Leukopenia (loo″ko-pe′ne-ah) Abnormally low white blood cell numbers in the blood.

Ligament (lig′ah-ment) Any tough, fibrous band connecting bones or supporting viscera.

Lipid (lip′id) Fat and fatlike compounds; insoluble in water and soluble in fat solvents.

Lumen (loo′men) The space inside of a tube or tubular organ; plural, lamina.

Luteum (loo″te-um′) Golden yellow; refers to the corpus luteum.

Lymph (limf) Clear fluid in the lymphatic vessels; tissue fluid.

Lymphocytes (lim′fo-sit) Individual cells of the immune system; originate in the bone marrow; one type of white blood cell.

Lysosomes (li′so-somz) Microscopic organelles in the cytoplasm; containing strong digestive enzymes.

Malignant (mah-lig′nant) Life threatening; cancerous.

Mammary glands (mam′er-e glandz) Milk-producing glands of the breasts.

Mastication (mas"ti-ka'shun) The act of chewing.

Matrix (ma'triks) The intercellular substance in which cells are embedded.

Medial (me'de-al) Pertaining to the middle; nearer the median plane.

Mediastinum (me"de-as-ti'num) The space in the center of the chest between the two lung cavities.

Medulla (me-dul'ah) The central portion of an organ in contrast to its cortex.

Meiosis (mi-o'sis) A special type of cell division occurring during the maturation of sex cells.

Membrane (mem'bran) A thin layer of tissue covering a surface or dividing a space of an organ, cell, or organelle.

Menarche (me-nar'ke) Beginning of the menstrual function.

Meninges (me-nin'jes) Three membranes that cover and protect the brain and spinal cord.

Menopause (men'o-pawz) Cessation of menstrual function, usually occurring between the ages of 50 and 55.

Menstruation (men"stroo-a'shun) A periodic, cyclic discharge of blood, secretions, tissue, and mucus from the mature female uterus in the absence of pregnancy.

Mesentery (mes'en-ter"e) Peritoneal fold attaching the intestine to the posterior abdominal wall.

Metabolic rate (met"a-bol'ik rat) The amount of energy expended by the body per unit time.

Metabolism (me-tab'o-lizm) The sum total of all chemical reactions occurring in the body.

Metacarpal (met"ah-kar'pal) one of the five bones of the palm of the hand.

Metastasis (me-tas'tah-sis) The spread of cancerous cells from a body part or organ into another not directly connected to it.

Metatarsal (met"ah-tar'sal) One of the five bones between the instep and the phalanges of the foot.

Microvilli (mi"kro-vil'i) Microscopic projections on the free surfaces of some epithelial cells; internal surface of the intestine.

Mineralocorticoid (min"er-al-o-kor'ti-koid) Hormone from the adrenal cortex particularly effective in causing retention of sodium and the loss of potassium.

Mitochondria (mi"to-kon'dre-ah) Cellular organelles that produce ATP molecules; powerhouse of the cell.

Mitosis (mi-to'sis) Cell division producing two identical daughter cells.

Molecule (mol'e-kul) A submicroscopic, individual unit of one type of substance; for instance, a sugar molecule; usually composed of a few to many thousands of atoms.

Monocyte (mon'o-sit) A type of white blood cell; transforms into a phagocyte after entering the tissues.

Monosaccharide (mon"o-sak'ah-rid) Any of several simple sugars; for instance, dextrose (glucose) and fructose.

Mucus (mu'kus) A sticky, thick liquid secreted by the mucous glands and mucous membranes.

Mucous membranes (mu'kus mem'branz) Line tracts and cavities of the body opening to the exterior; found in digestive, respiratory, urinary, and reproductive tracts.

Multiple sclerosis (mul'ti-pl skle-ro'sis) A chronic disease of the nervous system characterized by destruction of the myelin sheaths of neurons; leads to partial paralysis, changes in speech, inability to walk.

Muscular dystrophy (mus'ku-lar dis'tro-fe) A progressive disorder marked by atrophy and stiffness of the muscles.

Myelin sheaths (mi'e-lin sheth) Sheath around the nerve fibers; in peripheral nerves, formed by multiple wrappings of Schwann cells.

Myocardial infarction (mi"o-kar'de-al in-fark'shun) Area of dead tissue in the myocardium caused by interruption of blood supply; typically, the result of a heart attack.

Myocardium (mi"o-kar'de-um) The cardiac muscle layer of the wall of the heart.

Myopia (mi-o'pe-ah) Nearsightedness.

Myxedema (mik"se-de'mah) Condition caused by deficiency of thyroid hormone in adult.

Nares (na'rez) Nostrils.

Necrosis (ne-kro'sis) The death and disintegration of tissue caused by disease or injury.

Negative feedback The reverse stimulus; when appropriately balanced with the stimulus, the result is homeostasis.

Nephron (nef'ron) Basic functional unit of the kidney.

Nerve (nerv) A bundle of nerve fibers outside the brain or spinal cord; also, any one of those fibers.

Neuroglia (nu-rog'le-ah) Supportive cells of nervous tissues; non-neuronal; also called glia.

Neurohypophysis (nu"ro-hi-pof'i-sis) The posterior portion of the hypophysis or pituitary gland.

Neuron (nu'ron) Primary cell of nervous tissue that transmits impulses throughout the body.

Neurotransmitters (nu"ro trans'mit-erz) Chemical messengers that travel one way across the synapse between neurons.

Neutrophil (nu'tro-fil) The most abundant of the white blood cells; functions, in part, as a phagocyte.

Nucleus (nu'kle-us) The dense central body present in most cells; contains the genetic material.

Obesity (o-bes'i-te) The condition of a person extremely overweight.

Occlusion (o-kloo'zhun) Obstruction or closure.

Olfactory (ol-fak'to-re) The act of smelling; pertaining to the sense of smell.

Oogenesis (o"o-jen'e-sis) The process of development (maturation) of an egg (ova) within the ovary prior to its expulsion from the ovary.

Ophthalmic (of-thal'mik) Pertaining to the eye.

Optic (op'tik) Pertaining to the eye.

Oral (o'ral) Relating to the mouth.

Organelle (or"gan-el') A specialized microscopic structural and functional unit inside the cell; lysosomes, mitochondria.

Osmosis (oz-mo'sis) The natural diffusion (mixing) of a solvent through a semipermeable membrane from a dilute solution into a more concentrated one.

Osteocyte (os"te-o-sit") A mature bone cell.

Osteoporosis (os"te-o-po-ro'sis) A loss of bony substances, producing brittleness and softness of bones; often seen in people of very advanced age; more common in women.

Otic (o'tik) Pertaining to the ear.

Ovarian cycle (o-va're-an si'kl) The monthly cycle of follicle development and ovulation.

Ovary (o'vah-re) The female gonad in which ova (eggs) are produced (mature).

Ovulation (o" vu-la'shun) Release of an oocyte (ovum) through rupture of the mature follicle in the ovary.

Ovum (o'vum) The female egg; gamete or germ cell.

Oxidation (ok"si-da'shun) The chemical reaction wherein a substance combines with oxygen.

Oxytocin (ok"se-to'sin) Hormone from the posterior pituitary; stimulates contraction of the uterus during childbirth and the ejection of milk during nursing.

Palate (pal'at) Roof of the mouth.

Pancreas (pan'kre-as) A large gland located behind the stomach, producing both exocrine and endocrine secretions.

Paralysis (pah-ral'i-sis) Loss of voluntary muscle movement.

Paraplegia (par"ah-ple'je-ah) Paralysis of the lower limbs.

Parasympathetic (par"ah-sim"pah-thet'ik) A division of the autonomic nervous system.

Parathyroid glands (par"ah-thi'roid glandz) Small endocrine glands located on the posterior of the thyroid.

Parathyroid hormone Hormone from the parathyroid glands; helps to regulate blood calcium levels.

Parietal (pah-ri'e-tal) Of or pertaining to the walls of a cavity.

Parotid (pah-rot'id) Situated near the ear; as the parotid gland.

Patella (pah-tel'ah) The kneecap.

Pathogenesis (path"o-jen'e-sis) The development of a disease.

Pectoral (pek'to-ral) Pertaining to the breast or chest.

Pelvis (pel'vis) Any basinlike structure; particularly the basin-shaped ring of bone at the posterior extremity of the trunk.

Penis (pe'nis) The male organ of urination and copulation.

Pericardium (per"i-kar'de-um) The fibroserous sac that surrounds the heart.

Peripheral (pe-rif'er-al) **nervous system (PNS)** The system of nerves that connects the outer portions of the body with the central nervous system.

Peristalsis (per"i-stal'sis) The muscular waves of contraction propelling materials down a muscular tube; especially the digestive tract.

Peritoneum (per"i-to-ne'um) The serous membrane lining the abdominal (peritoneal) cavity.

Permeability (per"me-ah-bil'i-te) The property of membranes that allows ions and molecules to pass through.

pH Symbol designating hydrogen ion concentration.

Phagocyte (fag'o-sit) A cell capable of ingesting and digesting microorganisms, foreign materials, and cellular debris.

Phagocytosis (fag"o-si-to'sis) The ingestion, by phagocytes, of microorganisms, foreign materials, or cellular debris.

Phalanges (fah-lan'jez) The bones of the finger or toe.

Physiology (fiz"e-ol'o-je) The science of the functioning of living organisms.

Pinocytosis (pi"no-si-to'sis) The ingestion of liquids by cells.

Pituitary gland (pi-tu'i-tar"e gland) the neuroendocrine gland located beneath the brain; serves many important functions.

Plasma (plaz'mah) The fluid portion of the blood.

Platelet (plat'let) The small, colorless disks in circulating blood; important in the clotting process.

Pleura (ploor'ah) Double membranous sac enclosing the lungs and lining the chest cavity.

Pneumothorax (nu"mo-tho'raks) Air in the pleural cavity surrounding the lung.

Polycythemia (pol"e-si-the'me-ah) A disease characterized by too many red blood cells.

Polydipsia (pol"e-dip'se-ah) Excessive thirst.

Polymer (pol'i-mer) A compound formed by the combination of many simpler molecules all of the same type.

Polysaccharide (pol"e-sak'ah-rid) One of a group of carbohydrates composed of simple sugars; sugar polymers.

Posterior (pos-ter'e-or) Situated behind or toward the rear.

Posture (pos'chur) Position of the body.

Prepuce (pre'pus) The loose fold of skin that covers the glans penis or clitoris.

Process (pros'es) A prominence or projection; a series of actions for a specific purpose.

Progesterone (pro-jes'te-ron) Hormone that prepares the uterus for fertilized ovum.

Pronate (pro'nat) To turn the palm downward.

Prostaglandins (pros"tah-glan'dins) A group of naturally occurring fatty acids that affect many body functions.

Protein (pro'te-in) The main molecular building material of cells.

Proximal (prok'si-mal) Nearest; closest to any point of reference; opposite of distal.

Puberty (pu'ber-te) The age during which the reproductive organs first become functional.

Pulmonary (pul'mo-ner"e) Pertaining to the lungs.

Purkinje fibers (pur-kin'je fi'berz) Specialized fibers in the heart that conduct cardiac impulses into the walls of the ventricles.

Pus (pus) The fluid waste product of many infections; composed of dead white blood cells and dead tissue.

Quadriplegia (kwod"ri-ple'je-ah) The paralysis of all four limbs.

Receptor (re-sep'tor) Nerve ending sensitive to a specific stimulus; beginning of a dendrite.

Reflex (re'fleks) An involuntary (automatic) response to a stimulus.

Renal (re'nal) Pertaining to the kidney.

Ribonucleic acid (RNA) (ri"bo-nu'kle-ik as'id) Nucleic acid involved in protein synthesis.

Ribosomes (ri'bo-somz) Cytoplasmic organelles that are the sites of the protein assembly step of protein synthesis.

Rotate (ro'tat) To turn about an axis.

Sagittal (saj'i-tal) A plane or section parallel to the long axis of the body.

Saliva (sah-li'vah) The secretions of the salivary glands.

Sclera (skle'rah) The tough, white, outermost layer of the eyeball.

Scoliosis (sko"le-o'sis) A lateral curve in the vertebral column.

Scrotum (skro'tum) The external sac enclosing the testes.

Sebum (se'bum) The secretion of sebaceous glands.

Semen (se'men) Thick, whitish secretion of the reproductive organs of the male; composed of spermatozoa and secretions from several accessory glands.

Semilunar (sem"e-lu'nar) Resembling a crescent or half-moon.

Serous (se'rus) Pertaining to, characterized by, or resembling serum.

Serum (ser'um) Plasma minus clotting substances.

Sinus (si'nus) A recess, cavity, or hollow space.

Somatic (so-mat'ik) Pertaining to the framework of the body, as distinguished from the viscera.

Spermatogenesis (sper"mah-to-jen'e-sis) The process of meiosis in the male to produce sperm.

Spermatozoa (sper"mah-to-zo'ah) The mature male sex cells.

Sphincter (sfingk'ter) A ringlike muscle enclosing a natural orifice; for example, the anal sphincter.

Sputum (spu'tum) Matter ejected from the mouth, usually saliva mixed with mucus and other substances from the respiratory tract.

Squamous (skwa'mus) Pertaining to flat, thin cells that form the free surface of some epithelial tissues.

Steroids (ste'roidz) A large group of substances including certain hormones and cholesterol.

Stimulus (stim'u-lus) An excitant or irritant; a change in the environment producing a response.

Strabismus (strah-biz'mus) Inability to coordinate the movement of the two eyes; crossed eyes.

Stressor (stres'sor) Any injurious factor that produces biologic stress; for example, emotional trauma, infections, severe exercise.

Stroke (strok) The sudden rupture or clotting of a blood vessel to the brain.

Superior (soo-pe're-or) Refers to an area situated above.

Supination (soo"pi-na'shun) To turn the palm of the hand upward; opposite of pronate.

Sympathetic (sim"pah-thet'ik) Division of the autonomic nervous system; concerned with energy expenditure.

Synapse (sin'aps) Junctional region between two adjacent neurons.

Synarthrosis (sin"ar-tho'sis) Freely moveable joints.

Synovial fluid (si-no've-al) Viscous fluid secreted by synovial membrane to lubricate joint surfaces.

Synthesis (sin'the-sis) Putting together parts to form a more complex whole.

Systole (sis'to-le) The phase of heart activity during which the heart contracts and expels the contained blood; opposite of diastole.

Systolic pressure The pressure in the arteries during systole when the heart muscle is contracting.

Tachycardia (tak"e-kar'de-ah) Excessively rapid heart beat; abnormal; over 100 beats per minute.

Tarsal (tahr'sal) **bone** One of the seven bones that form the ankle and heel.

Tendon (ten'dun) A fibrous cord of connective tissue linking muscles and bones.

Testis (tes'tis) The primary male sex organ that produces sperm.

Thorax (tho'raks) That portion of the trunk above the diaphragm and below the neck.

Thrombin (throm'bin) The enzyme that induces clotting by converting fibrinogen to fibrin.

Thrombocyte (throm'bo-sit) A blood platelet; part of the blood clotting system.

Thrombus (throm'bus) A clot that is fixed or stuck to a vessel wall.

Thymus gland (thi'mus) An endocrine gland active in the immune response.

Thyroid gland (thi'roid gland) Large endocrine gland that produces thyroid hormones.

Tissue (tish'u) A group of similar cells forming a distinct structure.

Toxic (tok'sik) Harmful to the body; poisonous.

Trachea (tra'ke-ah) The windpipe.

Tract (trakt) A collection of nerve fibers in the central nervous system having the same origin, termination, and function.

Trauma (traw'mah) A wound or injury.

Tubal pregnancy (too'bal preg'nan-se) An ectopic pregnancy that occurs within a uterine tube.

Ulcer (ul'cer) An absence of the normal lining of a body surface in a limited area.

Umbilicus (um-bil'i-kus) The navel.

Urea (u-re'ah) The chief nitrogenous waste product in the urine, mainly from protein metabolism.

Ureter (u-re′ter)   The tube that carries urine from the kidney to the bladder.

Urethra (u-re′thrah)   The tube that carries the urine from the bladder to the outside of the body.

Varicose vein (var′i-kos van)   A dilated, enlarged vein whose valves are damaged.

Vas (vas)   A duct; vessel.

Vascular (vas′ku-lar)   Pertaining to the blood vessels.

Vasoconstriction (vas″o-kon-strik′shun)   Muscular contraction with narrowing of the blood vessels, leading to decreased flow of blood to the part.

Vasodilation (vas″o-di-la′shun)   Relaxation of the smooth muscles of the blood vessels producing dilation, leading to increased flow of blood to the part.

Vein (van)   A vessel carrying blood away from the tissues, toward the heart.

Ventral (ven′tral)   Anterior or front; opposite of dorsal.

Ventricle (ven′tri-kl)   Any small cavity; discharging chamber of the heart.

Venule (ven′-ul)   A small vein.

Viscera (vis′er-ah)   The internal organs.

Vitamin (vi′tah-min)   A variety of organic substances in foods necessary for the normal metabolic functioning of the body.

Vitreous humor (vit′re-us hu′mor)   Transparent, gelatinlike substances filling the posterior cavity of the eye (behind the lens).

Vulva (vul′va)   Female external genitalia.

White matter   The white substance of the central nervous system; the myelinated nerve fibers.

Zygote (zi′got)   A fertilized egg.

INDEX

Note: Page numbers in *italic* type refer to illustrations;
page numbers followed by the letter t refer to tables.

Peristalsis, definition of, 246, 305
  in large intestine, 248
  in ureters, 271
Peritoneum, definition of, 305
  layers of, 243
Pernicious anemia, 172
Petit mal seizure, 136
pH, definition of, 305
  of blood, control of, 235–236, 268
Phagocyte(s), definition of, 305
  description/function of, 210–211, 216
  immune subsystems relationship to, 218
  locomotion of, 211
  types of, 210–211
Phagocytosis, 18, 20, 305
Phalanges, 54, 58, 61, 64, 305
Pharynx, function of, 226
  in digestion, 243–245
Phosphoric acid, in DNA, 21, 22
Photomicrograph, 199
Physiology, anatomy and, 2
  definition of, 2, 2, 305
Pia mater, of meninges, 107, 109, 110
Pillae, of tongue, 132, 136
Pineal gland, description/function of, 145, 156
Pinna, of external ear, 125, 134
Pinocytosis, 18, 20, 305
Pituitary gland, 111–112, 113
  anterior lobe of, 146–148, 147–149
    disorders of, 149, 156–157
    estrogen/progesterone secretion by,
      290–291, 290
    follicle stimulating hormone secretion by,
      281
    functions of, 150–151
    hormones of, 146–149, 147, 281, 285,
      290–291, 290
    luteinizing hormone secretion by, 285
    Peyer's patch of, 247
  antidiuretic hormone and, 266–267
  autonomic nervous system and, 114
  definition of, 305
  description/function of, 146–149, 147–149
  disorders of, 148
  pineal gland function with, 156
  posterior lobe of, disorders of, 148, 157
    functions of, 147, 148
  water regulation by, 266–267, 269
Placenta, in uterus with fetus removed, 280
Plasma, definition of, 305
Plasma cells, 214
Plasma proteins, 166–167
Platelet(s), and blood composition, 164–165
  definition of, 305
  function of, 166
  plasma interaction with, 168, 169
Platelet block, formation of, 168, 169
Pleura, definition of, 305
Pleural cavity, structures of, 225, 225
Pleural membrane, 225
Pleurisy, 225
Plexuses, of spinal nerve, 116, 126–128
Pneumococcus, 238
Pneumonia, definition of, 238
  skin coloration and, 39
Pneumothorax, definition of, 305

Polycythemia, definition of, 305
Polydipsia, definition of, 305
Polymer, definition of, 305
Polypeptides, and protein digestion, 255
Polysaccharide, definition of, 305
Polyuria, 272
Pons, in respiration control, 236
  of hindbrain, 111, 111
Portal vein, 187
Posture, definition of, 305
Precapillary sphincters, 184
Pregnancy, calcium levels during, 45
  contraception/abortion and, 293
  ectopic, 286
  estrogen/progesterone secretion during, 285,
    290
  fetal position during, 280
  mammary glands during, 289
  Rh factor in, 171
  testing of, 292–293
Prepuce, definition of, 305
  female, 284
  of penis, 279, 283
Process, definition of, 305
Progesterone, 156
  definition of, 305
  function of, 290–291, 290
  in menstrual cycle, 291
  in milk production, 289, 291
  in oral contraceptives, 293
  in pregnancy, 290
  ovarian follicle cells production of, 147
  ovarian secretion of, 156, 284–285
Prolactin, function of, 148
  in milk production, 289
Prophase, of mitosis, 26, 27
Prostaglandins, definition of, 305
  description/function of, 155
Prostate gland, description/function of,
    282–284, 283–284
  prostaglandin secretion by, 155
  seminal fluid secretion by, 279
Protection, skin function of, 39
Protein, definition of, 305
  digestion of, 252–253, 255
  immune system function of, 210, 214–215
  manufacture of, 21–25, 25
    amino acid role in, 23, 25, 147–148, 153
    DNA role in, 22–23
    effects of growth hormone on, 147–148
  metabolism of, 258
  metabolism wastes of, 265
  return to blood of, 200
Proteoses, and protein digestion, 255
Prothrombin, conversion to thrombin of, 168, 169
  function of, 167
Psoriasis, 39
Puberty, definition of, 305
Pubis, 56, 62
Pulmonary artery(ies), 177–178, 177–178, 186
  angiograph of, 231
Pulmonary circulatory circuits, schematic
    drawing of, 197
Pulmonary edema, definition of, 238
Pulmonary flow, of circulatory system,
    186–187, 197